I0060891

The NLRP3 Inflammasome: An Attentive Arbiter of Inflammatory Response

Edited by

Puneetpal Singh
Department of Human Genetics
Punjabi University, Patiala
Punjab, India

The NLRP3 Inflammasome: An Attentive Arbiter of Inflammatory Response

Editor: Puneetpal Singh

ISBN (Online): 978-981-5223-94-1

ISBN (Print): 978-981-5223-95-8

ISBN (Paperback): 978-981-5223-96-5

© 2024, Bentham Books imprint.

Published by Bentham Science Publishers Pte. Ltd. Singapore. All Rights Reserved.

First published in 2024.

BENTHAM SCIENCE PUBLISHERS LTD.
End User License Agreement (for non-institutional, personal use)

This is an agreement between you and Bentham Science Publishers Ltd. Please read this License Agreement carefully before using the book/echapter/ejournal (**"Work"**). Your use of the Work constitutes your agreement to the terms and conditions set forth in this License Agreement. If you do not agree to these terms and conditions then you should not use the Work.

Bentham Science Publishers agrees to grant you a non-exclusive, non-transferable limited license to use the Work subject to and in accordance with the following terms and conditions. This License Agreement is for non-library, personal use only. For a library / institutional / multi user license in respect of the Work, please contact: permission@benthamscience.net.

Usage Rules:

1. All rights reserved: The Work is the subject of copyright and Bentham Science Publishers either owns the Work (and the copyright in it) or is licensed to distribute the Work. You shall not copy, reproduce, modify, remove, delete, augment, add to, publish, transmit, sell, resell, create derivative works from, or in any way exploit the Work or make the Work available for others to do any of the same, in any form or by any means, in whole or in part, in each case without the prior written permission of Bentham Science Publishers, unless stated otherwise in this License Agreement.
2. You may download a copy of the Work on one occasion to one personal computer (including tablet, laptop, desktop, or other such devices). You may make one back-up copy of the Work to avoid losing it.
3. The unauthorised use or distribution of copyrighted or other proprietary content is illegal and could subject you to liability for substantial money damages. You will be liable for any damage resulting from your misuse of the Work or any violation of this License Agreement, including any infringement by you of copyrights or proprietary rights.

Disclaimer:

Bentham Science Publishers does not guarantee that the information in the Work is error-free, or warrant that it will meet your requirements or that access to the Work will be uninterrupted or error-free. The Work is provided "as is" without warranty of any kind, either express or implied or statutory, including, without limitation, implied warranties of merchantability and fitness for a particular purpose. The entire risk as to the results and performance of the Work is assumed by you. No responsibility is assumed by Bentham Science Publishers, its staff, editors and/or authors for any injury and/or damage to persons or property as a matter of products liability, negligence or otherwise, or from any use or operation of any methods, products instruction, advertisements or ideas contained in the Work.

Limitation of Liability:

In no event will Bentham Science Publishers, its staff, editors and/or authors, be liable for any damages, including, without limitation, special, incidental and/or consequential damages and/or damages for lost data and/or profits arising out of (whether directly or indirectly) the use or inability to use the Work. The entire liability of Bentham Science Publishers shall be limited to the amount actually paid by you for the Work.

General:

1. Any dispute or claim arising out of or in connection with this License Agreement or the Work (including non-contractual disputes or claims) will be governed by and construed in accordance with the laws of Singapore. Each party agrees that the courts of the state of Singapore shall have exclusive jurisdiction to settle any dispute or claim arising out of or in connection with this License Agreement or the Work (including non-contractual disputes or claims).
2. Your rights under this License Agreement will automatically terminate without notice and without the

need for a court order if at any point you breach any terms of this License Agreement. In no event will any delay or failure by Bentham Science Publishers in enforcing your compliance with this License Agreement constitute a waiver of any of its rights.

3. You acknowledge that you have read this License Agreement, and agree to be bound by its terms and conditions. To the extent that any other terms and conditions presented on any website of Bentham Science Publishers conflict with, or are inconsistent with, the terms and conditions set out in this License Agreement, you acknowledge that the terms and conditions set out in this License Agreement shall prevail.

Bentham Science Publishers Pte. Ltd.
80 Robinson Road #02-00
Singapore 068898
Singapore
Email: subscriptions@benthamscience.net

BENTHAM SCIENCE

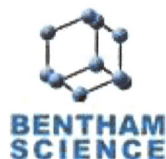

CONTENTS

PREFACE

The human body is an intricate and wondrous system, constantly engaged in a delicate balance of maintaining health and combating various threats. Inflammation, a fundamental process of the immune system, plays a critical role in the body's defense against infection and injury. While inflammation is an essential mechanism for maintaining tissue homeostasis, dysregulated or chronic inflammation can lead to the development and progression of numerous diseases. Within the realm of inflammation, the NLRP3 inflammasome has emerged as a captivating protagonist in recent years. This book, "The NLRP3 Inflammasome: An Attentive Arbiter of Inflammatory Response," delves deep into the intricate workings of this molecular complex and explores its pivotal role in shaping the inflammatory landscape.

Our understanding of the NLRP3 inflammasome has undergone significant advances since its initial discovery. This enigmatic protein complex, comprised of NLRP3 (NOD-like receptor family, pyrin domain-containing 3), ASC (apoptosis-associated speck-like protein containing a caspase recruitment domain), and pro-caspase-1, acts as a sensor of danger signals within the cell, orchestrating a cascade of events that culminate in the production and release of pro-inflammatory cytokines, particularly interleukin-1β (IL-1β) and IL-18.

"The NLRP3 Inflammasome: An Attentive Arbiter of Inflammatory Response" is a comprehensive exploration of the intricacies surrounding the NLRP3 inflammasome. Through the collaboration of esteemed scientists, researchers, and clinicians, this book seeks to shed light on the various aspects of NLRP3 biology, regulation, and its involvement in a wide array of diseases, ranging from metabolic disorders to neurodegenerative conditions.

In the first chapter, writer Dr. Rashmi Singh, along with her co-authors, has made a significant contribution to the understanding of the role of the NLRP3 inflammasome in airway inflammation and fibrosis. In their research, they have focused on elucidating the mechanisms of NLRP3 inflammasome activation and its impact on respiratory diseases such as asthma. Their work has highlighted the crucial role of NLRP3 in mediating caspase-1 activation and the secretion of proinflammatory cytokines, which contribute to the progression of asthma by promoting excessive inflammation, extracellular matrix accumulation, and airway remodeling. Moreover, they have identified endotoxin (lipopolysaccharide, LPS) as one of the activators of NLRP3, linking environmental factors to the incidence of asthma and allergic diseases. This chapter provides a comprehensive summary of their research findings, shedding light on the mechanisms underlying NLRP3 inflammasome activation and its regulation in asthmatic exacerbations.

In the second chapter, Dr. Sushweta Mahalanobish, along with co-authors Noyel Ghosh and Parames C. Sil, has made a significant contribution to the understanding of the role of NLRP3 inflammasome in pulmonary hypertension (PH). Their research focuses on the progressive pulmonary vasculopathy characterized by increased mean pulmonary arterial pressure, adverse vascular remodeling, and right ventricular failure. They explore the involvement of inflammation as a crucial factor in the onset and development of PH, specifically highlighting the NLRP3 inflammasome as a key mediator in the signaling cascade that regulates PH-associated conditions through inflammatory mechanisms. The activation of NLRP3 and the subsequent release of proinflammatory cytokines IL-1β and IL-18 contribute to adverse consequences on pulmonary vasculature and the onset of PH. The chapter delves into current PH therapies and their limitations and introduces the potential therapeutic targeting of NLRP3 inflammasomes to modulate inflammation in PH pathobiology. The authors provide a comprehensive insight into the role of NLRP3 inflammasome in PH and its implications for future therapeutic interventions.

Dr. Abhinav Kanwal and his team have provided a comprehensive exploration of the modulatory mechanism of the NLRP3 inflammasome in heart diseases. Despite significant advancements in therapy, heart failure remains a leading cause of mortality worldwide. The authors highlight the crucial role of the inflammasome in the progression of various cardiovascular diseases, including heart failure, abdominal aortic aneurysm, atherosclerosis, diabetic cardiomyopathy, hypertension, dilated cardiomyopathy, cardiac remodeling, and calcific aortic valve disease. Specifically, they focus on the NLRP3 inflammasome, a multi-protein signaling platform that tightly regulates inflammatory responses and antimicrobial host defense, leading to the generation of pro-inflammatory cytokines through the activation of caspase-1 and subsequent pyroptosis. By investigating the NLRP3 inflammasome in different cardiovascular diseases, the authors aim to uncover critical disease triggers and endogenous modulators with the aimof developing new therapeutic interventions in the future. The chapter provides a summary of recent literature, emphasizing the activation mechanism of the NLRP3 inflammasome and its implications in the pathophysiology of heart failure, shedding light on this complex and intriguing aspect of heart diseases.

In the fourth chapter, Monika Joon and Manisha Yadav explore the intricate relationship between Mycobacterium tuberculosis (Mtb) and the inflammasome. Mtb is known as a highly successful human pathogen, capable of evading the host immune response through the development of robust effectors. It can survive and multiply within the host's immune system, even in the presence of immune tools meant to eliminate it. Granuloma formation, a compensatory mechanism, offers partial benefits to both the host and the pathogen. While extensive research has been conducted on various mycobacterial virulence factors, the relatively newer concept of inflammasomes requires further investigation. Insights into the inflammasome-Mtb interaction may open up new avenues for the development of host-directed therapy (HDT) strategies to combat TB. By comprehending the intricate dynamics between the inflammasome and Mtb, novel approaches for managing this disease can be explored.

The fifth chapter by Syed Ehtaishamul Haque, Aamir Khan, and Ashif Iqubal deals with an overview of the NLRP3 inflammasome's activation mechanism, its association with cardiovascular complications, and the potential of NLRP3 inhibitors as cardioprotective agents. They highlight the positive correlation between NLRP3 inflammasome activation and various cardiovascular disorders, including hypertension, angina, arrhythmia, cardiac fibrosis, myocardial infarction, and heart failure. By discussing the structural components of the NLRP3 inflammasome and its molecular activation pathway, the authors underline its crucial role in the pathogenesis of cardiovascular diseases. Furthermore, they shed light on promising outcomes from studies exploring NLRP3 inflammasome inhibitors in cardiovascular disorders. Overall, the manuscript underscores the importance of targeting the NLRP3 inflammasome as a potential therapeutic approach for managing and treating cardiovascular diseases.

In the sixth chapter, Sonal Yadav examines the role of NLRP3 in protozoan parasitic infections. They discuss the activation of the NLRP3 inflammasome by various protozoan parasites, including *Giardia duodenalis*, *Entamoeba histolytica*, *Trichomonas vaginalis*, Plasmodium species, *Trypanosoma cruzi*, *Schistosomes*, *Toxoplasma gondii*, and Leishmania species. The authors highlight the protective effects of NLRP3 against certain infections, such as Giardia, *Trypanosoma cruzi*, and *Entamoeba histolytica*, while also noting its contribution to pathology in Schistosomes and Malaria parasite infections. They emphasize the need for further research to better understand the precise mechanisms and roles of NLRP3 in host defense and inflammatory pathology in parasitic protozoan infections, which could pave the way for the development of innovative treatment strategies.

The seventh chapter by Dr. Adekunle Babajide Rowaiye and his colleagues focuses on the NLRP3 inflammasome as a target for anti-inflammatory drugs. They highlight the crucial role of the NLRP3 inflammasome in the innate immune response and its association with various inflammation-related diseases. The authors discuss the activation of the NLRP3 inflammasome and the production of proinflammatory cytokines, emphasizing the importance of inhibitory mechanisms to decrease inflammation and inflammasome-mediated cell death. They further explore the potential of targeting signaling molecules along the NLRP3 inflammasome pathway as drug targets for effective inhibition and downregulation of proinflammatory cytokines. The chapter provides insights into the classes of NLRP3 inflammasome inhibitors, their anti-inflammatory effects, and underlying mechanisms of action.

Dr. Agnès Hamzaoui and co-authors, in the eighth chapter, investigate the potential value of sputum levels of Interleukin-38 (IL-38) and NLRP3 inflammasome in severe childhood asthma. Asthma is known to be an inflammatory airway disorder with varying expression of cytokines based on disease severity. The transition from exacerbation to remission involves a complex interplay between inflammatory and anti-inflammatory mediators. The authors focus on the expression of IL-38 and NLRP3 inflammasome in severe asthmatic children. They find that NLRP3 inflammasome is upregulated in severe asthma, while levels of IL-38 are low. The inflammatory profile of severe asthma in children is characterized by the expression of IL-17, IL-32, IL-1β, and NLRP3 inflammasome. This study sheds light on the potential role of IL-38 and NLRP3 inflammasome as biomarkers in severe childhood asthma. It contributes to a better understanding of the inflammatory mechanisms involved in the disease.

The ninth chapter by Lokesh Sharan, Anubrato Pal, Priya Saha, and Ashutosh Kumar explores the role of inflammasomes, specifically NLRP1, NLRP3, NLRC4, and AIM2, in inflammation and neuropathic pain. These inflammasomes play a crucial role in the development of autoimmune and metabolic disorders, cancer, and various inflammatory conditions. The activation of inflammasomes is triggered by molecular changes, such as mitochondrial dysfunction, neuroinflammation, lysosomal damage, oxidative stress, sensitization, and disinhibition, leading to the activation of proinflammatory pathways and subsequent development of inflammasome-related neuropathic pain. Among these inflammasomes, NLRP3 has been extensively studied and identified as a key player in neuropathy. This chapter provides an overview of the involvement of inflammasomes, particularly NLRP3, in neuropathic pain. Based on available evidence, targeting inflammasome activity is proposed as a potential cutting-edge approach for the successful treatment of neuropathic pain. The understanding of inflammasome-mediated mechanisms in neuropathic pain may pave the way for the development of novel therapeutic strategies in the future.

The chapters in this book provide in-depth analyses of the mechanisms underlying NLRP3 inflammasome activation, the signaling pathways involved, and the interplay between NLRP3 and other cellular processes. Additionally, the authors delve into the consequences of dysregulated NLRP3 activation, highlighting the implications for disease pathogenesis and potential therapeutic interventions. From the role of NLRP3 in sterile inflammation to its contribution to the pathogenesis of autoimmune disorders, each chapter offers valuable insights into this captivating field of research.

I hope that "The NLRP3 Inflammasome: An Attentive Arbiter of Inflammatory Response" serves as a valuable resource for scientists, clinicians, and students alike, fostering a deeper understanding of the NLRP3 inflammasome and its impact on human health. It is our sincere belief that by unraveling the mysteries surrounding this vigilant arbiter of inflammation, we can unlock novel therapeutic strategies that harness its potential for the betterment of patients worldwide.

I would like to express my sincere gratitude to Mr. Nitin Kumar for his invaluable assistance in the editing and refining of the book. I am also immensely thankful to Ms. Humaira Hashmi, In-charge of the eBook Department, and Ms. Asma Ahmed, Manager of the eBooks Publication Department for her support in publishing this book and Mr. Mahmood Alam, Director of Publications at Bentham Science Publishers, for their unwavering support, encouragement, and assistance. Their contributions have been instrumental in bringing this book to fruition.

Puneetpal Singh
Department of Human Genetics
Punjabi University, Patiala
Punjab, India

List of Contributors

Anju Jaiswal	Department of Zoology, MMV, Banaras Hindu University, Varanasi-221002, India
Asha Kumari	Department of Pathology, University of Alabama at Birmingham, USA
Abhinav Kanwal	Department of Pharmacology, All India Institute of Medical Sciences, Bathinda, Punjab, India
Aamir Khan	Department of Pharmacology, School of Pharmaceutical Education and Research, Jamia Hamdard, New Delhi-110062, India
Agnès Hamzaoui	Tunis El Manar University, Medicine Faculty of Tunis, Department of Paediatric and Respiratory Diseases, Abderrahman Mami Hospital, Pavillon B, Ariana, Research Laboratory 19SP02 "Chronic Pulmonary Pathologies: From Genome to Management", Tunisia
Anubrato Pal	Department of Pharmacology and Toxicology, National Institute of Pharmaceutical Education and Research (NIPER), Kolkata 700054, West Bengal, India
Ashutosh Kumar	Department of Pharmacology and Toxicology, National Institute of Pharmaceutical Education and Research (NIPER)-SAS Nagar, Mohali, Punjab, 160062, India
Anchal Arora	Department of Pharmacology, All India Institute of Medical Sciences, Bathinda, Punjab, India
Ashif Iqubal	Department of Pharmacology, School of Pharmaceutical Education and Research, Jamia Hamdard, New Delhi-110062, India
Adekunle Babajide Rowaiye	Department of Agricultural Biotechnology, National Biotechnology Development Agency, Abuja, Nigeria Department of Pharmaceutical Science, North Carolina Central University, Durham, NC 27707, USA
Gunpreet Kaur	University Centre of Excellence in Research, Baba Farid University of Health Sciences, Faridkot, Punjab, India
Harpreet Kaur	Department of Medical Parasitology (PGIMER), Chandigarh, India
Kamel Hamzaoui	Tunis El Manar University, Medicine Faculty of Tunis, Department of Paediatric and Respiratory Diseases, Abderrahman Mami Hospital, Pavillon B, Ariana, Research Laboratory 19SP02 "Chronic Pulmonary Pathologies: From Genome to Management", Tunisia
Lokesh Sharan	Department of Pharmacology and Toxicology, National Institute of Pharmaceutical Education and Research (NIPER), Kolkata 700054, West Bengal, India
Lorretha Chinonye Emenyeonu	Bioresources Development Centre, Owode, National Biotechnology Development Agency, Abuja, Nigeria
Monika Joon	Government College Bahadurgarh, Affiliated to MDU, Rohtak, Haryana, India
Manisha Yadav	Dr. B. R. Ambedkar Centre for Biomedical Research (ACBR), University of Delhi, Delhi-110007, India

Manisha Yadav	Dr. B. R. Ambedkar Centre for Biomedical Research (ACBR), University of Delhi, Delhi-110007, India
Noyel Ghosh	Division of Molecular Medicine, Bose Institute, P-1/12, CIT Scheme VII M, Kolkata-700054, West Bengal, India
Navjot Kanwar	University Institute of Pharmaceutical Sciences, Punjab University, Chandigarh, India
Oni Solomon Oluwasunmibare	Bioresources Development Centre, Isanlu, National Biotechnology Development Agency, Abuja, Nigeria
Parames C. Sil	Division of Molecular Medicine, Bose Institute, P-1/12, CIT Scheme VII M, Kolkata-700054, West Bengal, India
Parveen Bansal	University Centre of Excellence in Research, Baba Farid University of Health Sciences, Faridkot, Punjab, India
Priscilla Aondona	Department of Medical Biotechnology, National Biotechnology Development Agency, Abuja, Nigeria
Priya Saha	Department of Pharmacology and Toxicology, National Institute of Pharmaceutical Education and Research (NIPER)-SAS Nagar, Mohali, Punjab, 160062, India
Rashmi Singh	Department of Zoology, MMV, Banaras Hindu University, Varanasi-221002, India
Ravinder Sharma	University Institute of Pharmaceutical Sciences and Research, BFUHS, Faridkot, Punjab, India
Rakesh Singh Dhanda	Celluleris AB, VentureLab, Scheelevägen 15, 223 70 Lund, Sweden
Sushweta Mahalanobish	Division of Molecular Medicine, Bose Institute, P-1/12, CIT Scheme VII M, Kolkata-700054, West Bengal, India
Syed Ehtaishamul Haque	Department of Pharmacology, School of Pharmaceutical Education and Research, Jamia Hamdard, New Delhi-110062, India
Sonal Yadav	Dr. B. R. Ambedkar Centre for Biomedical Research (ACBR), University of Delhi, Delhi-110007, India
Sabrine Louhaichi	Tunis El Manar University, Medicine Faculty of Tunis, Department of Paediatric and Respiratory Diseases, Abderrahman Mami Hospital, Pavillon B, Ariana, Research Laboratory 19SP02 "Chronic Pulmonary Pathologies: From Genome to Management", Tunisia
Tarimoboere Agbalalah	Department of Medical Biotechnology, National Biotechnology Development Agency, Abuja, Nigeria Department of Anatomy, Faculty of Basic Medical Sciences, Baze University, Abuja, Nigeria
Umar Suleiman Abubakar	Bioresources Development Centre, Kano, National Biotechnology Development Agency, Abuja, Nigeria
Vikas Gupta	University Centre of Excellence in Research, Baba Farid University of Health Sciences, Faridkot, Punjab, India

CHAPTER 1

Role of NLRP3 Inflammasome in Airway Inflammation and Fibrosis

Anju Jaiswal[1]**, Asha Kumari**[2] **and Rashmi Singh**[1,*]

[1] *Department of Zoology, MMV, Banaras Hindu University, Varanasi-221002, India*

[2] *Department of Pathology, University of Alabama at Birmingham, USA*

Abstract: The NLRP3 inflammasome is a critical component of the innate immune system that mediates caspase-1 activation and the secretion of proinflammatory cytokines IL-1β/IL-18 in response to microbial infection and cellular damage. Nucleotide-binding oligomerization domain (NOD)-like receptor family pyrin domain 3 (NLRP3), one of the members of the NLR family, consists of NLRP3, the adaptor molecule, apoptosis-associated speck-like protein containing a caspase and recruitment domain (ASC) and an inflammatory caspase-1 that causes excessive inflammasome activation in respiratory diseases like asthma and could exacerbate the progression of asthma by considerably contributing to ECM accumulation and airway remodeling. NLRP3 is closely associated with airway inflammation and asthma exacerbations as endotoxin (lipopolysaccharide, LPS) is one of its activators present in the environment. Asthma is a complex immunological and inflammatory disease characterized by the presence of airway inflammation, airway wall remodeling and bronchial hyperresponsiveness (BHR). Symptomatic attacks of asthma can be caused by a myriad of situations, including allergens, infections, and pollutants, which cause the rapid aggravation of respiratory problems. The presence of LPS in the environment is positively correlated with the incidence of asthma and allergic diseases. In this chapter, we summarize our current understanding of the mechanisms of NLRP3 inflammasome activation by multiple signaling events in asthmatic exacerbations and their regulation.

Keywords: Caspases and NLRP3 regulators, Fibrosis, Inflammation, Inflammasomes, Pyroptosis, ROS.

INTRODUCTION

The fundamental elements of the innate immune system are physical as well as chemical obstacles to infection and a number of cellular components that identify invasive pathogens and trigger antimicrobial immune responses. The mucosal surfaces with antimicrobial secretions, vascular endothelium, ciliated respiratory

---

[*] **Corresponding author Rashmi Singh:** Department of Zoology, MMV, Banaras Hindu University, Varanasi-221002, India; E-mails: singhras@bhu.ac.in, rashmisinghmmv@gmail.com

Puneetpal Singh (Ed.)
All rights reserved-© 2024 Bentham Science Publishers

epithelium, and epidermis all serve as examples of physical and chemical defensive systems. The air, along with a mixture of gases, carries other substances, such as dust particles, smoke and biological contaminants, such as dust mites, fungi, bacteria, spores, pollen grains and viruses. Lungs remain in continuous contact with the environmental air and several stimuli; hence, the quality of breathing air has a great impact on the health of an individual (Fig. **1**). The overall risk assessment of respiratory diseases is further complicated by socioeconomic status, lifestyle, age, nutritional status, environmental exposure to pollutants and genetic factors of the individual. These factors altogether may predispose or alter the prognosis of the disease (Fig. **2**). The extent of lung damage is also determined by the toxicity, intensity, duration and route of exposure as well as the physical state, such as the size or characteristics of the inhaled substances.

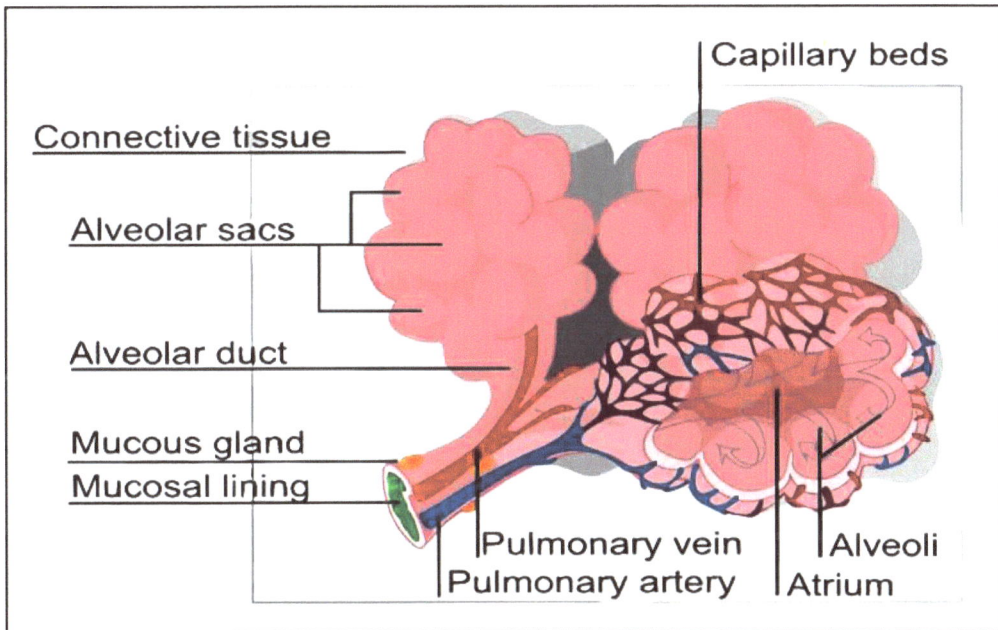

Fig. (1). Structure of lungs showing internal anatomy. Lungs are divided into smaller subunits *i.e.*, alveolar sacs confined with fine capillaries (www.wikipedia.org).

INNATE IMMUNE SYSTEM AND PATTERN RECOGNITION RECEPTORS (PPRs)

Apart from acting as the first line of protection, innate immunity is also essential for the initiation of adaptive responses, which guard against recurrent infections caused by the same pathogen [1]. The cellular elements of innate immunity also include T lymphocytes, cytotoxic natural killer (NK) cells, phagocytic macrophages and granulocytes, and DCs that deliver antigens. By using autophagy, phagocytosis, complement activation, and immunological stimulation by several families of PRRs, the innate immune system is initially able to identify and restrict microorganisms in an infection [2]. To identify the evolutionarily conserved features of pathogens, referred to as pathogen-associated molecular patterns (PAMPs), the innate immune reactions require a small number of pattern recognition receptors (PRRs), which are encoded in the germ line [3]. In addition, PRRs identify host elements as "danger" signals if they are found in atypical biological macromolecules or on areas of either infection, inflammation or any kind of cellular stress. Several different categories of PRRs were identified by a particular pathogen *via* diverse PAMPs. Host PRRs recognize microbes with extremely diverse biochemical compositions by nearly identical mechanisms. A transmembrane protein called TLRs and cytosolic NLRs are the two PRR families with the best-described members. The induction of specific genes and the formation of a wide variety of chemicals, such as cytokines, cell adhesion molecules, chemokines, and immunoreceptors, are the final effects of PRR-induced signal transduction processes. These molecules work with each other to synchronize the initial infection-related response from the host in addition to serving as a crucial link to the adaptive immune response. The two most important PAMPs are thought to be viral RNA and bacterial endotoxins. One of the strongest PAMPs ever discovered is LPS, a bacterial endotoxin that causes inflammation.

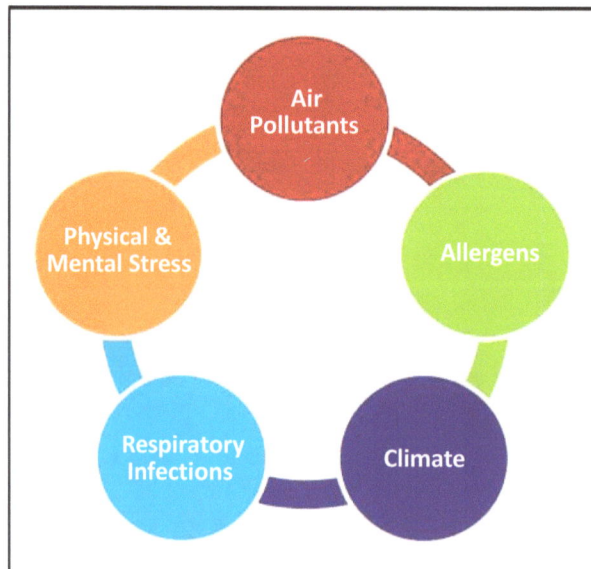

Fig. (2). Common inducers of respiratory diseases among thousands of known factors (www.wikipedia.org).

LPS INDUCED RESPIRATORY DISEASES

Endotoxin or Lipopolysaccharide (LPS) is the most ubiquitous pro-inflammatory factor present in almost all types of living environments (rural, urban or larger cities). Being a major component of bioaerosols, LPS is a common cause of airborne-associated lung diseases all over the world. It is an integral component of the outer wall of gram-negative bacteria, with potent immune stimulatory capacity due to the presence of Lipid A moiety (Fig. **3**).

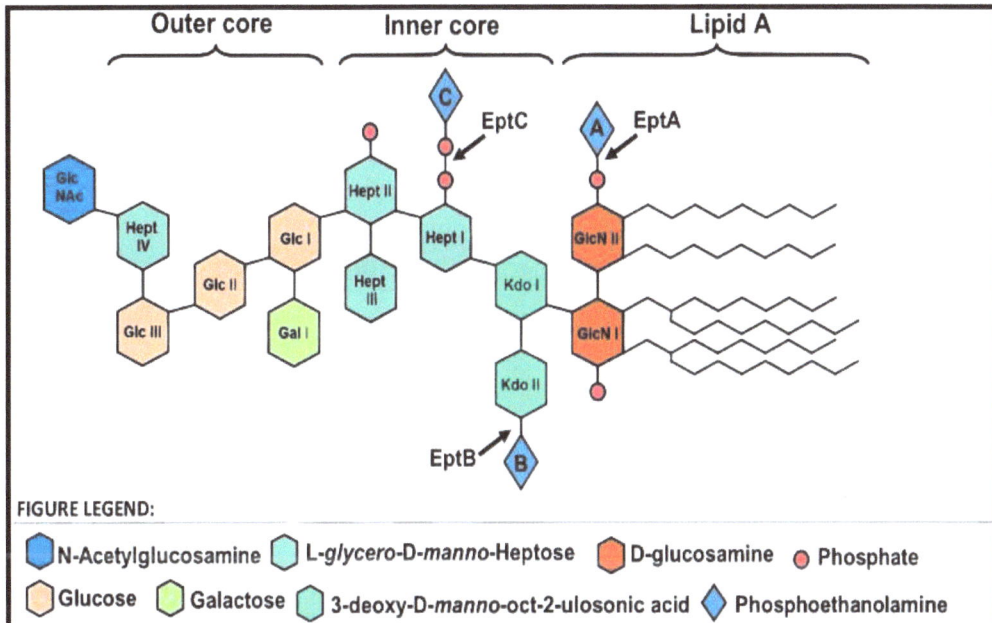

Fig. (3). Structure of Lipopolysaccharide [10].

In addition to the cytoplasmic membrane, the gram-negative bacterial cell wall also has an outer membrane made of LPS, proteins, and phospholipids as well as a thin coating of peptidoglycan. The lipid A moiety is connected to the core polysaccharide by an O-linked polysaccharide, which is what makes up LPS [4]. LPS binds to the TLR4 receptor to initiate several signaling cascades, including inflammation. LPS has a potent immunostimulatory capacity that stimulates immune cells to initiate inflammatory response characterized by proinflammatory cytokines, such as tumor necrosis factor (TNF-α), IL-1, IL-6 and interferon gamma (IFN-γ) [5]. Increasing incidences of allergic and asthmatic diseases in developing countries have been explained by the "hygiene hypothesis", where low level of endotoxin exposure at an early age is responsible for protection from allergic diseases as compared to exposure at later phases of life. Hygienic practices also contribute to more episodes of allergic diseases in the later phases of life [6] (Strachan, 1989). On the other hand, in recent years, studies have shown that the presence of LPS in a living environment was positively correlated with the incidence of asthma and allergic diseases [7]. In another study, lower doses of LPS exposure have been found to cause asthmatic exacerbations in mice models [8]. Recent studies have linked the risk of developing asthma to skewed Th2 response to an allergen and an imbalance between Th1 and Th2 response [9].

LPS Induced Asthmatic Exacerbations

Asthma is a complex disease of the airways affecting almost all ages, genders and races worldwide. The major symptoms include wheezing, coughing and shortness of breath, leading to sleepless nights and missed school and workdays. It is associated with enormous healthcare expenditures, and despite the advances in effective therapies, the economic burden associated with disease control and morbidity continues to increase. It represents multiple phenotypes depending upon the frequency and severity of the inducer (Figs. **4** and **5**).

Airway hyperresponsiveness is a pathological hallmark of asthma, where airways become highly sensitive and responsive to inhaled constrictor agonists, such as methacholine, histamine or cold air [11]. It is defined as an ease with which the airways respond to a stimulator, such as the sensitivity and reactivity to a given stimuli. Histamine, prostaglandins and leukotriene altogether mediate the constriction and narrowing of the airway passage. They promote smooth muscle contraction, increased vascular permeability in small blood vessels and mucus secretion, and also help in further recruitment of leukocytes to airways [12].

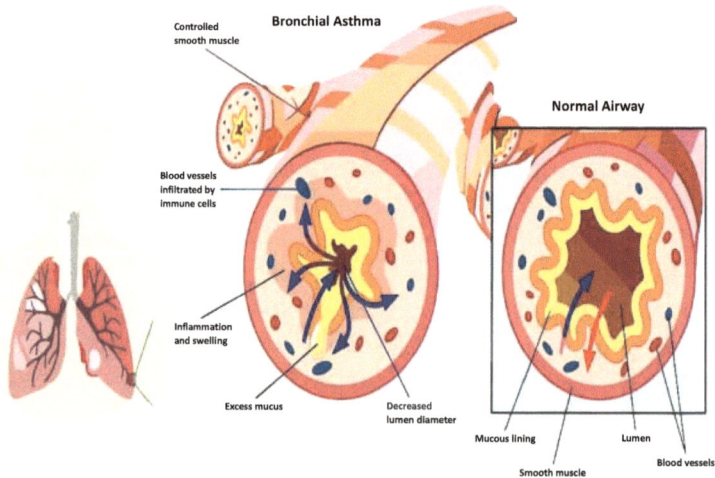

Fig. (4). Pathological changes in bronchial asthma (www.kabs.com).

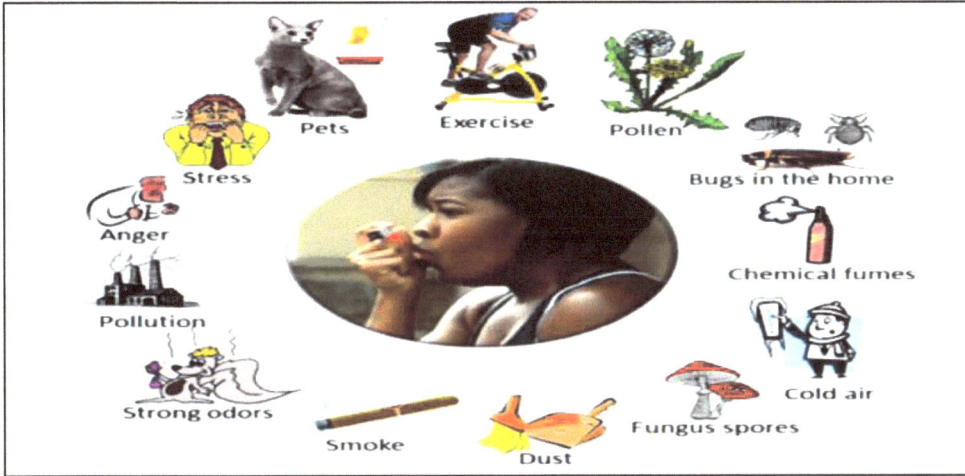

Fig. (5). Factors responsible for inducing and exacerbating asthma (www.wikipedia.org).

Asthmatic inflammation is mainly driven by Th2-specific cytokines, such as IL-4, IL-5 and IL-13. IL-5 regulates the genes responsible for cell proliferation and maturation of eosinophils, whereas IL-4 promotes class switching of IgG to IgE production. Interleukin-13 mediates airway hyperresponsiveness, mucus production and sub-epithelial fibrosis [13]. Inflammation can be of two types, acute and chronic. Acute inflammation can be caused by toxic pollutants, microbial intrusion, or tissue injury. The most noticeable aspect of the remodeling of the airways is fibrosis, which is the end phase of chronic inflammatory processes, and excessive extracellular matrix (ECM) deposition is one of its defining characteristics. Structural changes in the asthmatic airways, irreversible or reversible, are referred to as airway remodeling. These changes result in airway wall thickening associated with a rapid decline in the lung function and severity of the disease. It is characterized by epithelial cell alterations, sub-epithelial fibrosis, sub-mucosal gland hyperplasia, increased airway smooth muscle mass and airway vascularization [14, 15].

Inflammasome: An Important Aspect of Innate Immune System

The word "Inflammasome" was first used in 2002 by a scientific team led, Jurg Tschopp. It is a complex consisting of multiple proteins made up of a Nod sensor that can trigger an inflammatory caspase called caspase 1 [16]. The human genome has 23 NLR genes, compared to 34 NLR genes in the mouse genome [17]. Various inflammasomes have various activation patterns, and NLRs participate in a variety of signaling pathways. Based on the commonalities in their domain topologies and the unique roles they play, these receptors are further split into three different subfamilies. The three subfamilies are made up of the NLRPs also known as NALPs, the IPAFs (also called NLRC4,) and the NODs [18]. The biggest and most well-studied NLRP subfamily that possesses the PYRIN (PYD) domain is the NLRP3 inflammasome [19]. The nucleotide-binding domain and leucine-rich repeat protein 3 (NLRP3) inflammasome are now the most studied of the four inflammasome subtypes. NLRP3 inflammasomes are vast multiprotein complexes formed inside cells that participate in exacerbating inflammatory response in the lungs after activating pro-inflammatory cytokine IL-1β and IL-18, and a lytic form of programmed cell death. An increasing body of research has shown that pathogen-associated molecular patterns (PAMPs) and danger-associated molecular patterns (DAMPs), which are known to enhance asthmatic symptoms, trigger the activation of NLRP3 inflammasome. LPS-induced respiratory illness can be of several types, like lung inflammation, injury, disseminated Intracellular Coagulation (DIC) and oxidative damage. But all of these lead to an exacerbated response in airway disease conditions.

The most significant and researched class of PRRs is the Toll like receptor (TLR) family. TLRs were initially identified primarily due to their resemblance to the Toll protein of *Drosophila melanogaster*, which was involved in antifungal response as well as dorsoventral patterning during embryogenesis of *Drosophila* [20, 21]. TLRs are receptors that are positioned at cell or endosome membranes. They recognize PAMPs through their LRR domain and use their TIR domain to transmit signals to the intracellular space [22]. Numerous distinct signaling pathways are activated when TLR4 is engaged by particular PAMPs. TLR4 either activates the toll/interferon response factor (TRIF)-dependent signaling pathway or the myeloid differentiation factor 88 (MyD88)-dependent and independent signaling pathway to produce type I interferons (IFNs) and proinflammatory cytokines [23]. The activation of MAPK and early-phase NF-B contributes to the development of a proinflammatory reaction that is brought in by the MyD88-dependent pathway [3]. The MyD88-independent pathway leads to the induction of IFN and IFN-inducible genes. A significant number of cytosolic PRRs are responsible for TLR4-independent pathogen recognition [24].

The human cias1 gene, which has 9 coding exons and is found on chromosome 1q44, is the source of the 1016 amino acid protein NLRP3 [25]. NLRP3 inflammasome is a multimeric protein complex made up of the adapter protein ASC, the caspase-1 enzyme, and the sensor molecule NLR3 [26]. NLRP3 has a core NACHT domain, a carboxy-terminal LRR, and a PYD domain at its amino-terminal region interacting in association with the PYD domain of ASC in a homotypic manner [26].

Activation Mechanism of the NLRP3 Inflammasome

The NLRP3 inflammasome is activated by a wide range of stimuli, both pathogenic and sterile [27]. There are two categories of inflammasome effects: "conventional" and "non-conventional" impacts [28]. The first stage of the process is a reaction that involves the activation of certain cytokines or TLR4 receptors (through a PRR-mediated signal), which can increase the NF-kb mediated transcription of NLRP3, pro-IL-1 and pro-IL-18 [29]. The complex's oligomerization phase, in which the adaptor proteins ASC and inflammatory pro-caspase-1 are recruited, represents the second stage of the canonical route. The complex is then activated, and the conversion of pro-IL-1 and pro-IL-18 into their activated version takes place. Also, the subsequent caspase-1 activation causes a breakdown of Gasdermin D (GSMD), which causes pyroptosis, a sort of programmed form of cell death [30]. It is characterized by cell enlargement, accompanied by lysis and the discharge of internal contents, including proinflammatory cytokines like IL1 and IL18. The non-canonical pathway is dependent on either caspase-4/5 or caspase-11 in mice (for humans) instead of caspase-1 [28]. Ion flux, mitochondrial malfunction, and the formation of reactive oxygen species (ROS), as well as lysosomal disruption, are among the various processes reported to cause inflammasome activation. Uncertainty still exists on how these circumstances contribute to inflammasome activation. An intracellular potassium ion efflux is one activation process that seems to be conserved by numerous activators. Extracellular ATP can activate the P2X7, a purinergic receptor (ATP-gated ion channel,) causing potassium efflux, that is required for the activation of the inflammasome [19]. LPS priming causes the formation of NLRP3, which is essential for pro-inflammatory cytokine and ATP release *via* the P2X7 receptor [31].

ROS generation represents a stress-related signal, which is also a key step in NLRP3 inflammasome activation by acting on a target that is upstream of it [32]. By preventing NLRP3 activation, ROS inhibition can decrease the release of IL-1β [33]. DAMPs, such as crystalline or particulate matter, can cause lysosomal membrane damage, releasing lysosomal substances (such as cathepsin B) into the cytosol and activating NLRP3 [34]. IL-1β exerts its physiological impacts by initiating a cascade of signaling that includes p38, JNK (Jun N-terminal kinase) and NF-kB activation (Fig. **6**) [29, 35].

NLRP3 Inflammasome and Airway Inflammation

Innate immunity and inflammation appear to be significantly influenced by the inflammasome. The contribution of NLRP3 inflammasome to airway inflammation is expanding [36]. There is debate about the extent of the contribution of NLRP3 inflammasome in the setting of respiratory disease because it is a relatively novel idea that involves airway inflammation. In contrast to other lung conditions like COPD, asthmatic airway inflammation has received significant attention in terms of research . Airway inflammation is one of the most obvious symptoms of asthma, characterized by cellular infiltration that includes a large number of mast cells, eosinophils, neutrophils, lymphocytes, and macrophages. Th2-cells that release interleukin IL-4, IL-5, and IL-13 are the main source of lymphocytic inflammation [37]. Mucus metaplasia, subepithelial fibrosis, and infiltration of inflammatory cells, such as macrophages and eosinophils, are all caused by IL-13. The overexpression of IL-4 and IL-5 induces subepithelial fibrosis, a significant airway eosinophilia and mucus production. It is frequently believed that asthmatic airway inflammation is the cause of airway remodeling. In comparison to healthy controls, the thickening of the airway wall increases by 50–230% in fatal asthma, although it increases by 25–150% in nonfatal asthma. These modifications occur as a consequence of altered epithelial cells, mucus gland hyperplasia, subepithelial fibrosis, and more formation of blood vessels [38].

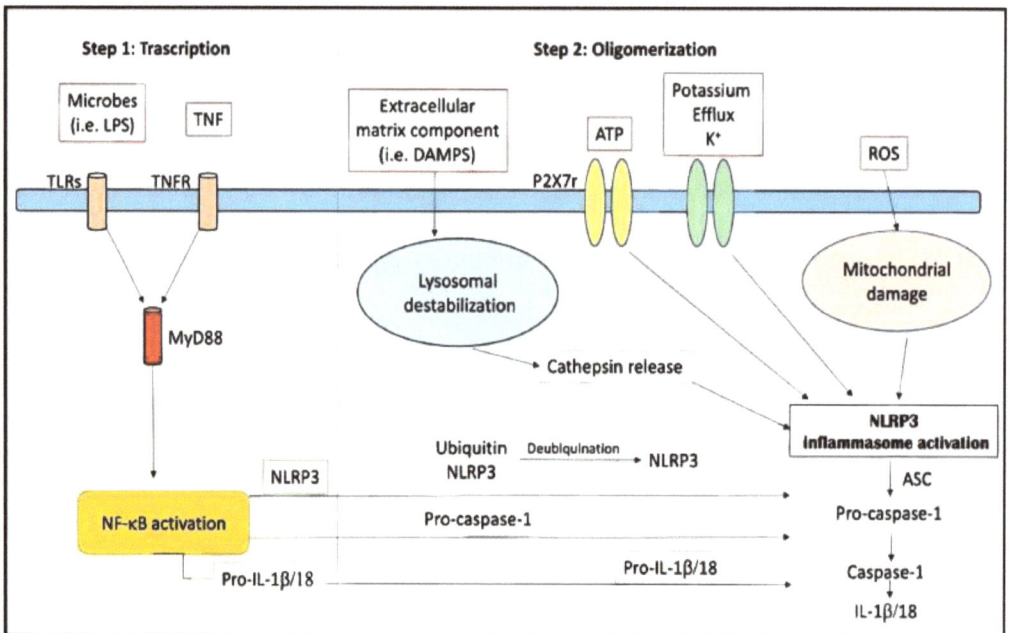

Fig (6). NLRP3inflammasome assembly and activation mechanism [35].

A complex, long-lasting inflammatory condition called allergic asthma causes inflammation in the conducting airways, a loss in respiratory function, and tissue remodeling [39]. The smooth muscle, submucosal layer, epithelium, and vascular structures are the elements of the airway wall thatare affected by the structural alterations seen in asthma [39]. Type 2 asthma, which is primarily characterized by T helper type 2 (Th2) cell-mediated inflammation, and non-type 2 asthma, which is linked to Th1 and/or Th17 cell inflammation, are two different asthma endotypes that are classified according to the immune cell reactions that are involved in the pathophysiology [37, 40, 41]. Since there is now no appropriate approach for treating fibrotic disorders, more studies on the function of inflammasomes in such conditions are crucial for the development of novel diagnostic medications.

Role of NLRP3 Inflammasome in Chronic Airway Inflammation

Both bacteria and viruses have been linked to asthma exacerbations. Viruses have been found in 45–80% of adult and 80% of pediatric asthma exacerbations, but bacterial infections are now more widely acknowledged to show a significant impact [43]. There is considerable debate over the contribution of NLRP3 inflammasomes in allergic asthmatic inflammation, and more research is necessary to clear the contradictions. Clinical and animal investigations showed that NLRP3 inflammasome protein was up-regulated in asthma patients and in an OVA-induced animal model of asthma [44, 45], indicating that NLRP3 inflammasome performed a prominent function in the pathogenesis of asthma after increased mRNA and protein expression of NLRP3, ASC, and Caspase-1 in U937 cells after LPS stimulation in lung tissues of asthmatic mice. NLRP3 knockout mice displayed decreased inflammatory cell infiltration and cytokine generation. These mice also showed a significant decrease in IgE production and mucus generation in the lungs after being challenged with OVA [46]. In addition, IL-1R1 or IL-1β- knockout mice displayed dramatically lowered expression of cytokines related to Th2 cells, such IL-5, IL-13, and IL-33 [46]. The OVA-induced murine model showed active caspase-1 together with dramatically increased serum concentrations of TNF-a and IL-1β [47]. Also, translocation of IL-1β and IL-18 to the epithelium apical surface was observed in inflamed airways of mice, while healthy epithelium stored these cytokines in their cytoplasm [47]. Purinergic receptor-mediated activation of the NLRP3 inflammasome, as shown by a number of *in vitro* studies, was found to be effective in mediating uric acid-induced airway inflammation [48]. This theory was confirmed *in vivo* in experimental mouse models of lung damage and asthma. The involvement of P2X7 receptors in many asthma models has been established, and both clinical samples and all these animals exhibit enhanced P2X7 expression levels [49]. Additionally, in allergic asthma models, it was demonstrated that danger signals like uric acid and alum support adaptive Th2 cell immunity [46]. Contrary to the findings mentioned above, which showed a detrimental effect of NLRP3 on airway inflammation in asthmatic models, mice lacking PYCARD,

NLRP3, or Caspase showed no influence on the Th2 cell immunity and thus did not depend on NLRP3 inflammasome activation [50]. This finding was also confirmed by a study comparing inflammatory response and airway hyperreactivity in wild-type mice *vs* NLRP3 deficient mice with allergic asthma model, which showed that no difference was observed in NLRP3-deficient mice as compared to wild-type mice in their pathophysiological characteristics, such as eosinophils counts, mucus secretion, and hyper-responsiveness [51]. Reports suggested that IL-1β has the capacity to stimulate the synthesis of a diverse range of additional chemokines and cytokines at the site of inflammation. They have the potential to strongly influence Th17 development, which is a process that is probably a major factor in the pathogen-induced aggravation. It should be noted that IL-1β has been demonstrated to support TH17 differentiation and IL-17 production, which are essential for the emergence of asthma with steroid resistance and allergic asthma aggravation [42, 52]. The effect of caspase-1 activation products on Th17 cells may turn out to be the most significant effect of NLRP3 inflammasome involvement in respiratory illness. Th17 cells are a unique group of CD4 T lymphocytes that are distinguished by the generation of strong immunoregulatory cytokines, particularly members of the IL-17 family. IL-17A has a strong impact on atopy [53] and asthma [54]. Current findings have shown that inflammasome activity affects innate immune responses in persons with atopic asthma and that infection-related exacerbations result in excessive inflammasome activation. Our findings also confirmed the earlier reports, which suggest that inflammasomes are responsible for the heightened inflammatory response, which has been associated with respiratory infections and asthma exacerbations [42, 55].

In bronchoalveolar lavage fluid (BALF) of LPS-/OVA-treated animals lacking NLRP3 and ASC, a decreased concentration of the pro-inflammatory cytokines, IL-1, IL-5, and IFN-γ, was observed. Anakinra, an IL-1R antagonist, and genetic deletion of IL-1R1 both resulted in lower eosinophil counts, indicating that IL-1 may be the primary factor in the recruitment of eosinophils in asthma [56]. In allergic airway inflammation models, NLRP3-inflammasome- dependent IL-1β release was associated with Th17 promotion. Besides neutrophilic asthma, the importance of IL-1β and IL-17A may also promote eosinophilic asthma [42]. Additionally, it had been discovered that BAL fluid of asthmatic patients had elevated levels of NLRP3 and caspase-1 than healthy people. Identical results in rodent models of AAI (LPS and ovalbumin therapy) and neutrophilic asthma (LPS and ovalbumin treatment) [47] supported these research work on humans. NLRP3 Inflammasomes not only aid in the proteolytic activation of IL-1β, but they also take part in caspase-1induced pyroptosis, promoting the release of a lot of inflammatory mediators in extracellular medium, due to whichthey are recognized for their importance in asthma [42]. It has been demonstrated that therapy with anti-IL-1 antibodies, caspase-1 inhibitors (Ac-YVAD-cho), or NLRP3 inhibitors (MCC950) reduces IL-1 synthesis and airway hyperresponsiveness *in vivo* in steroid-resistant asthma [56].

Airway Fibrosis

Fibrosis is caused by unresolved inflammation or poor stimulus clearance that leads to a prolonged inflammatory response [57]. The lungs, kidney, liver, and heart are just a few of the many fibroblast-containing organs that can develop fibrosis. It is characterized by ECM deposition, including the development of collagen, fibronectin, and glycoproteins, which ultimately destroys the structural integrity of the lungs and causes airway obstruction resulting in a high mortality rate [58]. Inflammasome has been linked to fibrosis in a growing number of research studies in the last few years. A study was conducted to look into the relationship between pulmonary fibrosis and inflammasome, involving the IL-1 receptor and MyD88 signaling [59]. The profibrotic drug bleomycin resulted in reduced response in mice lacking the ASC protein. Mice lacking in both, MyD88 and IL-1R1, displayed worse reactions to bleomycin. Additionally, recombinant mouse IL-1β administered directly to the lungs of wild-type mice caused a significant rise in tissue oxidation, inflammation, and collagen accumulations. The introduction of IL-1βneutralizing antibodies was not found to be as successful in reducing fibrosis in the wild-types as compared to IL-1 receptor antagonists [59]. Extracellular matrix proteins, including matrix metalloproteases-9 (MMP-9) and MMP-12, which are responsible for ECM degradation and consequent airway remodeling in asthma, can be produced when IL-1β concentration increases in the lungs [42]. IL-1β (and IL-18) can increase collagen synthesis in a dose-dependent way, according to *in vitro* experiments [60]. The mechanism behind the involvement of IL-1β in the progression of fibrosis is thought to be its connection to TGF-β [61]. TGF-β1 and platelet-derived growth factors are then significantly increased in epithelial cells of airways, which lead to collagen accumulation in the lungs [62]. While IL-1β can activate its own genes, prolonged inflammasome stimulation could culminate in ongoing IL-1βcleavage, which could function as a positive feedback mechanism to maintain a high amount of active TGF-β1 proteins and promote fibrosis. According to a report, the action of TGF-β is inhibited after a very short-term contact *via* NF-κB and the Smad pathway [63]. These genes are responsible for the transcription of TGF-β. Thus, the TGF-/Smad signaling, which is connected to fibrosis, is intimately linked to the inflammasome as well. AKT, phosphatidylinositol-3 kinase (PI3K), p38 MAPK, the extracellular signal-regulated kinases (ERKs), Rho family GTPases, and c-Jun amino-terminal kinase (JNK) are just a few of the non-Smad signaling pathways that TGF-β may activate. The contribution of EMT in lung fibrosis is a subject of growing concern [64, 65]. NLRP3 Inflammasome signaling cascade and its function in EMT have subsequently been the subject of some investigations. High levels of TGF-β, which initiates EMT activities in epithelial cells, were secreted by myofibroblasts. Any slight defect in this process could stimulate the production of excessive amounts of extracellular matrix components by myofibroblast, which would accelerate the generation of wounds and compromise the tissue functioning ability. Research has suggested that the activation of NLRP3 inflammasome through the IL-1b/IL-1Rs/MyD88/NF-kB signaling caused the transformation of epithelial cells into mesenchymal cells, resultingin fibrosis in the lungs [66]. Lung fibroblasts are the major cells involved in pulmonary fibrosis, and it has been reported that IL-1β participated in pulmonary fibrogenesis when fibroblast cells were isolated from mice and exposed to bleomycin. NLRP3 inflammasome controlled IL-1β *via* miR-155, resulting in fibrosis in the lungs [67, 68]. According to a report, NLRP3 inflammasome silencing resulted in a considerable drop in IL-1β and TGF-β levels in a bleomycin-induced lung injury model [69]. Additionally, the expression of α-SMA increased noticeably, whereas E-cadherin levels were dramatically reduced. As a result, the NLRP3 inflammasome in alveolar epithelial cells was activated, which suggests that TGF-β may control EMT [69]. Various results lead us to hypothesize that the NLRP3 inflammasome and all these signal transduction pathways interact extensively as fibrosis develops. The profuse release of IL-1 and IL-18, as well as the beginning of pyroptosis, are all key factors in the development of fibrotic pathologies and are caused by the chronic activation of inflammasomes. These cytokines can exacerbate fibrosis progression and finally result in structural changes and organ failure. IL-1 has the capacity to mediate the interaction between fibrosis and inflammation to create a positive feedback loop. The NLRP3 inflammasome, which has been associated with immunological response against bacteria, viruses, fungi, and parasites, has received the greatest attention these days [70]. The inflammasome/ASC/caspase-1/IL-1/IL-18 pathway induces inflammation, which is a key precondition for fibrosis. Additionally, while NF-kB is crucial for the stimulation and formation of the inflammasome, it also regulates inflammasome activation and exacerbates harmful inflammation. The inflammasome is also intimately linked to TGF-/Smad signaling, which is connected to fibrosis [71].

Immunomodulation

Treatment of severe asthma is based on the administration of anti-inflammatory medications (inhaled corticosteroids) for the prevention of symptoms and relief medication (bronchodilators β2 agonists) during exacerbations [72]. Long-term use of inhaled corticosteroid treatment may lead to detrimental effects, such as cataracts, osteoporosis in old age patients and stunting of growth in children. While some patients with severe asthma respond well to high-dose inhaled corticosteroids in combination with a long-acting β-agonist, a significant proportion of patients that require oral corticosteroids to control the symptoms also show adverse effects. Studies have suggested that the preventive treatment of severe asthma is cost-effective, especially in more severe and uncontrolled cases. Herbs and plants naturally contain many active constituents, thus drugs derived from such sources can have multiple health benefits. Due to the presence of these compounds, they are an ideal candidate for the treatment of a variety of symptoms. The idea of using plant-derived molecules for the treatment of allergic diseases is not a new concept. In fact, some commonly used conventional drugs are derived from plants. The current approach to the management of severe asthma is predominantly based on the use of inhaled bronchodilators and corticosteroids. The plant-based medicines in asthma may prove to be a better and safe alternative approach [73]. In nature, many medicinal plants exist that possess immunomodulatory properties, and their ingredients are used as immunomodulatory agents to treat various ailments. The restorative and rejuvenating power of these herbal remedies might be due to their action on the immune system. Some of the medicinal plants are believed to enhance the natural resistance of the body against infections. Plant-derived materials, such as proteins, lectines, polysaccharides, *etc.*, have been shown to stimulate the immune system. Ayurveda and other Indian literature have mentioned the use of medicinal plants in the treatment of various human ailments. There are a number of plants which have been reported to have immunomodulatory activities. Some important medicinal plants with immunomodulatory properties are *Allium sativum, Aloe vera, Andrographis panticulator, Azadirachta indica, Boerhauvia diffusa, Boswelli- aserrata, Curcuma longa, Centella astiatica, Curica papaya, Datura quercifolia, Emblica officinalis, Hydrastis Canadensis, Hypericum perforatum, Ocimum sanctum, Panax ginsangi, Piper longum, Withania somnifera etc*. These immunomodulatory properties have been studied through different mechanisms and are found to modulate alteration in total and differential cell count, delayed-type hypersensitivity reaction, phagocytosis, nitric oxide production, expression of co-stimulatory molecules *etc* [73, 74].

CURCUMIN AS IMMUNOMODULATORY AGENT

The anti-inflammatory action of curcumin has been extensively studied against several diseases. It targets several well-known transcription factors, AP-1 and NF-kβ, the well-known master switch of cells, thus inhibiting the downstream secretion of proinflammatory cytokines, such as TNF-α, IL-10, IL-1, IL-2, IL-6, IL-8 and IL-12. Curcumin is a potent immunomodulatory agent that can modulate the activation of T cells, B cells, macrophages, neutrophils, natural killer cells and dendritic cells [75]. The anti-inflammatory action of curcumin was also evaluated against acute as well chronic asthmatic murine models, where intranasal curcumin pretreatment at much lower doses (5 mg/ml) was effective in suppressing nitric oxide, IL-4, IL-5, IFN-γ and IgE antibodies [76, 77]. Curcumin protects against airway hyperresponsiveness in the sensitized guinea pigs, which was demonstrated by a constant volume body plethysmograph, thus significantly inhibiting airway constriction and hyperactivity in the guinea pigs.

Curcumin, when administered through the intraperitoneal route (20 mg/kg), lowered the protein expressions of p38, JNK, NF-κB, IL-6, IL-8 and TNF-α. This way, curcumin suppressed both LPS induced lung injury and neutrophil activation and injury [78]. The anti-inflammatory effects of curcumin have also been evaluated in murine as well as in cell lines, where curcumin effectively suppressed microRNAs, neutrophils accumulation, cytokine secretion and major transcription factors [79]. Curcumin was reported to inhibit lung inflammation and fibrosis when fed orally at 300 mg/kg for 10 days and by gastric incubation at 200 mg/kg in bleomycin and amiodarone-induced rat models [80, 81]. We reported earlier about the involvement of multiple pathways by which intranasal curcumin inhibits inflammatory response and LPS-induced asthma exacerbations, such as, PI3KAkt, HIF-1, TNF, MAPK and NF-κB pathway [82, 83]. We have recently reported the impact of intranasal curcumin on LPS-exposed airway inflammation and remodeling by regulating TLR4/NFkB/ NLRP3 inflammasome signaling, where oxidative stress was also modulated by intranasal curcumin, which was comparable to dexamethasone alone and in combination as well (Fig. 7). Further, it attenuated IL-5 and IL-17 secretion and remodeling in lungs, thereafter, reduced the severity of asthma by ameliorating pyroptosis *via* Gasdermin D inhibition [42].

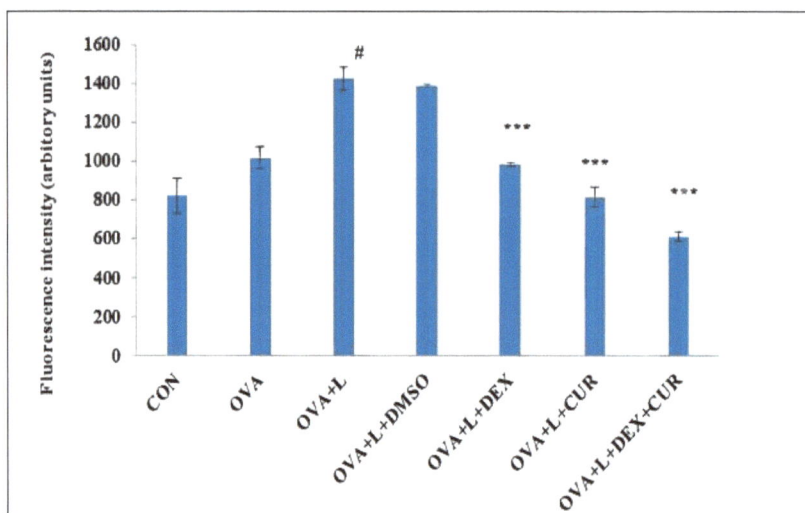

Fig. (7). Detection of reactive oxygen species (ROS) in BALF cells of LPS-exposed and OVA-induced mice where ROS is reduced significantly after curcumin and combined treatment (Cur + Dex) [42].

CONCLUDING REMARKS

The NLRP3 inflammasome is present in the cytoplasm of different immune cells as well as structural cells but not in any particular organelle. Regarding the function, signaling pathways, and its part in pathogenicity, it is one of the most well-studied inflammasome complexes. We have reported reduced NLRP3 inflammasome activation, cleaved caspase-1 induction, and consequently decreased IL-1β secretion through TLR4/NF-κB pathways after intranasal curcumin administration where its impact was studied alone and in combination with dexamethasone, a known corticosteroid. Further studies may help in finding an effective candidate for relaxing inflammation and airway remodeling that might be a better alternative for mild to severe lung diseases in the future.

ACKNOWLEDGEMENT

The authors are thankful to the Technology Development Program (TDP division), Science and Engineering Research Board (SERB), the Department of Science and Technology, New Delhi, India, in part for financial assistance.

REFERENCES

[1]   Råberg L, Vestberg M, Hasselquist D, Holmdahl R, Svensson E, Nilsson JÅ. Basal metabolic rate and the evolution of the adaptive immune system. Proc Biol Sci 2002; 269(1493): 817-21.
[http://dx.doi.org/10.1098/rspb.2001.1953] [PMID: 11958713]

[2]   Schmid-Schönbein GW. Analysis of inflammation. Annu Rev Biomed Eng 2006; 8(1): 93-151.
[http://dx.doi.org/10.1146/annurev.bioeng.8.061505.095708] [PMID: 16834553]

[3]   Mogensen TH. Pathogen recognition and inflammatory signaling in innate immune defenses. Clin Microbiol Rev 2009; 22(2): 240-73.
[http://dx.doi.org/10.1128/CMR.00046-08] [PMID: 19366914]

[4]   Trent MS, Stead CM, Tran AX, Hankins JV. Diversity of endotoxin and its impact on pathogenesis. J Endotoxin Res 2006; 12(4): 205-23.
[http://dx.doi.org/10.1179/096805106X118825] [PMID: 16953973]

[5]   Bone RC. The pathogenesis of sepsis. Ann Intern Med 1991; 115(6): 457-69.
[http://dx.doi.org/10.7326/0003-4819-115-6-457] [PMID: 1872494]

[6]   Strachan DP. Hay fever, hygiene, and household size. BMJ 1989; 299(6710): 1259-60.
[http://dx.doi.org/10.1136/bmj.299.6710.1259] [PMID: 2513902]

[7]   Thorne PS, Kulhánková K, Yin M, Cohn R, Arbes SJ Jr, Zeldin DC. Endotoxin exposure is a risk factor for asthma: the national survey of endotoxin in United States housing. Am J Respir Crit Care Med 2005; 172(11): 1371-7.
[http://dx.doi.org/10.1164/rccm.200505-758OC] [PMID: 16141442]

[8]   Dong L, Li H, Wang S, Li Y. Different doses of lipopolysaccharides regulate the lung inflammation of asthmatic mice *via* TLR4 pathway in alveolar macrophages. J Asthma 2009; 46(3): 229-33.
[http://dx.doi.org/10.1080/02770900802610050] [PMID: 19373628]

[9]   Busse WW. Anti-immunoglobulin E (omalizumab) therapy in allergic asthma. Am J Respir Crit Care Med 2001; 164(8 Pt 2) (Suppl. 1): S12-7.
[http://dx.doi.org/10.1164/ajrccm.164.supplement_1.2103026] [PMID: 11704612]

[10]   Raetz CRH, Whitfield C. Lipopolysaccharide endotoxins. Annu Rev Biochem 2002; 71(1): 635-700.
       [http://dx.doi.org/10.1146/annurev.biochem.71.110601.135414] [PMID: 12045108]

[11]   Postma DS, Kerstjens HAM. Characteristics of airway hyperresponsiveness in asthma and chronic
       obstructive pulmonary disease. Am J Respir Crit Care Med 1998; 158(5 Pt 3): S187-92.
       [http://dx.doi.org/10.1164/ajrccm.158.supplement_2.13tac170] [PMID: 9817744]

[12]   Ishmael FT. The inflammatory response in the pathogenesis of asthma. J Am Osteopath Assoc 2011;
       111(11) (Suppl. 7): S11-7.
       [PMID: 22162373]

[13]   Barnes PJ. Th2 cytokines and asthma: An introduction. Respir Res 2001; 2(2): 64-5.
       [http://dx.doi.org/10.1186/rr39] [PMID: 11686866]

[14]   Nelson HS, Davies DE, Wicks J, Powell RM, Puddicombe SM, Holgate ST. Airway remodeling in
       asthma: New insights. J Allergy Clin Immunol 2003; 111(2): 215-25.
       [http://dx.doi.org/10.1067/mai.2003.128] [PMID: 12589337]

[15]   Lambert RK, Wiggs BR, Kuwano K, Hogg JC, Paré PD. Functional significance of increased airway
       smooth muscle in asthma and COPD. J Appl Physiol 1993; 74(6): 2771-81.
       [http://dx.doi.org/10.1152/jappl.1993.74.6.2771] [PMID: 8365980]

[16]   Martinon F, Burns K, Tschopp J. The inflammasome. Mol Cell 2002; 10(2): 417-26.
       [http://dx.doi.org/10.1016/S1097-2765(02)00599-3] [PMID: 12191486]

[17]   Kanneganti TD, Lamkanfi M, Núñez G. Intracellular NOD-like receptors in host defense and disease.
       Immunity 2007; 27(4): 549-59.
       [http://dx.doi.org/10.1016/j.immuni.2007.10.002] [PMID: 17967410]

[18]   Zhao Y, Shao F. The NAIP – NLRC 4 inflammasome in innate immune detection of bacterial flagellin
       and type III secretion apparatus. Immunol Rev 2015; 265(1): 85-102.
       [http://dx.doi.org/10.1111/imr.12293] [PMID: 25879286]

[19]   He Y, Hara H, Núñez G. Mechanism and regulation of NLRP3 inflammasome activation. Trends
       Biochem Sci 2016; 41(12): 1012-21.
       [http://dx.doi.org/10.1016/j.tibs.2016.09.002] [PMID: 27669650]

[20]   Medzhitov R, Preston-Hurlburt P, Janeway CA Jr. A human homologue of the Drosophila Toll protein
       signals activation of adaptive immunity. Nature 1997; 388(6640): 394-7.
       [http://dx.doi.org/10.1038/41131] [PMID: 9237759]

[21]   Lemaitre B, Nicolas E, Michaut L, Reichhart JM, Hoffmann JA. The dorsoventral regulatory gene
       cassette spätzle/Toll/cactus controls the potent antifungal response in Drosophila adults. Cell 1996;
       86(6): 973-83.
       [http://dx.doi.org/10.1016/S0092-8674(00)80172-5] [PMID: 8808632]

[22]   O'Neill LAJ, Bowie AG. The family of five: TIR-domain-containing adaptors in Toll-like receptor
       signalling. Nat Rev Immunol 2007; 7(5): 353-64.
       [http://dx.doi.org/10.1038/nri2079] [PMID: 17457343]

[23]   Burns K, Martinon F, Esslinger C, *et al.* MyD88, an adapter protein involved in interleukin-1
       signaling. J Biol Chem 1998; 273(20): 12203-9.
       [http://dx.doi.org/10.1074/jbc.273.20.12203] [PMID: 9575168]

[24]   Iwasaki A, Medzhitov R. Toll-like receptor control of the adaptive immune responses. Nat Immunol
       2004; 5(10): 987-95.
       [http://dx.doi.org/10.1038/ni1112] [PMID: 15454922]

[25]   Lamkanfi M, Kanneganti TD. Nlrp3: An immune sensor of cellular stress and infection. Int J Biochem
       Cell Biol 2010; 42(6): 792-5.
       [http://dx.doi.org/10.1016/j.biocel.2010.01.008] [PMID: 20079456]

[26]   Sutterwala FS, Haasken S, Cassel SL. Mechanism of NLRP3 inflammasome activation. Ann N Y

Acad Sci 2014; 1319(1): 82-95.
[http://dx.doi.org/10.1111/nyas.12458] [PMID: 24840700]

[27]   Howrylak JA, Nakahira K. Inflammasomes: Key mediators of lung immunity. Annu Rev Physiol 2017; 79(1): 471-94.
[http://dx.doi.org/10.1146/annurev-physiol-021115-105229] [PMID: 28192059]

[28]   Jo EK, Kim JK, Shin DM, Sasakawa C. Molecular mechanisms regulating NLRP3 inflammasome activation. Cell Mol Immunol 2016; 13(2): 148-59.
[http://dx.doi.org/10.1038/cmi.2015.95] [PMID: 26549800]

[29]   Latz E, Xiao TS, Stutz A. Activation and regulation of the inflammasomes. Nat Rev Immunol 2013; 13(6): 397-411.
[http://dx.doi.org/10.1038/nri3452] [PMID: 23702978]

[30]   Ramos-Junior ES, Morandini AC. Gasdermin: A new player to the inflammasome game. Biomed J 2017; 40(6): 313-6.
[http://dx.doi.org/10.1016/j.bj.2017.10.002] [PMID: 29433834]

[31]   Franchi L, Eigenbrod T, Núñez G. Cutting edge: TNF-α mediates sensitization to ATP and silica *via* the NLRP3 inflammasome in the absence of microbial stimulation. J Immunol 2009; 183(2): 792-6.
[http://dx.doi.org/10.4049/jimmunol.0900173] [PMID: 19542372]

[32]   Shimada K, Crother TR, Karlin J, *et al.* Oxidized mitochondrial DNA activates the NLRP3 inflammasome during apoptosis. Immunity 2012; 36(3): 401-14.
[http://dx.doi.org/10.1016/j.immuni.2012.01.009] [PMID: 22342844]

[33]   Cruz CM, Rinna A, Forman HJ, Ventura ALM, Persechini PM, Ojcius DM. ATP activates a reactive oxygen species-dependent oxidative stress response and secretion of proinflammatory cytokines in macrophages. J Biol Chem 2007; 282(5): 2871-9.
[http://dx.doi.org/10.1074/jbc.M608083200] [PMID: 17132626]

[34]   Zheng R, Tao L, Jian H, *et al.* NLRP3 inflammasome activation and lung fibrosis caused by airborne fine particulate matter. Ecotoxicol Environ Saf 2018; 163: 612-9.
[http://dx.doi.org/10.1016/j.ecoenv.2018.07.076] [PMID: 30092543]

[35]   Fusco R, Siracusa R, Genovese T, Cuzzocrea S, Di Paola R. Focus on the role of NLRP3 inflammasome in diseases. Int J Mol Sci 2020; 21(12): 4223.
[http://dx.doi.org/10.3390/ijms21124223] [PMID: 32545788]

[36]   Cassel SL, Joly S, Sutterwala FS. The NLRP3 inflammasome: A sensor of immune danger signals. Semin Immunol 2009; 21(4): 194-8.
[http://dx.doi.org/10.1016/j.smim.2009.05.002] [PMID: 19501527]

[37]   Samitas K, Delimpoura V, Zervas E, Gaga M. Anti-IgE treatment, airway inflammation and remodelling in severe allergic asthma: Current knowledge and future perspectives. Eur Respir Rev 2015; 24(138): 594-601.
[http://dx.doi.org/10.1183/16000617.00001715] [PMID: 26621973]

[38]   Shifren A, Witt C, Christie C, Castro M. Mechanisms of remodelling in asthmatic airways. J Allergy 2012; 316049.

[39]   Holgate ST, Holloway J, Wilson S, *et al.* Understanding the pathophysiology of severe asthma to generate new therapeutic opportunities. J Allergy Clin Immunol 2006; 117(3): 496-506.
[http://dx.doi.org/10.1016/j.jaci.2006.01.039] [PMID: 16522446]

[40]   Robinson D, Humbert M, Buhl R, *et al.* Revisiting T ype 2-high and T ype 2-low airway inflammation in asthma: current knowledge and therapeutic implications. Clin Exp Allergy 2017; 47(2): 161-75.
[http://dx.doi.org/10.1111/cea.12880] [PMID: 28036144]

[41]   Santus P, Saad M, Damiani G, Patella V, Radovanovic D. Current and future targeted therapies for severe asthma: Managing treatment with biologics based on phenotypes and biomarkers. Pharmacol Res 2019; 146: 104296.

[http://dx.doi.org/10.1016/j.phrs.2019.104296] [PMID: 31173886]

[42] Jaiswal A, Dash D, Singh R. Intranasal curcumin and dexamethasone combination ameliorates inflammasome (NLRP3) activation in lipopolysachharide exposed asthma exacerbations. Toxicol Appl Pharmacol 2022; 436: 115861.
[http://dx.doi.org/10.1016/j.taap.2021.115861] [PMID: 34998855]

[43] Hayden FG. Rhinovirus and the lower respiratory tract. Rev Med Virol 2004; 14(1): 17-31.
[http://dx.doi.org/10.1002/rmv.406] [PMID: 14716689]

[44] Rossios C, Pavlidis S, Hoda U, *et al.* Sputum transcriptomics reveal upregulation of IL-1 receptor family members in patients with severe asthma. J Allergy Clin Immunol 2018; 141(2): 560-70.
[http://dx.doi.org/10.1016/j.jaci.2017.02.045] [PMID: 28528200]

[45] Kim RY, Pinkerton JW, Essilfie AT, *et al.* Role for NLRP3 inflammasome–mediated, IL-1β–dependent responses in severe, steroid-resistant asthma. Am J Respir Crit Care Med 2017; 196(3): 283-97.
[http://dx.doi.org/10.1164/rccm.201609-1830OC] [PMID: 28252317]

[46] Besnard AG, Guillou N, Tschopp J, *et al.* NLRP3 inflammasome is required in murine asthma in the absence of aluminum adjuvant. Allergy 2011; 66(8): 1047-57.
[http://dx.doi.org/10.1111/j.1398-9995.2011.02586.x] [PMID: 21443539]

[47] Tran HB, Lewis MD, Tan LW, *et al.* Immunolocalization of NLRP3 inflammasome in normal murine airway epithelium and changes following induction of ovalbumin-induced airway inflammation. J Allergy 2012; 2012: 1-13.
[http://dx.doi.org/10.1155/2012/819176] [PMID: 22523501]

[48] Idzko M, Hammad H, van Nimwegen M, *et al.* Extracellular ATP triggers and maintains asthmatic airway inflammation by activating dendritic cells. Nat Med 2007; 13(8): 913-9.
[http://dx.doi.org/10.1038/nm1617] [PMID: 17632526]

[49] Müller T, Vieira RP, Grimm M, *et al.* A potential role for P2X7R in allergic airway inflammation in mice and humans. Am J Respir Cell Mol Biol 2011; 44(4): 456-64.
[http://dx.doi.org/10.1165/rcmb.2010-0129OC] [PMID: 20508067]

[50] Kool M, Willart MAM, van Nimwegen M, *et al.* An unexpected role for uric acid as an inducer of T helper 2 cell immunity to inhaled antigens and inflammatory mediator of allergic asthma. Immunity 2011; 34(4): 527-40.
[http://dx.doi.org/10.1016/j.immuni.2011.03.015] [PMID: 21474346]

[51] Allen IC, Jania CM, Wilson JE, *et al.* Analysis of NLRP3 in the development of allergic airway disease in mice. J Immunol 2012; 188(6): 2884-93.
[http://dx.doi.org/10.4049/jimmunol.1102488] [PMID: 22323538]

[52] McKinley L, Alcorn JF, Peterson A, *et al.* TH17 cells mediate steroid-resistant airway inflammation and airway hyperresponsiveness in mice. J Immunol 2008; 181(6): 4089-97.
[http://dx.doi.org/10.4049/jimmunol.181.6.4089] [PMID: 18768865]

[53] Milner JD. IL-17 producing cells in host defense and atopy. Curr Opin Immunol 2011; 23(6): 784-8.
[http://dx.doi.org/10.1016/j.coi.2011.09.006] [PMID: 22019285]

[54] Wang YH, Wills-Karp M. The potential role of interleukin-17 in severe asthma. Curr Allergy Asthma Rep 2011; 11(5): 388-94.
[http://dx.doi.org/10.1007/s11882-011-0210-y] [PMID: 21773747]

[55] Lee TH, Song HJ, Park CS. Role of inflammasome activation in development and exacerbation of asthma. Asia Pac Allergy 2014; 4(4): 187-96.
[http://dx.doi.org/10.5415/apallergy.2014.4.4.187] [PMID: 25379478]

[56] Kim SR, Kim DI, Kim SH, *et al.* NLRP3 inflammasome activation by mitochondrial ROS in bronchial epithelial cells is required for allergic inflammation. Cell Death Dis 2014; 5(10): e1498-8.
[http://dx.doi.org/10.1038/cddis.2014.460] [PMID: 25356867]

[57]   Gallo J, Raska M, Kriegova E, Goodman SB. Inflammation and its resolution and the musculoskeletal system. J Orthop Translat 2017; 10: 52-67.
[http://dx.doi.org/10.1016/j.jot.2017.05.007] [PMID: 28781962]

[58]   Wynn TA, Ramalingam TR. Mechanisms of fibrosis: Therapeutic translation for fibrotic disease. Nat Med 2012; 18(7): 1028-40.
[http://dx.doi.org/10.1038/nm.2807] [PMID: 22772564]

[59]   Gasse P, Mary C, Guenon I, *et al.* IL-1R1/MyD88 signaling and the inflammasome are essential in pulmonary inflammation and fibrosis in mice. J Clin Invest 2007; 117(12): 3786-99.
[http://dx.doi.org/10.1172/JCI32285] [PMID: 17992263]

[60]   Postlethwaite AE, Raghow R, Stricklin GP, Poppleton H, Seyer JM, Kang AH. Modulation of fibroblast functions by interleukin 1: increased steady-state accumulation of type I procollagen messenger RNAs and stimulation of other functions but not chemotaxis by human recombinant interleukin 1 alpha and beta. J Cell Biol 1988; 106(2): 311-8.
[http://dx.doi.org/10.1083/jcb.106.2.311] [PMID: 2828381]

[61]   Alyaseer AAA, de Lima MHS, Braga TT. The role of NLRP3 inflammasome activation in the epithelial to mesenchymal transition process during the fibrosis. Front Immunol 2020; 11: 883.
[http://dx.doi.org/10.3389/fimmu.2020.00883] [PMID: 32508821]

[62]   Kolb M, Margetts PJ, Anthony DC, Pitossi F, Gauldie J. Transient expression of IL-1β induces acute lung injury and chronic repair leading to pulmonary fibrosis. J Clin Invest 2001; 107(12): 1529-36.
[http://dx.doi.org/10.1172/JCI12568] [PMID: 11413160]

[63]   Luo DD, Fielding C, Phillips A, Fraser D. Interleukin-1 beta regulates proximal tubular cell transforming growth factor beta-1 signalling. Nephrol Dial Transplant 2009; 24(9): 2655-65.
[http://dx.doi.org/10.1093/ndt/gfp208] [PMID: 19420104]

[64]   Ning ZW, Luo XY, Wang GZ, *et al.* MicroRNA-21 mediates angiotensin II-induced liver fibrosis by activating NLRP3 inflammasome/IL-1β axis *via* targeting Smad7 and Spry1. Antioxid Redox Signal 2017; 27(1): 1-20.
[http://dx.doi.org/10.1089/ars.2016.6669] [PMID: 27502441]

[65]   Gong Z, Zhou J, Zhao S, *et al.* Chenodeoxycholic acid activates NLRP3 inflammasome and contributes to cholestatic liver fibrosis. Oncotarget 2016; 7(51): 83951-63.
[http://dx.doi.org/10.18632/oncotarget.13796] [PMID: 27924062]

[66]   Song C, He L, Zhang J, *et al.* Fluorofenidone attenuates pulmonary inflammation and fibrosis *via* inhibiting the activation of NALP 3 inflammasome and IL -1β/ IL -1R1/MyD88/ NF -κB pathway. J Cell Mol Med 2016; 20(11): 2064-77.
[http://dx.doi.org/10.1111/jcmm.12898] [PMID: 27306439]

[67]   Wang X, Sun B, Liu S, Xia T. Structure activity relationships of engineered nanomaterials in inducing NLRP3 inflammasome activation and chronic lung fibrosis. NanoImpact 2017; 6: 99-108.
[http://dx.doi.org/10.1016/j.impact.2016.08.002] [PMID: 28480337]

[68]   Artlett CM, Sassi-Gaha S, Hope JL, Feghali-Bostwick CA, Katsikis PD. Mir-155 is overexpressed in systemic sclerosis fibroblasts and is required for NLRP3 inflammasome-mediated collagen synthesis during fibrosis. Arthritis Res Ther 2017; 19(1): 144.
[http://dx.doi.org/10.1186/s13075-017-1331-z] [PMID: 28623945]

[69]   Tian R, Zhu Y, Yao J, *et al.* NLRP3 participates in the regulation of EMT in bleomycin-induced pulmonary fibrosis. Exp Cell Res 2017; 357(2): 328-34.
[http://dx.doi.org/10.1016/j.yexcr.2017.05.028] [PMID: 28591554]

[70]   Strowig T, Henao-Mejia J, Elinav E, Flavell R. Inflammasomes in health and disease. Nature 2012; 481(7381): 278-86.
[http://dx.doi.org/10.1038/nature10759] [PMID: 22258606]

[71]   Chen TT, Xiao F, Li N, *et al.* Inflammasome as an effective platform for fibrosis therapy. J Inflamm

Res 2021; 14: 1575-90.
[http://dx.doi.org/10.2147/JIR.S304180] [PMID: 33907438]

[72]   Bousquet J, Jeffery PK, Busse WW, Johnson M, Vignola AM. Asthma. Am J Respir Crit Care Med 2000; 161(5): 1720-45.
[http://dx.doi.org/10.1164/ajrccm.161.5.9903102] [PMID: 10806180]

[73]   Das S, Bordoloi R, Newar N. A review on immune modulatory effect of some traditional medicinal herbs. J Pharm Chem Biol Sci 2014; 2: 33-42.

[74]   Mukherjee PK, Nema NK, Bhadra S, *et al.* Immunomodulatory leads from medicinal plants. Indian J Tradit Knowl 2014; 13: 235-56.

[75]   Jagetia GC, Aggarwal BB. "Spicing up" of the immune system by curcumin. J Clin Immunol 2007; 27(1): 19-35.
[http://dx.doi.org/10.1007/s10875-006-9066-7] [PMID: 17211725]

[76]   Shubhasini, Chauhan PS. Kumari S, *et al.*, Intranasal curcumin and its evaluation in murine model of asthma. Int Immunopharmacol 2013; 17: 733-43.
[http://dx.doi.org/10.1016/j.intimp.2013.08.008]

[77]   Chauhan PS, Subhashini, Dash D, Singh R. Intranasal curcumin attenuates airway remodeling in murine model of chronic asthma. Int Immunopharmacol 2014; 21(1): 63-75.
[http://dx.doi.org/10.1016/j.intimp.2014.03.021] [PMID: 24746751]

[78]   Jeong H, Yun C. Effect of curcumin on LPS-induced neutrophil activation and acute lung injury. Eur Respir J 2012; 40: 4635.

[79]   Ma F, Liu F, Ding L, *et al.* Anti-inflammatory effects of curcumin are associated with down regulating microRNA-155 in LPS-treated macrophages and mice. Pharm Biol 2017; 55(1): 1263-73.
[http://dx.doi.org/10.1080/13880209.2017.1297838] [PMID: 28264607]

[80]   Punithavathi D, Venkatesan N, Babu M. Curcumin inhibition of bleomycin-induced pulmonary fibrosis in rats. Br J Pharmacol 2000; 131(2): 169-72.
[http://dx.doi.org/10.1038/sj.bjp.0703578] [PMID: 10991907]

[81]   Punithavathi D, Venkatesan N, Babu M. Protective effects of curcumin against amiodarone-induced pulmonary fibrosis in rats. Br J Pharmacol 2003; 139(7): 1342-50.
[http://dx.doi.org/10.1038/sj.bjp.0705362] [PMID: 12890714]

[82]   Kumari A, Dash D, Singh R. Lipopolysaccharide (LPS) exposure differently affects allergic asthma exacerbations and its amelioration by intranasal curcumin in mice. Cytokine 2015; 76(2): 334-42.
[http://dx.doi.org/10.1016/j.cyto.2015.07.022] [PMID: 26239413]

[83]   Kumari A, Singh DK, Dash D, Singh R. Intranasal curcumin protects against LPS-induced airway remodeling by modulating toll-like receptor-4 (TLR-4) and matrixmetalloproteinase-9 (MMP-9) expression *via* affecting MAP kinases in mouse model. Inflammopharmacology 2019; 27(4): 731-48.
[http://dx.doi.org/10.1007/s10787-018-0544-3] [PMID: 30470954]

CHAPTER 2

NLRP3 Inflammasome: A Novel Mediator in Pulmonary Hypertension

Sushweta Mahalanobish[1], **Noyel Ghosh**[1] and **Parames C. Sil**[1,*]

[1] Division of Molecular Medicine, Bose Institute, P-1/12, CIT Scheme VII M, Kolkata-700054, West Bengal, India

Abstract: Pulmonary hypertension (PH) is marked by elevated mean pulmonary arterial pressure, unfavorable vascular remodeling and right ventricular failure. Current enormous amounts of clinical and preclinical data suggest the role of inflammation as a crucial factor for PH onset and development by modulating both innate and adaptive immune responses. In this context, NLRP3 inflammasome appears as a key step in the signaling cascade that negatively regulates various PH-associated conditions by inducing inflammatory outbursts. The activation of NLRP3 by pathogen-associated molecular pattern molecules/damage-associated molecular pattern molecules and caspase-1 mediated release of proinflammatory cytokines IL-1β and IL-18 are the key molecular events associated with NLRP3 inflammasomal pathway. Released IL-1β and IL-18 bring about adverse consequences on the pulmonary vasculature and the resulting onset of PH. Within this section, we will provide an in-depth understanding of present pulmonary hypertension (PH) treatments and their shortcomings. We will also discuss the contribution of NLRP3 inflammasomes in promoting inflammation within the context of PH pathobiology, as well as explore potential therapeutic approaches to target them.

Keywords: Inflammasome, Interleukin, Lung, NLRP3, Pulmonary hypertension.

INTRODUCTION

The main purpose of the immune system of our body is to safeguard against bacterial infections, eliminate carcinogenic cells, and arouse immune responses during cellular damage. During innate immunity, germline-encoded signaling receptors [pattern recognition receptors (PRRs)] recognize the microbial agents [pathogen-associated molecular patterns (PAMPs)] or agents released from injured host cells [damage-associated molecular patterns (DAMPs)]. Their interactions evoke the inflammatory responses against microbial agents or injured

*Corresponding author Parames C. Sil: Division of Molecular Medicine, Bose Institute, P-1/12, CIT Scheme VII M, Kolkata-700054, West Bengal, India; E-mails: parames@jcbose.ac.in, parames_95@yahoo.co.in

Puneetpal Singh (Ed.)
All rights reserved-© 2024 Bentham Science Publishers

cells and reinstate cellular homeostasis. Interestingly, as various commensal microbes are present in different organs (like gut and lung), a specific mechanism in the tissue selectively discriminates such local microflora from the foreign pathogens and hence helps to sustain a balanced immune response.

Several infectious agents, as well as exogenous particulates, are inhaled into our respiratory tract during inspiration. Innate immunity protects our respiratory machinery from these unpleasant substances,. In the lungs, specialized PRRs such as NOD-like receptors (NLRs), Retinoic acid-inducible gene I (RIG-I)-like receptors (RLRs), and Toll-like receptors (TLRs) stimulate the inflammatory response and induce immune cells to secret different chemokines like Monocyte chemoattractant protein-1 (MCP-1) or cytokines like interleukin-8 (IL-8), Tumor necrosis factor (TNF) and promote the involvement of various immune cells (like lymphocytes, neutrophils, *etc.*). Various cytokines, including IL-1β as well as IL-18, can trigger lung inflammation. Both of them are capable of exhibiting proteolytic activity, regulated by various innate immune receptors that assemble into a multiprotein composite called inflammasome [1]. Inflammasome activation is not only pathogen dependent but also dysregulated metabolism or damaged tissue triggers the onset of inflammasome-induced immune response. Evidence suggest that the NLRP3 inflammasome activation is required for viral or bacterial infections. Prolonged stimulation of this signaling factor causes the onset of various respiratory disorders like idiopathic pulmonary fibrosis (IPF), asthma, pulmonary hypertension (PH), and so on.

PH is a severely ruinous disorder where the mean arterial pressure of the pulmonary system remains more than 25 mm Hg at resting condition [2]. According to the World Health Organization, pulmonary arterial hypertension (PAH) is a Group 1 PH, which refers to increased pulmonary vascular resistance along with vascular remodeling of lung tissue [3]. The remodeling occurs in all the 3 layers of the vessel —the intima, media and adventitia, which cause enhanced resistance of pulmonary vasculature, functional impairment of the right ventricle and resulting mortality [4]. Recently, the role of inflammation on PH onset has received greater attention. Immune cells like macrophages, neutrophils, B-lymphocytes as well as T-lymphocytes inside the vessels have been found to be associated with both animal and human PH. In addition to the existence of autoantibodies, higher amounts of cytokines related to the inflammasomal pathway have been detected in the blood of PAH patients [5]. The presence of inflammasomal effectors and blockade of cytokines related to the inflammasomal pathway suggest the possible therapeutic approach to target inflammasome in PAH therapy. In this context, our initial focus is directed towards comprehending the activation of the NLR family pyrin domain-containing 3 (NLRP3) inflammasome, subsequently delving into its role in regulating pulmonary hypertension (PH).

Overview of NLRP3 Inflammasome

The NLRP3 inflammasome is composed of a multiprotein complex that stimulates the activation and maturation of inflammatory cytokines IL-1β and IL-18 [6]. NLRP3 belongs to the NOD-like receptor family, having three domains: a carboxy-terminal leucine-rich repeat domain (LRR), a middle nucleotide-binding domain (NACHT), and an amino-terminal pyrin domain (PYD). When the LRR domain senses a PAMP or a DAMP, the NLRP3 NACHT domain leads the process of oligomerization, and then the PYD domain interacts with the PYD domain of the adaptor molecule apoptosis-associated speck-like protein containing a CARD (ASC). Subsequently, the ASC CARD domain interacts with the pro-caspase-1 CARD domain that ultimately causes caspase-1 cleavage. The resulting activation of caspase-1 induces pro-IL-1β and pro-IL-18 cleavage to active IL-1β and IL-18 form and subsequent inflammation. Moreover, functional caspase-1 mediated gasdermin D activation triggers the onset of programmed cell death, *i.e.*, pyroptosis [7].

Effectors of NLRP3 Inflammasome Activation

The formation of NLRP3 inflammasome involves the requirement of a broad range of inducers like exogenous as well as endogenous activators. Exogenous activators are generally environmental particulates (silica crystals, asbestos fibers, *etc.*). The accumulation of endogenous activator molecules during metabolic disbalance or alteration of cellular homeostasis triggers the formation of NLRP3 inflammasome. It has been found that uric acid presents as a nontoxic soluble form under normal conditions. However, a high concentration of uric acid causes the formation of monosodium urate crystals that trigger the formation of NLRP3 inflammasome and induce IL-1β-mediated chronic inflammation. Likewise, intracellular ATP plays an important role in normal cellular homeostasis. During tissue damage, extracellular ATP interacts with P2X purinoreceptor 7 (P2X7) and causes NLRP3 activation [8]. As the formation of the NLRP3 inflammasome relies on a diverse range of signals, these stimuli do not engage with receptors. Alternatively, NLRP3 interacts with general upstream activators. Various types of intracellular events can lead to NLRP3 activation, like alteration of the redox system, ion concentration, and lysosomal stability.

Oxidative Stress and Reactive Oxygen Species (ROS)

The onset of oxidative stress triggers the production of exaggerated ROS, which is responsible for the activation of NLRP3 [9]. Although the involvement of the NADPH oxidase system is considered a prerequisite for NLRP3 activation, NLRP3 activation in mouse and human cell lines in the absence of NADPH oxidase suggests NADPH oxidase-independent NLRP3 formation [10, 11]. Furthermore, mitochondria-mediated ROS causes NLRP3 activation [12 - 14]. The necessity of ROS is crucial in the transcriptional priming of NLRP3 instead of the post-translational modifications of NLRP3 [15].

Lysosomal Activity

Activation of immune cells and cell-mediated phagocytosis of fibrillar protein or crystalline structures and lysosome-mediated destruction causes the release of cathepsins like proteases [16 - 18], which in turn causes the activation of NLRP3 inflammasome. However, the significance of lysosomal activity in NLRP3 activation has not been extensively investigated, and additional research in this area is required.

Fluctuation of Ion Concentration

Any kind of change in ion concentration (like increase and decrease of $Ca+2$ or K^+ concentration) causes NLRP3 activation [19, 20]. Following the verification of various types of upstream activators of NLRP3, it has been deduced that the participation of potassium (K^+) efflux holds paramount importance in the process of NLRP3 activation [21]. Interestingly, damaged mitochondria-mediated release of several factors acts as a common mediator for NLRP3 activation. Initially, activated NLRP3 is attached to mitochondria *via* mitochondrial antiviral signaling protein (MAVS) [22, 23]. Mitochondrial K^+ efflux induces mitochondrial ROS production [24]. Furthermore, phagolysosome-mediated Ca^{2+} mobilization causes mitochondrial damage-induced NLRP3 activation [25]. Interestingly, Ca^{2+}-induced mitochondrial damage results in mitochondrial ROS production and subsequent release of different mitochondrial components, which are sensed by NLRP3. The released cardiolipin from the mitochondrial membrane by NLRP3 activators interacts with the LRR domain of NLRP3, leading to the activation of NLRP3 in macrophages [26]. Overall, it indicates the involvement of dysfunctional mitochondrial cardiolipin in regulating NLRP3 activity. (Fig. **1**) represents the activation of NLRP3 inflammasome.

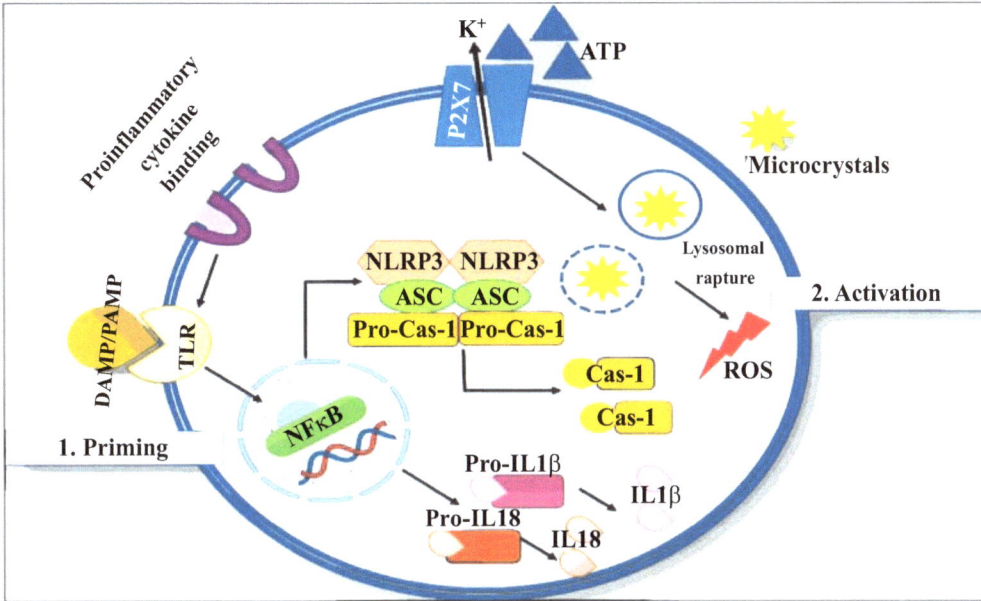

Fig. (1). Possible mechanism of NLRP3-mediated inflammasome activation.

Multistep Regulatory Mechanism of NLRP3 Inflammasome

The activity of NLRP3 is regulated at several levels, *i.e.*, from transcription to post-translational alteration.

Transcriptional Regulation

Inside a macrophage, NLRP3 is unable to evoke the inflammasomal response, and therefore, it depends upon NF-κB-mediated transcriptional priming to induce NLRP3 response. Interestingly, various immune signaling receptors (such as TLRs and TNFR) can control the NLRP3 induction [27 - 29]. It has been noticed that macrophages need continuous stimulation to build up enough amount of NLRP3 protein for inflammasome activation.

Post-transcriptional Regulation

Evidence-based studies have suggested that the expression of NLRP3 is controlled by micro-RNA (miRNA) in myeloid origin (CD11bþ) at the post-transcriptional level [30, 31]. The interaction of miR-223 with NLRP3 untranslated region decreases the rate of NLRP3 translation. It has been found that the expression of miR-223 is not controlled by pro-inflammatory cytokines, but the expression level of miR-223 changes between myeloid cells. Neutrophils exhibit a high level of expression and a modest expression level by macrophages, whereas dendritic cells (DCs) show a relatively low amount of expression. Therefore, this distinct expression profile of miR-223 refers to cell-specific sensitivity and necessitates additional transcriptional regulation to counteract the aberrant activation of the NLRP3 inflammasome.

Post-translational Alteration

Before inflammasome formation, various post-translational alterations occur in the NLRP3 protein level. Exposing macrophages to lipopolysaccharide for ten minutes causes caspase-1 activation. Increased mitochondrial ROS production in LPS posttreatment leads to NLRP3 deubiquitination, resulting in its activation. The enzymatic activity of BRCC3 leads to deubiquitination on NLRP3 [32, 33].

Other than deubiquitination, several types of alterations can also induce the formation of NLRP3. Although, no evidence has been reported to support direct NLRP3 phosphorylation, several experimental studies have indicated the role of kinase in inducing NLRP3 activation. Tyrosine kinase Syk triggers the function of NLRP3 while *Candida albicans* mediates the infection. The recognition of *C. albicans* and the resulting activation of Syk by Tyrosine-based activation motif (ITAM)-coupled receptors induce the formation of NLRP3 inflammasome [34]. Protein kinase R (PKR) directly interacts with NLRP3, NLRP1, and NLRC4, and therefore, blocks the function of the kinase domain of PKR, thus inhibiting the inflammasome-induced caspase-1 activation [35]. Moreover, the presence of TGF-β-activated kinase 1 (TAK1) inhibitor (5Z-7-oxozeaenol) blocks the formation of NLRP3 inflammasome, which suggests the involvement of TAK1 in inflammasome regulation [36]. Remarkably, the mobilization of intracellular Ca^{2+} during cell swelling leads to TAK1-induced NLRP3 activation [37]. All these outcomes provide strong support for the involvement of Syk, PKR, and TAK1-mediated NLRP3 activation to form a functional inflammasome.

Role of Inflammation in PH

Inflammation and immunity are the major inducing factors in PH pathogenesis [38]. Recent research have suggested the involvement of inflammation in the pathogenesis of vascular disorders involving PH. PH is characterized by dysfunction in endothelial cells, excessive cellular proliferation, along with impaired apoptosis. Germline mutations of bone morphogenic protein receptor (BMPR) II have been found in patients with familial and sporadic primary PH [39]. The connection between pulmonary hypertension (PH) and modified immunity has been affirmed through the observation that group 1 PH includes pulmonary arterial hypertension (PAH) linked to autoimmune conditions such as systemic sclerosis and systemic lupus erythematosus [40]. Patients suffering from systemic inflammatory diseases are susceptible to PH, and PH is often associated with autoimmune disorders and human immunodeficiency virus symptoms [41 - 43]. Increased concentration of proinflammatory cytokines and chemokines like MCP-1, IL-6 and IL-1 in the plasma of patients leads to idiopathic PH [44 - 46]. A study showed elevated levels of IL-1 and IL-6 in the plasma of PH patients where the administration of IL-1 antagonist alleviated the onset of monocrotaline-induced PH in rat models [47]. Diverse perivascular inflammatory cells, particularly monocytes and macrophages, along with the presence of RANTES, have been identified in the lungs of individuals with PH [48]. Surprisingly, the development of PH does not occur in all of the BMPRII mutant family members, which suggests the requirement of additional factors for PH development in this group. Interestingly, mutated BMPRII enhances the chance of inflammation in the pulmonary vasculature. Therefore, inflammation is a "second hit" for PH development in BMPRII mutated patients [49, 50]. These explanations have highlighted the role of inflammation in PH. Additionally, PH patients exhibit signs of chronic inflammation in the absence of immune disorders, along with an increased number of perivascular infiltrates and high levels of circulating cytokines [51]. Hence, for advanced therapeutic purposes, researchers must identify the alternative pathways that may involve remodeling (Fig. **2**).

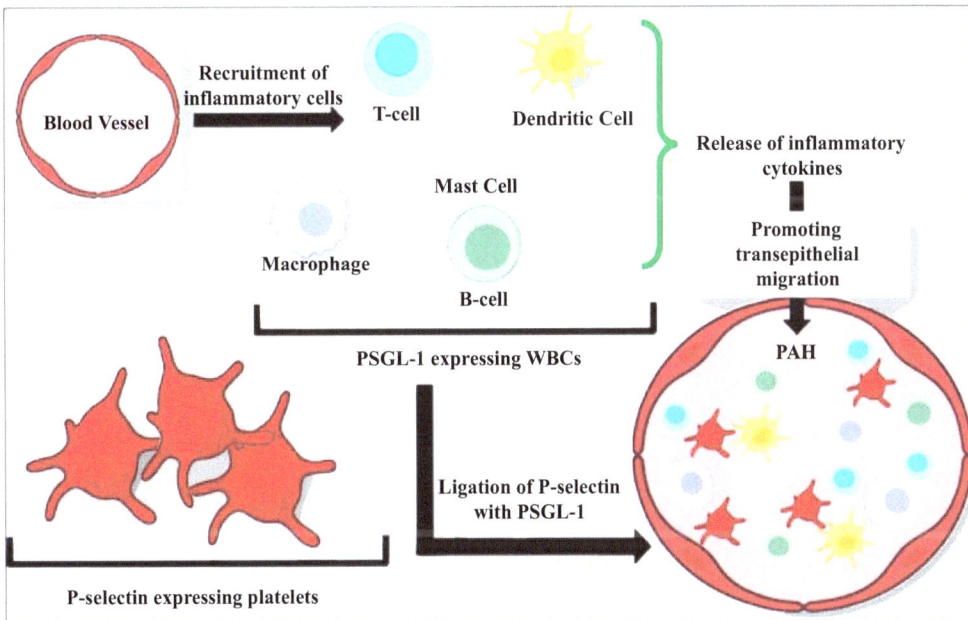

Fig. (2). Role of inflammation in PH.

Role of NLRP3 Inflammasome in Pulmonary Hypertension Onset

The involvement of NLRP3 inflammasome, along with its downstream signaling cascades in various pulmonary diseases like asthma, COPD and cystic fibrosis, has been investigated [52 - 54]. Different *in vitro* and *in vivo* evidence indicate the involvement of inflammasomes in PAH pathogenesis. During long-term hypoxia, mice without inflammasome adaptor molecules- ASC were saved from raised right ventricular hypertrophy and right ventricular systolic pressure (RVSP) [55]. Additionally, ASC null mice did not exhibit upregulated expression of caspase-1, IL-18, or IL-1β as compared to wildtype. Unexpectedly, mice with NLRP3 knockout were suspected of developing the disease at a similar extent to wildtype, without any remarkable difference in cytokine levels or RVSP. These data indicate that ASC loss (which is a prerequisite for many NLRP3 functions) but not NLRP3 is protective. It has been found that downstream signaling molecules participate in PH onset in rodents to activate inflammasomes like IL-1β, and its receptor, IL-1R,. After hypoxia onset, IL-1β, IL-1R, and MyD88 (IL-1R adaptor) are increased in the lungs of mice [56]. IL-1R or MyD88 knockout mice are saved from hypoxic PH, similar to those treated with the IL-1R receptor blocker, anakinra [56, 57]. In pulmonary artery smooth muscle cells, IL-1β treatment induced the growth of these cells in a MyD88 and IL-1R-mediated way [56, 57]. These results suggest the involvement of IL-1R in PH. Blocking the IL-1β expression can inhibit the upstream expression of inflammasome. Several possibilities are present behind this effect. Besides the presence of an upstream negative feedback loop, NF-κB and MyD88 are also involved in the amplification of inflammasome signaling. Similar to TLR, the receptor of IL-1β also engages NF-κB and MyD88, leading to the upregulation of IL-1β in a paracrine as well as autocrine manner. The use of the IL-1R blocker disrupts this cycle, thereby damaging the system. In the inflammasomal pathway, TLR signaling opens up various signaling mechanisms for PAH development. It has been found that TLR4, downstream of HMGB1, is involved in the development of PAH in different models [57, 58]. Moreover, downstream of TLR4 and MyD88, NF-κB stimulates IL-6 expression, which drives the development of PH in mice [59]. Finally, the "gut-lung axis" plays an important role where gut-derived bacterial lipopolysaccharide induces PAH, resulting in heart failure [60]. All these converging signaling pathways indicate that the disruption of this chain by using inflammasome inhibitors can target PAH related pathogenic signaling cascade. In the canonical inflammasome pathway, ASC and caspase-1 induce further cleavage of downstream substrates. During viral infection, Type 1 interferons upregulate the expression of double-stranded RNA kinase (PKR) [61]. PKR directly interacts with NLRP3, and PKR inhibition suppresses IL-1β, IL-18, and HMGB1 release [62]. It has been observed that PKR can activate pulmonary vessels of both Sugen-hypoxia and monocrotaline-treated rats [63]. Inhibition of PKR has been observed to prevent the development of PH in these models, block ASC activation and inhibit the release of HMGB1 and IL-1β [63]. It has been found that in endothelial cells, PKR is involved in the release of HMGB1 and cytokine and stimulates the cocultured smooth muscle cell proliferation [63]. This highlights the significance of a crucial regulatory protein in the inflammasome pathway, offering a potential clinical target. The inhibition of Caspase-1 in PH models shows that where caspase-1 knockout mice are moderately not affected by PH, caspase-1 induces the proliferation of smooth muscle cells [64]. In caspase-1 knockouts, re-administration of exogenous IL-1β and IL-18 restores PH phenotype, suggesting the importance of caspase-1 in downstream cytokine release. Therefore, the inhibition of canonical inflammasomes suppresses the release of diverse proteins in PH models, hence subjected to extensive clinical and translational analysis (Fig. **3**).

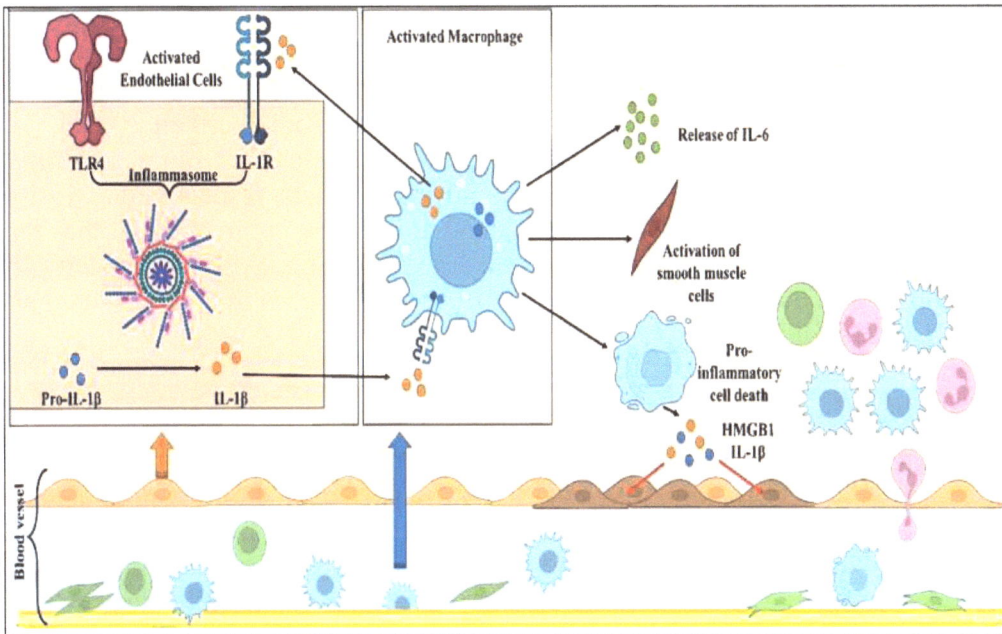

Fig. (3). Role of Inflammasome-mediated inflammation in PH.

Targeting NLRP3 for Pulmonary Hypertension Prevention

Role of Synthetic Inhibitors

The importance of inflammasome in PAH progression has been cleared from biomarkers and interventional studies. During PAH, high levels of HMGB1 were found in patients suffering from congenital or idiopathic heart disease associated with PAH [65, 66]. High levels of IL-1β in PAH patients' serum are related to worse outcomes [67]. It has been observed that the blockade of IL-1β with canakinumab in atherosclerosis patients reduces recurrent cardiac events and the inflammation outcome [68]. This approach is applied to patients with PAH and right ventricular failure, where they are treated with anakinra, an IL-1R antagonist. Although no hemodynamic change is observed over a three-month period, a significant improvement has been noticed in heart failure with reduced C-reactive protein levels [69]. In recent years, various approaches have been adopted for the clinical translation of inflammasome-based therapies. Different types of drugs are poised for trial, and some of them have been entered into trials previously. During the inflammasome priming stage, toll-like receptor-mediated activation of NF-κB is required [70]. Therefore, bardoxolone (NF-κB inhibitor) has been examined in Phase 3 trials in PAH patients. However due to some safety issues, this trial has been recently stopped (NCT 02657356). MCC-950, an NLRP3 inhibitor, can be used as a drug as it shows efficacy in aortic diseases, cardiac ischemia, and other inflammatory diseases [71, 72]. Pro-drug VX-765 can target the catalytic activity of caspase-1 [73]. Moreover, the use of necrosulfonamide or disulfiram can inhibit the activity of further downstream molecule-gasdermin D (the effector pore of inflammasome activation) [73, 74]. The activity of effector molecules like IL-1β or IL-6 released from gasdermin D can be inhibited by using canakinumab and tocilizumab, respectively. Most of these drugs, which target the inflammasomal activity by controlling all the steps in the pathway, are under extensive clinical investigation. Still, their specificity, tolerability, and overall immunosuppressive properties need to be considered and monitored carefully.

Role of Natural Inhibitors

Natural products are a promising source for therapeutic purposes [75 - 78]. Only a few reports have been found on how natural compounds can downregulate the NLRP3 inflammasomal activity in PAH. Ellagic acid (EA) is known for its anti-inflammatory, anti-oxidative, and anti-proliferative features. EA administration in rats decreases the systolic pressure of the right ventricle, wall thickness/external diameter ratio of pulmonary arteries and right ventricular hypertrophy in MCT-induced PAH. EA also reduces the MCT-mediated oxidative stress and the release of NLRP3, caspase-1, and IL-β in the lungs. It increases the amount of inflammatory cytokines and brain natriuretic peptides in serum [79]. Arctigenin, another bioactive component of *Arctium lappa,* shows efficacy in preventing PAH development. The treatment with (50 mg/ kg/day, intra-peritoneally) improves pulmonary arterial remodeling and right ventricular systolic pressure, reduces inflammatory cytokines expression, and suppresses pulmonary vascular smooth muscle cells proliferation in the lungs. Arctigenin effectively suppresses MCT-mediated upregulation of NLRP3, caspase-1 and IL-1β expression in the lungs

[80]. NLRP3 inflammasome formation is a multistep process, and some of the basic findings still need to be identified [81]. Further research is required to investigate the significance of natural bioactive compounds in PH alleviation, as natural bioactive compounds are cheap, easily available and free from side effects.

CONCLUSION

The activation of inflammasome during PAH brings out several important consequences. The release of various pro-inflammatory cytokines, lytic cell death, and infiltration of leukocytes, along with endothelial dysfunction, are associated with inflammasome activation. Therefore, this field requires extensive research in basic and translational science and clinical trials. By using several pharmacological interventions, targeting inflammasome is one of the therapeutic options for PAH patients in the future. PH represents a collection of syndromes with a broad range of etiologies. Determining the precise populations to apply inflammasome targeted therapy is one of the key challenges. A lot of important work, like the characterization of biomarkers in inflammasome-activated patients suffering from PAH, needs to be done. Once a comprehensive evaluation framework is established, the initiation of clinical trials within specific populations will yield advantages through translational therapies.

REFERENCES

[1]   Martinon F, Pétrilli V, Mayor A, Tardivel A, Tschopp J. Gout-associated uric acid crystals activate the NALP3 inflammasome. Nature 2006; 440(7081): 237-41.
        [http://dx.doi.org/10.1038/nature04516] [PMID: 16407889]

[2]   Goldenberg NM, Rabinovitch M, Steinberg BE. Inflammatory basis of pulmonary arterial hypertension. Anesthesiology 2019; 131(4): 898-907.
        [http://dx.doi.org/10.1097/ALN.0000000000002740] [PMID: 31094755]

[3]   Sysol JR, Machado RF. Classification and pathophysiology of pulmonary hypertension. Contin Cardiol Educ 2018; 4(1): 2-12.
        [http://dx.doi.org/10.1002/cce2.71]

[4]   Rabinovitch M, Guignabert C, Humbert M, Nicolls MR. Inflammation and immunity in the pathogenesis of pulmonary arterial hypertension. Circ Res 2014; 115(1): 165-75.
        [http://dx.doi.org/10.1161/CIRCRESAHA.113.301141] [PMID: 24951765]

[5]   Hu Y, Chi L, Kuebler WM, Goldenberg NM. Perivascular inflammation in pulmonary arterial hypertension. Cells 2020; 9(11): 2338.
        [http://dx.doi.org/10.3390/cells9112338] [PMID: 33105588]

[6]   Wen H, Gris D, Lei Y, *et al.* Fatty acid–induced NLRP3-ASC inflammasome activation interferes with insulin signaling. Nat Immunol 2011; 12(5): 408-15.
        [http://dx.doi.org/10.1038/ni.2022] [PMID: 21478880]

[7]   Swanson KV, Deng M, Ting JPY. The NLRP3 inflammasome: Molecular activation and regulation to therapeutics. Nat Rev Immunol 2019; 19(8): 477-89.
        [http://dx.doi.org/10.1038/s41577-019-0165-0] [PMID: 31036962]

[8]   Pelegrin P, Surprenant A. Pannexin-1 couples to maitotoxin- and nigericin-induced interleukin-1β release through a dye uptake-independent pathway. J Biol Chem 2007; 282(4): 2386-94.

[http://dx.doi.org/10.1074/jbc.M610351200] [PMID: 17121814]

[9]   Mahalanobish S, Dutta S, Saha S, Sil PC. Melatonin induced suppression of ER stress and mitochondrial dysfunction inhibited NLRP3 inflammasome activation in COPD mice. Food Chem Toxicol 2020; 144: 111588.
[http://dx.doi.org/10.1016/j.fct.2020.111588] [PMID: 32738376]

[10]   Latz E. NOX-free inflammasome activation. Blood 2010; 116(9): 1393-4.
[http://dx.doi.org/10.1182/blood-2010-06-287342] [PMID: 20813905]

[11]   van Bruggen R, Köker MY, Jansen M, *et al.* Human NLRP3 inflammasome activation is Nox1-4 independent. Blood 2010; 115(26): 5398-400.
[http://dx.doi.org/10.1182/blood-2009-10-250803] [PMID: 20407038]

[12]   Zhou R, Yazdi AS, Menu P, Tschopp J. A role for mitochondria in NLRP3 inflammasome activation. Nature 2011; 469(7329): 221-5.
[http://dx.doi.org/10.1038/nature09663] [PMID: 21124315]

[13]   Wen H, Gris D, Lei Y, *et al.* Fatty acid–induced NLRP3-ASC inflammasome activation interferes with insulin signaling. Nat Immunol 2011; 12(5): 408-15.
[http://dx.doi.org/10.1038/ni.2022] [PMID: 21478880]

[14]   Nakahira K, Haspel JA, Rathinam VAK, *et al.* Autophagy proteins regulate innate immune responses by inhibiting the release of mitochondrial DNA mediated by the NALP3 inflammasome. Nat Immunol 2011; 12(3): 222-30.
[http://dx.doi.org/10.1038/ni.1980] [PMID: 21151103]

[15]   Bauernfeind F, Bartok E, Rieger A, Franchi L, Núñez G, Hornung V. Cutting edge: reactive oxygen species inhibitors block priming, but not activation, of the NLRP3 inflammasome. J Immunol 2011; 187(2): 613-7.
[http://dx.doi.org/10.4049/jimmunol.1100613] [PMID: 21677136]

[16]   Hornung V, Bauernfeind F, Halle A, *et al.* Silica crystals and aluminum salts activate the NALP3 inflammasome through phagosomal destabilization. Nat Immunol 2008; 9(8): 847-56.
[http://dx.doi.org/10.1038/ni.1631] [PMID: 18604214]

[17]   Halle A, Hornung V, Petzold GC, *et al.* The NALP3 inflammasome is involved in the innate immune response to amyloid-β. Nat Immunol 2008; 9(8): 857-65.
[http://dx.doi.org/10.1038/ni.1636] [PMID: 18604209]

[18]   Duewell P, Kono H, Rayner KJ, *et al.* NLRP3 inflammasomes are required for atherogenesis and activated by cholesterol crystals. Nature 2010; 464(7293): 1357-61.
[http://dx.doi.org/10.1038/nature08938] [PMID: 20428172]

[19]   Fernandes-Alnemri T, Wu J, Yu J-W, *et al.* The pyroptosome: A supramolecular assembly of ASC dimers mediating inflammatory cell death *via* caspase-1 activation. Cell Death Differ 2007; 14(9): 1590-604.
[http://dx.doi.org/10.1038/sj.cdd.4402194] [PMID: 17599095]

[20]   Pétrilli V, Papin S, Dostert C, Mayor A, Martinon F, Tschopp J. Activation of the NALP3 inflammasome is triggered by low intracellular potassium concentration. Cell Death Differ 2007; 14(9): 1583-9.
[http://dx.doi.org/10.1038/sj.cdd.4402195] [PMID: 17599094]

[21]   Muñoz-Planillo R, Kuffa P, Martínez-Colón G, Smith BL, Rajendiran TM, Núñez G. K$^+$ efflux is the common trigger of NLRP3 inflammasome activation by bacterial toxins and particulate matter. Immunity 2013; 38(6): 1142-53.
[http://dx.doi.org/10.1016/j.immuni.2013.05.016] [PMID: 23809161]

[22]   Misawa T, Takahama M, Kozaki T, *et al.* Microtubule-driven spatial arrangement of mitochondria promotes activation of the NLRP3 inflammasome. Nat Immunol 2013; 14(5): 454-60.
[http://dx.doi.org/10.1038/ni.2550] [PMID: 23502856]

[23] Subramanian N, Natarajan K, Clatworthy MR, Wang Z, Germain RN. The adaptor MAVS promotes NLRP3 mitochondrial localization and inflammasome activation. Cell 2013; 153(2): 348-61.
[http://dx.doi.org/10.1016/j.cell.2013.02.054] [PMID: 23582325]

[24] Malinska D, Mirandola SR, Kunz WS. Mitochondrial potassium channels and reactive oxygen species. FEBS Lett 2010; 584(10): 2043-8.
[http://dx.doi.org/10.1016/j.febslet.2010.01.013] [PMID: 20080090]

[25] Shimada K, Crother TR, Karlin J, *et al.* Oxidized mitochondrial DNA activates the NLRP3 inflammasome during apoptosis. Immunity 2012; 36(3): 401-14.
[http://dx.doi.org/10.1016/j.immuni.2012.01.009] [PMID: 22342844]

[26] Iyer SS, He Q, Janczy JR, *et al.* Mitochondrial cardiolipin is required for Nlrp3 inflammasome activation. Immunity 2013; 39(2): 311-23.
[http://dx.doi.org/10.1016/j.immuni.2013.08.001] [PMID: 23954133]

[27] Franklin BS, Bossaller L, De Nardo D, *et al.* The adaptor ASC has extracellular and 'prionoid' activities that propagate inflammation. Nat Immunol 2014; 15(8): 727-37.
[http://dx.doi.org/10.1038/ni.2913] [PMID: 24952505]

[28] Bauernfeind F, Bartok E, Rieger A, Franchi L, Núñez G, Hornung V. Cutting edge: reactive oxygen species inhibitors block priming, but not activation, of the NLRP3 inflammasome. J Immunol 2011; 187(2): 613-7.
[http://dx.doi.org/10.4049/jimmunol.1100613] [PMID: 21677136]

[29] Franchi L, Eigenbrod T, Núñez G. Cutting edge: TNF-α mediates sensitization to ATP and silica *via* the NLRP3 inflammasome in the absence of microbial stimulation. J Immunol 2009; 183(2): 792-6.
[http://dx.doi.org/10.4049/jimmunol.0900173] [PMID: 19542372]

[30] Ferhani N, Letuve S, Kozhich A, *et al.* Expression of high-mobility group box 1 and of receptor for advanced glycation end products in chronic obstructive pulmonary disease. Am J Respir Crit Care Med 2010; 181(9): 917-27.
[http://dx.doi.org/10.1164/rccm.200903-0340OC] [PMID: 20133931]

[31] Mortaz E, Folkerts G, Nijkamp FP, Henricks PAJ. ATP and the pathogenesis of COPD. Eur J Pharmacol 2010; 638(1-3): 1-4.
[http://dx.doi.org/10.1016/j.ejphar.2010.04.019] [PMID: 20423711]

[32] Py BF, Kim MS, Vakifahmetoglu-Norberg H, Yuan J. Deubiquitination of NLRP3 by BRCC3 critically regulates inflammasome activity. Mol Cell 2013; 49(2): 331-8.
[http://dx.doi.org/10.1016/j.molcel.2012.11.009] [PMID: 23246432]

[33] Juliana C, Fernandes-Alnemri T, Kang S, Farias A, Qin F, Alnemri ES. Non-transcriptional priming and deubiquitination regulate NLRP3 inflammasome activation. J Biol Chem 2012; 287(43): 36617-22.
[http://dx.doi.org/10.1074/jbc.M112.407130] [PMID: 22948162]

[34] Gross O, Poeck H, Bscheider M, *et al.* Syk kinase signalling couples to the Nlrp3 inflammasome for anti-fungal host defence. Nature 2009; 459(7245): 433-6.
[http://dx.doi.org/10.1038/nature07965] [PMID: 19339971]

[35] Lu B, Nakamura T, Inouye K, *et al.* Novel role of PKR in inflammasome activation and HMGB1 release. Nature 2012; 488(7413): 670-4.
[http://dx.doi.org/10.1038/nature11290] [PMID: 22801494]

[36] Gong YN, Wang X, Wang J, *et al.* Chemical probing reveals insights into the signaling mechanism of inflammasome activation. Cell Res 2010; 20(12): 1289-305.
[http://dx.doi.org/10.1038/cr.2010.135] [PMID: 20856264]

[37] Compan V, Baroja-Mazo A, López-Castejón G, *et al.* Cell volume regulation modulates NLRP3 inflammasome activation. Immunity 2012; 37(3): 487-500.
[http://dx.doi.org/10.1016/j.immuni.2012.06.013] [PMID: 22981536]

[38]   Foley A, Steinberg BE, Goldenberg NM. Inflammasome activation in pulmonary arterial hypertension. Front Med 2022; 8: 826557.
[http://dx.doi.org/10.3389/fmed.2021.826557] [PMID: 35096915]

[39]   Lane KB, Machado RD, Pauciulo MW, *et al.* Heterozygous germline mutations in BMPR2, encoding a TGF-β receptor, cause familial primary pulmonary hypertension. Nat Genet 2000; 26(1): 81-4.
[http://dx.doi.org/10.1038/79226] [PMID: 10973254]

[40]   Bazan IS, Mensah KA, Rudkovskaia AA, *et al.* Pulmonary arterial hypertension in the setting of scleroderma is different than in the setting of lupus: A review. Respir Med 2018; 134: 42-6.
[http://dx.doi.org/10.1016/j.rmed.2017.11.020] [PMID: 29413506]

[41]   Marchesi C, Paradis P, Schiffrin EL. Role of the renin–angiotensin system in vascular inflammation. Trends Pharmacol Sci 2008; 29(7): 367-74.
[http://dx.doi.org/10.1016/j.tips.2008.05.003] [PMID: 18579222]

[42]   Dorfmüller P, Perros F, Balabanian K, Humbert M. Inflammation in pulmonary arterial hypertension. Eur Respir J 2003; 22(2): 358-63.
[http://dx.doi.org/10.1183/09031936.03.00038903] [PMID: 12952274]

[43]   Opravil M, Pechère M, Speich R, *et al.* HIV-associated primary pulmonary hypertension. A case control study. Swiss HIV Cohort Study. Am J Respir Crit Care Med 1997; 155(3): 990-5.
[http://dx.doi.org/10.1164/ajrccm.155.3.9117037] [PMID: 9117037]

[44]   Humbert M, Monti G, Brenot F, *et al.* Increased interleukin-1 and interleukin-6 serum concentrations in severe primary pulmonary hypertension. Am J Respir Crit Care Med 1995; 151(5): 1628-31.
[http://dx.doi.org/10.1164/ajrccm.151.5.7735624] [PMID: 7735624]

[45]   Itoh T, Nagaya N, Ishibashi-Ueda H, *et al.* Increased plasma monocyte chemoattractant protein-1 level in idiopathic pulmonary arterial hypertension. Respirology 2006; 11(2): 158-63.
[http://dx.doi.org/10.1111/j.1440-1843.2006.00821.x] [PMID: 16548900]

[46]   Balabanian K, Foussat A, Dorfmüller P, *et al.* CX(3)C chemokine fractalkine in pulmonary arterial hypertension. Am J Respir Crit Care Med 2002; 165(10): 1419-25.
[http://dx.doi.org/10.1164/rccm.2106007] [PMID: 12016106]

[47]   Tuder RM, Cool CD, Geraci MW, *et al.* Prostacyclin synthase expression is decreased in lungs from patients with severe pulmonary hypertension. Am J Respir Crit Care Med 1999; 159(6): 1925-32.
[http://dx.doi.org/10.1164/ajrccm.159.6.9804054] [PMID: 10351941]

[48]   Dorfmüller P, Zarka V, Durand-Gasselin I, *et al.* Chemokine RANTES in severe pulmonary arterial hypertension. Am J Respir Crit Care Med 2002; 165(4): 534-9.
[http://dx.doi.org/10.1164/ajrccm.165.4.2012112] [PMID: 11850348]

[49]   Upton PD, Morrell NW. TGF-β and BMPR-II pharmacology—implications for pulmonary vascular diseases. Curr Opin Pharmacol 2009; 9(3): 274-80.
[http://dx.doi.org/10.1016/j.coph.2009.02.007] [PMID: 19321386]

[50]   Song Y, Coleman L, Shi J, *et al.* Inflammation, endothelial injury, and persistent pulmonary hypertension in heterozygous BMPR2-mutant mice. Am J Physiol Heart Circ Physiol 2008; 295(2): H677-90.
[http://dx.doi.org/10.1152/ajpheart.91519.2007] [PMID: 18552156]

[51]   Stacher E, Graham BB, Hunt JM, *et al.* Modern age pathology of pulmonary arterial hypertension. Am J Respir Crit Care Med 2012; 186(3): 261-72.
[http://dx.doi.org/10.1164/rccm.201201-0164OC] [PMID: 22679007]

[52]   Kim RY, Pinkerton JW, Essilfie AT, *et al.* Role for NLRP3 inflammasome–mediated, IL-1β–dependent responses in severe, steroid-resistant asthma. Am J Respir Crit Care Med 2017; 196(3): 283-97.
[http://dx.doi.org/10.1164/rccm.201609-1830OC] [PMID: 28252317]

[53]   Iannitti RG, Napolioni V, Oikonomou V, *et al.* IL-1 receptor antagonist ameliorates inflammasome-dependent inflammation in murine and human cystic fibrosis. Nat Commun 2016; 7(1): 10791.
[http://dx.doi.org/10.1038/ncomms10791] [PMID: 26972847]

[54]   Dostert C, Pétrilli V, Van Bruggen R, Steele C, Mossman BT, Tschopp J. Innate immune activation through Nalp3 inflammasome sensing of asbestos and silica. Science 2008; 320(5876): 674-7.
[http://dx.doi.org/10.1126/science.1156995] [PMID: 18403674]

[55]   Cero FT, Hillestad V, Sjaastad I, *et al.* Absence of the inflammasome adaptor ASC reduces hypoxia-induced pulmonary hypertension in mice. Am J Physiol Lung Cell Mol Physiol 2015; 309(4): L378-87.
[http://dx.doi.org/10.1152/ajplung.00342.2014] [PMID: 26071556]

[56]   Parpaleix A, Amsellem V, Houssaini A, *et al.* Role of interleukin-1 receptor 1/MyD88 signalling in the development and progression of pulmonary hypertension. Eur Respir J 2016; 48(2): 470-83.
[http://dx.doi.org/10.1183/13993003.01448-2015] [PMID: 27418552]

[57]   Goldenberg NM, Hu Y, Hu X, *et al.* Therapeutic targeting of high-mobility group box-1 in pulmonary arterial hypertension. Am J Respir Crit Care Med 2019; 199(12): 1566-9.
[http://dx.doi.org/10.1164/rccm.201808-1597LE] [PMID: 30939030]

[58]   Bauer EM, Shapiro R, Billiar TR, Bauer PM. High mobility group Box 1 inhibits human pulmonary artery endothelial cell migration *via* a Toll-like receptor 4- and interferon response factor 3-dependent mechanism(s). J Biol Chem 2013; 288(2): 1365-73.
[http://dx.doi.org/10.1074/jbc.M112.434142] [PMID: 23148224]

[59]   Steiner MK, Syrkina OL, Kolliputi N, Mark EJ, Hales CA, Waxman AB. Interleukin-6 overexpression induces pulmonary hypertension. Circ Res 2009; 104(2): 236-244, 28p, 244.
[http://dx.doi.org/10.1161/CIRCRESAHA.108.182014] [PMID: 19074475]

[60]   Ranchoux B, Bigorgne A, Hautefort A, *et al.* Gut–lung connection in pulmonary arterial hypertension. Am J Respir Cell Mol Biol 2017; 56(3): 402-5.
[http://dx.doi.org/10.1165/rcmb.2015-0404LE] [PMID: 28248132]

[61]   Kang R, Tang D. PKR-dependent inflammatory signals. Sci Signal 2012; 5(247): pe47.
[http://dx.doi.org/10.1126/scisignal.2003511] [PMID: 23092889]

[62]   Lu B, Nakamura T, Inouye K, *et al.* Novel role of PKR in inflammasome activation and HMGB1 release. Nature 2012; 488(7413): 670-4.
[http://dx.doi.org/10.1038/nature11290] [PMID: 22801494]

[63]   Li Y, Li Y, Li L, Yin M, Wang J, Li X. PKR deficiency alleviates pulmonary hypertension *via* inducing inflammasome adaptor ASC inactivation. Pulm Circ 2021; 11(4): 1-13.
[http://dx.doi.org/10.1177/20458940211046156] [PMID: 34540200]

[64]   Udjus C, Cero FT, Halvorsen B, *et al.* Caspase-1 induces smooth muscle cell growth in hypoxia-induced pulmonary hypertension. Am J Physiol Lung Cell Mol Physiol 2019; 316(6): L999-L1012.
[http://dx.doi.org/10.1152/ajplung.00322.2018] [PMID: 30908936]

[65]   Bauer EM, Shapiro R, Billiar TR, Bauer PM. High mobility group Box 1 inhibits human pulmonary artery endothelial cell migration *via* a Toll-like receptor 4- and interferon response factor 3-dependent mechanism(s). J Biol Chem 2013; 288(2): 1365-73.
[http://dx.doi.org/10.1074/jbc.M112.434142] [PMID: 23148224]

[66]   Huang Y Y, Su W, Zhu Z W. Elevated serum HMGB1 in pulmonary arterial hypertension secondary to congenital heart disease. Vascul Pharmacol 2016; 85: 66-72.
[http://dx.doi.org/10.1016/j.vph.2016.08.009]

[67]   Soon E, Holmes AM, Treacy CM, *et al.* Elevated levels of inflammatory cytokines predict survival in idiopathic and familial pulmonary arterial hypertension. Circulation 2010; 122(9): 920-7.
[http://dx.doi.org/10.1161/CIRCULATIONAHA.109.933762] [PMID: 20713898]

[68]   Ridker PM, Everett BM, Thuren T, *et al.* Antiinflammatory therapy with canakinumab for atherosclerotic disease. N Engl J Med 2017; 377(12): 1119-31.
[http://dx.doi.org/10.1056/NEJMoa1707914] [PMID: 28845751]

[69]   Trankle CR, Canada JM, Kadariya D, *et al.* IL-1 blockade reduces inflammation in pulmonary arterial hypertension and right ventricular failure: A single-arm, open-label, phase IB/II Pilot Study. Am J Respir Crit Care Med 2019; 199(3): 381-4.
[http://dx.doi.org/10.1164/rccm.201809-1631LE] [PMID: 30418047]

[70]   Swanson KV, Deng M, Ting JPY. The NLRP3 inflammasome: Molecular activation and regulation to therapeutics. Nat Rev Immunol 2019; 19(8): 477-89.
[http://dx.doi.org/10.1038/s41577-019-0165-0] [PMID: 31036962]

[71]   van Hout GPJ, Bosch L, Ellenbroek GHJM, *et al.* The selective NLRP3-inflammasome inhibitor MCC950 reduces infarct size and preserves cardiac function in a pig model of myocardial infarction. Eur Heart J 2016; ehw247.
[http://dx.doi.org/10.1093/eurheartj/ehw247] [PMID: 27432019]

[72]   Ren P, Wu D, Appel R, *et al.* Targeting the NLRP3 inflammasome with inhibitor MCC950 prevents aortic aneurysms and dissections in mice. J Am Heart Assoc 2020; 9(7): e014044.
[http://dx.doi.org/10.1161/JAHA.119.014044] [PMID: 32223388]

[73]   Scott TE, Kemp-Harper BK, Hobbs AJ. Inflammasomes: A novel therapeutic target in pulmonary hypertension? Br J Pharmacol 2019; 176(12): 1880-96.
[http://dx.doi.org/10.1111/bph.14375] [PMID: 29847700]

[74]   Hu JJ, Liu X, Xia S, *et al.* FDA-approved disulfiram inhibits pyroptosis by blocking gasdermin D pore formation. Nat Immunol 2020; 21(7): 736-45.
[http://dx.doi.org/10.1038/s41590-020-0669-6] [PMID: 32367036]

[75]   Mahalanobish S, Saha S, Dutta S, Sil PC. Mangiferin alleviates arsenic induced oxidative lung injury *via* upregulation of the Nrf2-HO1 axis. Food Chem Toxicol 2019; 126: 41-55.
[http://dx.doi.org/10.1016/j.fct.2019.02.022] [PMID: 30769048]

[76]   Mahalanobish S, Saha S, Dutta S, Ghosh S, Sil PC. Melatonin counteracts necroptosis and pulmonary edema in cadmium-induced chronic lung injury through the inhibition of angiotensin II. J Biochem Mol Toxicol 2022; 36(10): e23163.
[http://dx.doi.org/10.1002/jbt.23163] [PMID: 35844137]

[77]   Dutta S, Mahalanobish S, Saha S, Ghosh S, Sil PC. Natural products: An upcoming therapeutic approach to cancer. Food Chem Toxicol 2019; 128: 240-55.
[http://dx.doi.org/10.1016/j.fct.2019.04.012] [PMID: 30991130]

[78]   Mahalanobish S, Saha S, Dutta S, Ghosh S, Sil PC. Anti-inflammatory efficacy of some potentially bioactive natural products against rheumatoid arthritis. Discovery and Development of Anti-Inflammatory Agents from Natural Products. Elsevier 2019; pp. 61-100.
[http://dx.doi.org/10.1016/B978-0-12-816992-6.00003-6]

[79]   Tang B, Chen G, Liang M, Yao J, Wu Z. Ellagic acid prevents monocrotaline-induced pulmonary artery hypertension *via* inhibiting NLRP3 inflammasome activation in rats. Int J Cardiol 2015; 180: 134-41.
[http://dx.doi.org/10.1016/j.ijcard.2014.11.161] [PMID: 25438234]

[80]   Jiang WL, Han X, Zhang YF, Xia QQ, Zhang JM, Wang F. Arctigenin prevents monocrotaline-induced pulmonary arterial hypertension in rats. RSC Advances 2019; 9(1): 552-9.
[http://dx.doi.org/10.1039/C8RA07892K] [PMID: 35521617]

[81]   Mahalanobish S, Ghosh N, Sil PC. NLRP3 inflammasome-assisted pathogenesis in chronic obstructive pulmonary disorder. immune function is depressed with aging while inflammation is heightened: An enigma. Nova 2022; 57: 37-65.

CHAPTER 3

Modulatory Mechanism of NLRP3 Inflammasome in Heart Diseases: "An Enigma Wrapped in a Riddle"

Anchal Arora[1], **Ravinder Sharma**[2], **Navjot Kanwar**[3], **Vikas Gupta**[4], **Gunpreet Kaur**[4], **Parveen Bansal**[4] and **Abhinav Kanwal**[1,*]

[1] *Department of Pharmacology, All India Institute of Medical Sciences, Bathinda, Punjab, India*

[2] *University Institute of Pharmaceutical Sciences and Research, BFUHS, Faridkot, Punjab, India*

[3] *University Institute of Pharmaceutical Sciences, Punjab University, Chandigarh, India*

[4] *University Centre of Excellence in Research, Baba Farid University of Health Sciences, Faridkot, Punjab, India*

Abstract: Despite breakthroughs in therapy over the prior two decades, heart failure is considered the foremost cause of mortality globally. The inflammasome plays a pivotal role in the advancement of heart failure, abdominal aortic aneurysm, atherosclerosis, diabetic cardiomyopathy, hypertension, dilated cardiomyopathy, cardiac remodeling and calcific aortic valve disease. The NLRP3 inflammasome is a crucial multi-protein signaling platform that tightly regulates inflammatory responses. It regulates antimicrobial host defense, which causes pyroptosis through caspase-1 activation by the eventual production of pro-inflammatory cytokines. The investigation of the NLRP3 inflammasome in various cardiovascular diseases may reveal critical disease triggers and endogenous modulators, leading to the development of new therapeutic interventions in the future. The target of this chapter is to summarise the recent literature describing the activation mechanism of the NLRP3 inflammasome by implicating different inflammatory pathways in the pathophysiology of heart failure.

Keywords: Caspase-1, Heart failure, IL-1β, Inflammation, NLRP3 inflammasome.

INTRODUCTION

Heart failure (HF) is a leading cause of morbidity and mortality in the United States, with rising prevalence of obesity, diabetes, hypertension, *etc.*, throughout the world. In the United States, about 6 million people have been officially diagnosed with heart failure. Additionally, many others have a condition called

* **Corresponding author Abhinav Kanwal:** Department of Pharmacology, All India Institute of Medical Sciences, Bathinda, Punjab, India; E-mail: abhinavkanwal@gmail.com

Puneetpal Singh (Ed.)
All rights reserved-© 2024 Bentham Science Publishers

asymptomatic left ventricular insufficiency, which means their hearts are not working quite right, and they are at risk of developing heart failure. Unfortunately, heart failure causes over half a million deaths every year in the United States. For people with severe heart failure, more than 50% of them do not survive past one year. This information is extracted from the American Heart Association 2003 guidelines. Heart failure presents with symptoms such as dyspnea, peripheral edema, orthopnea, paroxysmal nocturnal dyspnea, and bendopnea [1]. Nevertheless, significant breakthroughs in the insight of HF at the body system and cellular-molecular levels have prompted significant progress in heart failure medication that has changed clinical practice. Although symptomatic relief and reliability of life improvement are still essential goals, it is now feasible to start therapy with the assumption that disease progression can be slowed and, in many cases, survival can be extended.

The main components of this disease, volume overload (congestion) and myocardial dysfunction (heart failure), have historically been the focus of pharmacological therapy. The use of diuretics and cardiac glycosides has traditionally been highlighted in treatment plans, with research efforts focused on the creation of novel medicines that enhance contractile function. Such treatments have not been shown to increase survival while being successful in alleviating symptoms and stabilizing patients with hemodynamic decompensation. Further recent research has shed more light on the origins and progression of CHF, offering a conceptual framework that views the condition as the result of disturbed circulatory dynamics and pathologic cardiac remodeling. The way blood moves in the body and the changes that take place in the heart when it is not healthy have improved a lot. These improvements have helped doctors to take care of heart failure better. Before we talk about how a thing called the NLRP3 inflammasome is connected to heart failure, first make sure we understand how NLRP3 is linked to treating heart failure [2].

Innate immunity and adaptive immunity are key components in mammals to provide protection against internal and external dangers in the host. Endogenous and exogenous pathogens are sensed by the utilization of pattern recognition receptors or sensor proteins (PRRs) of the innate immune response. In 2002, the novel PRR, *i.e.*, inflammasome, was reported for the first time. PRR is a protein complex with a high molecular weight that triggers pro-interleukin-1 (pro-IL-1) to be processed as well as the stimulation of inflammatory caspase. Inflammasomes are the critical components of innate immunity because they function as signaling platforms exceedingly proficient in tackling a wide variety of harmful microorganisms, pathogens and cell-related products linked to stress and damage [3]. Five distinct members of the nucleotide-binding oligomerization domain (NOD) family, which includes NLRP1, NLRP3, and NLRC4, along with absent-in-melanoma 2 (AIM2) and pyrin, have been demonstrated to play a role in inflammasome formation [4]. Additionally, findings of the formation of the inflammasome by other PRR members comprising NLRP2, NLRP6, NLRP7, NLRP12, and IFI16 (interferon-γ inducible nuclear gene) have been documented in the literature [5, 6]. Through recognition receptors (PRRs) such NLRP1, NLRP3, AIM2 and pyrin, an apoptosis-associated speck-like protein with a caspase-recruitment domain (ASC) is essential for engaging pro-caspase-1 in the inflammasome complex. The LRR (leucine-rich repeat) domain senses the danger signal and causes NLRP3 monomer oligomerization *via* the NACHT domains and is accompanied by the link between the PYD domains of NLRP3 and ASC. Eventually, ASC, which functions as an adapter protein, enlists procaspase-1 into the assembly through its CARD domain [7].

The structure of the recombinant complex of the mitotic Ser/Thr kinase NEK7 and the NLRP3 protein without the pyrin domain was recently identified by Sharif *et al.* An earring-shaped structure made up of curved LRR and spherical NACHT domains was visible on the cryo-EM map. The C-terminal lobe of NEK7 interacts with the NBD (nucleotide-binding domain), LRR and HD2 (helical domain 2) domains of NEK7 (NIMA-related kinase 7). This structure implies that NEK7 may form bipartite contacts with neighboring NLRP3 subunits to activate the NLRP3 inflammasome [8]. The NLRP3 inflammasome-mediated increase in IL-1 and IL-18 production is linked to the beginning of atherosclerotic plaque formation in both atherosclerotic patients and animal models [9]. Both experimental autoimmune encephalomyelitis (EAE) in animal models and multiple sclerosis (MS) in humans have been linked to the NLRP3 inflammasome as their cause [10].

The activation of the NLRP3 inflammasome is also associated with various other conditions, including inflammatory bowel disease (IBD), ulcerative colitis, and Crohn's disease [11]. Malignancies related to the NLRP3 inflammasome include gastrointestinal cancers, melanoma, hepatitis C virus-associated hepatocellular carcinoma, breast cancer, and colon cancer [12]. Over and above NLRP3 activation anomalies, cryopyrin-associated periodic disorders (CAPS) are the genetic NLRP3 abnormalities [13]. Mutations within the NLRP3 gene lead to a gain-of-function outcome, which causes CAPS diseases, which are characterized by increased IL-1β secretion and other symptoms that are unique to CAPS [14].

TRIGGERING OF NLRP3 INFLAMMASOME

A number of triggers, including pathogen-associated RNA, adenosine triphosphate (ATP), heme, potassium ionophores (K^+), particulate matter, and bacterial and fungal toxins, can stimulate NLRP3. Since NLRP3 is yet to be seen to interrelate with any of these agonists, it is thought that they produce a shared cellular signal due to their biochemical dissimilarity. The activation of the NLRP3 inflammasome has been demonstrated to result from various mechanisms, which include cascades of events that lead to ionic imbalances, mitochondrial functioning imbalance, more reactive oxygen species and lysosomal damage (Fig. 1).

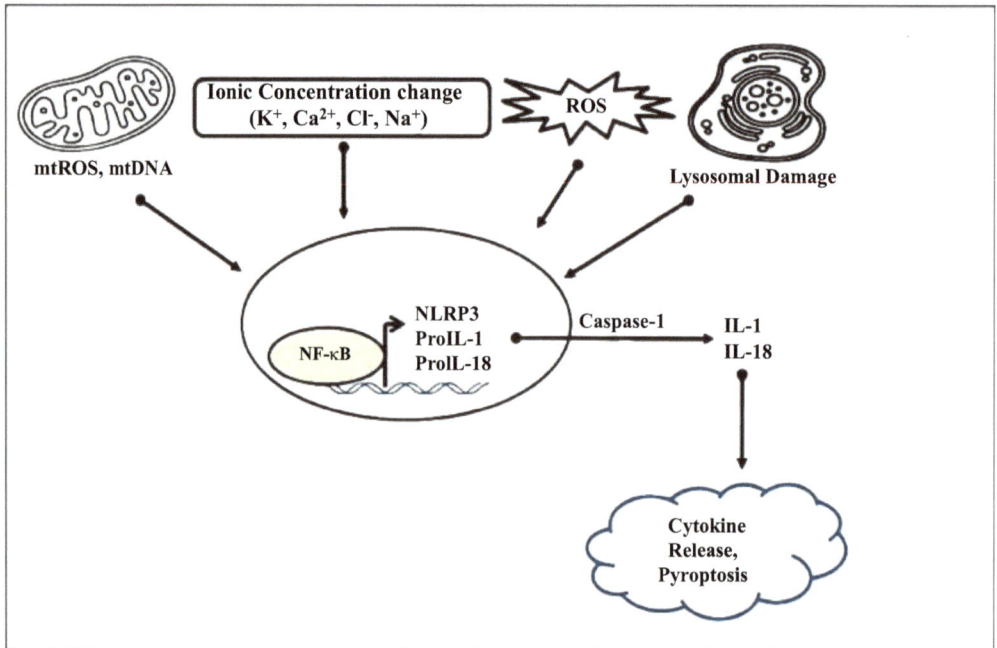

Fig. (1). Activation of NLRP3 inflammasome.

Ionic Flux/ Ionic Activation

In treated cells, NLRP3 stimulus elicits ionic flux phenomena such as K^+, Cl^- efflux, and Ca^{2+} Na^+ influx, which are involved in activating the NLRP3 inflammasome [15].

K^+ Efflux

It has long been known that the majority of NLRP3 stimuli cause cells to experience K^+ efflux, a frequent ionic event. In response to nigericin or ATP, macrophages and monocytes cause IL-1β maturation and release, which were discovered to be mediated by cytosolic K^+ depletion in experiments conducted before the discovery of inflammasome, which are now recognized for being NLRP3 stimuli. Furthermore, NLRP3 can be activated by K^+ efflux solely, and an increased level of K^+ extracellular inhibits the NLRP3 activation but does not lead to the inhibition of inflammasomes, such as AIM2 or NLRC4. Therefore, it has been assumed that a drop in intracellular K^+ is the typical trigger for the activation of NLRP3 inflammasome. Furthermore, the efflux of potassium is dispensable for the alternative NLRP3 inflammasome pathway, whereas it plays a crucial role in mediating the caspase-11 within the cascade of non-canonical inflammasome. Moreover, potassium efflux triggers Ca^{2+}-independent phospholipase A2, which facilitates the maturation of IL-1β [16, 17].

Recent investigations have demonstrated that distinct small chemical entities like CL097, GB111-NH2, and imiquimod possess the ability to trigger NLRP3 activation autonomously from K^+ efflux. This suggests that either NLRP3 inflammasome activation is prompted by a subsequent occurrence following K^+ efflux or alternative pathways for NLRP3 inflammasome activation exist, independent of K^+ efflux. Additionally, mice macrophages with the Muckle-Wells syndrome-related NLRP3 mutation (NLRP3R258W) activate the inflammasome even in the absence of K^+ efflux following simple LPS (lipopolysaccharide) activation. Based on these statistics, potassium ion efflux is not merely essential but also obligatory for the activation of the NLRP3 inflammasome. These results also unveil that a reduction in intracellular potassium levels could potentially induce conformational changes in NLRP3 akin to those brought about by small molecules, signals originating from the alternative inflammasome pathway, or mutations that activate NLRP3. Further investigation is required to determine the mechanisms by which NLRP3 identifies fluctuations in intracellular potassium concentrations. It is also essential to explore potential regulatory proteins involved in this process and elucidate the activation mechanisms triggered by the efflux of potassium ions (K^+) [16 - 18].

Ca^{2+} Mobilization

Even while Ca^{2+} influx is a common feature of many intracellular signaling pathways, its significance in NLRP3 inflammasome stimulation is still debatable. The chemical BAPTA-AM, which helps control calcium ions (Ca^{2+}) in cells, can stop the release of IL-1β. This suggests that calcium movement is involved in making the NLRP3 inflammasome work [19]. Additionally, it has been demonstrated that a variety of NLRP3 stimuli, including adenosine triphosphate, nigericin, and particulate matter, alter the intracellular concentration of calcium ions. It has been suggested that a variety of Ca^{2+} sources actually contribute to the spike in intracellular Ca^{2+} that occurs when the stimulation of NLRP3 ensues Phospholipase C, GPRC6A, and the calcium-sensing receptor (CaSR) serve as stimuli for NLRP3 activation of G-protein-coupled receptors (GPCRs) downstream, leading to the hydrolysis of phosphatidylinositol 4, 5-bisphosphate

(PIP2) to generate inositol 1, 4, 5-triphosphate (IP3). The IP3 receptor (IP3R) is an ion channel that is ligand-gated and causes Ca^{2+} efflux from the endoplasmic reticulum (ER) lumen to the cytosol in response to IP3. Additionally, NLRP3 activation and Ca^{2+} flow are prevented by the 2-aminoethoxy diphenylborinate (2APB) suppression of IP3R.

The development of NLRP3 inhibitors is now based on the discovery of how 2APB can block the NLRP3 activation independent of its capacity to limit calcium mobilization. Similarly, an elevation in cytosolic calcium (Ca^{2+}) concentrations arises from the interaction between Ca^{2+} and channels like TRPV2, TRPM7, TRPM2, and P2RX7 situated along the plasma membrane [20]. The lysosome is indeed thought to be a source of Ca^{2+} that might help activate the NLRP3 inflammasome. This surge in cytosolic Ca^{2+}, despite its origin, has been demonstrated to be essential for NLRP3 inflammasome expression since stimulation of NLRP3 leads to the activation of caspase 1. The secretion of IL-1 is reduced when ER or plasma membrane Ca^{2+} channels are blocked. It is still not known how an upsurge in cytosolic Ca^{2+} encourages NLRP3 inflammasome activation. According to research, Ca^{2+} directly controls NLRP3 inflammasome activation because it can enhance the association of ASC and NLRP3 in macrophages. As an alternative, it is hypothesized that the rise in cytosolic Ca^{2+} results in mitochondrial Ca^{2+} overloading, which promotes mitochondrial malfunction and activates the NLRP3 inflammasome.

In contradistinction to those findings, an alternate study illustrates that the activation of the inflammasome is impeded by BAPTA-AM, irrespective of its capacity to sequester calcium ions. This research also shows that the activation of the NLRP3 inflammasome is triggered by a range of stimuli, encompassing ATP, nigericin, and the lysosomotropic peptide Leu-Leu-OMe. Further pieces of evidence suggest that the external Ca^{2+} pool is not necessary for NLRP3 inflammasome activation, which is concluded from the fact that K^+ efflux-inducing stimuli can cause macrophages that have been cultured in Ca2+free media to become activated. Ca^{2+} mobilization may not be required for the NLRP3 inflammasome to activate, but it may occasionally serve a regulatory role in this process [19 - 21].

Na^+ Influx and Cl^- Efflux

Two significant ionic measures associated with NLRP3 inflammasome stimulation are Na^+ inflow and Cl^- efflux. Gramicidin, nigericin, or potassium ion-free medium all cause the NLRP3 inflammasome to activate, however it is activated by silica, ATP, or aerolysin when the sodium ion inflow is blocked by lowering extracellular sodium ion. It was observed that a reduction in Na^+ influx elevated the potassium ion efflux threshold, which is necessary to trigger NLRP3 activation in the low-potassium ion environment. Furthermore, investigations have shown that delivering monosodium urate crystals (MSU) to lysosomes causes a rise in intracellular sodium ions, which causes cellular content expansion and water inflow, resulting in a decline in intracellular potassium levels. To induce NLRP3 inflammasome activation, sodium ions (Na^+) could potentially decrease the intracellular potassium (K^+) concentration below the threshold of 90 mM. The activation of the NLRP3 inflammasome does not solely result from the influx of sodium ions (Na^+), a phenomenon driven by Na+ ionophores [15]. Hence, the entry of sodium ions (Na^+) seems to regulate the initiation of the NLRP3 inflammasome, possibly by influencing the efflux of potassium ions (K^+) triggered by stimuli. A prior investigation, which demonstrated an increase in ATP-induced IL-1 maturation and secretion due to heightened extracellular chloride ion (Cl^-) concentration (from 130 mM to 9 mM), initially prompted the notion that the influx of chloride ions (Cl^-) could potentially play a role in the activation of the NLRP3 inflammasome.

However, when there is more chloride (Cl^-) outside the cell, it can actually reduce the release of IL-1. Using certain substances that block chloride channels, like indanyloxyacetic acid, 4,40-diisothiocyano-2,20-stilbenedisulfonic acid, mefenamic acid, flufenamic acid, and 5-nitro-2-(3-phenylpropylamino) benzoic acid, can slow down the activation of the NLRP3 inflammasome [22]. However, the NLRC4 or, according to reports, chloride channels, such as the chloride intracellular channels (CLICs) and volume-regulated anion channel (VRAC), control the activation of the NLRP3 inflammasome.

Due to mitochondrial dysfunction, CLICs translocate to the plasma membrane. This relocation results in chloride ion (Cl^-) efflux, which subsequently governs the activation of the NLRP3 inflammasome by facilitating the interaction between NLRP3 and Nek7. Nevertheless, the mechanism through which Cl^- efflux enhances the interaction between NLRP3 and Nek7 remains unclear. Remarkably, the inhibition of CLICs leads to reduced pro-IL-1 mRNA production and ASC speck formation, while NLRP3 protein levels remain unaffected. Moreover, it has been observed that Cl^- efflux can trigger the formation of ASC specks, yet without K^+ efflux, it fails to activate the NLRP3 inflammasome [23 - 25]. It is necessary to conduct more research to determine how Cl^- efflux interacts with other ionic events to activate the NLRP3 inflammasome.

Reactive Oxygen Species

ROS is generated by aerobic metabolism, and research has indicated that ROS are responsible for activating NLRP3 in treated cells, with NOX serving as the primary ROS generator. Notably, NLRP3 inflammasome activation in both human and animal cells appears largely unaffected by NOX inhibition. However, in certain mouse models, such as those involving ischemic stroke followed by brain injury, inhibition of NOX2 may potentially exert an impact.

Furthermore, NADPH oxidase 4 (NOX4) assists in fatty acid oxidation, which contributes to the activation of NLRP3 [21]. Bauernfeind *et al*. provided a new outlook on how ROS functioned by demonstrating that ROS inhibitors also prevented the signal that primed NLRP3 activation. According to the findings presented above, the ROS pathway is crucial to the activation of NLRP3.The components are intricate and need detailed research to ascertain how they differ from one another.

Mitochondrial Dysfunction

Within mitochondria, the respiratory process operates as a cascading sequence. Upon disruption of the sequential mechanism, mitochondrial ROS (mtROS), which is oxygen used in the respiratory chain, may start to build. Nakahira *et al*. earlier established that mtROS was necessary for NLRP3's response to ATP and LPS [22]. Mice deficient in the mitochondrial protective protein exhibited elevated levels of mitochondrial reactive oxygen species (mtROS) and amplified the production of IL-1 and IL-18 under septic conditions [23]. MtDNA is another byproduct of mitochondrial malfunction.

It was observed during the research that the dysfunctional mitochondria released mtDNA not only linked with NLRP3 but also carried out oxidation and was crucial for activation. Further research provided more proof that the TLR (Toll-like receptors) signal pathway, which induces the production of mtDNA, is essential for the activation process.

Lysosomal Damage

It has been discovered that particulate matter encourages macrophage NLRP3 inflammasome activation. Due to the inability of these particles to be broken down by active lysosomal enzymes, lysosomes are disrupted, which causes the acidification of the lysosomes and oozing of contents of lysosomes to the cytoplasm. A proton pump called H^+ ATPase maintains hydrogen equilibrium in the cytosol and lysosomes. The inhibition of H^+ ATPase by bafilomycin A similarly leads to a reduction in particulate matter-induced NLRP3 inflammasome activation, underscoring the significant impact of lysosomal acidification on the activation mechanism. Another plausible explanation for particulate matter-induced NLRP3 activation is the potential leakage of active lysosomal enzymes [19]. Notably, cathepsin B, an exceptional lysosomal enzyme, was found to be essential for IL-1 release but did not affect pro-IL-1 production. Comparable outcomes were observed in studies concerning cathepsins X, L, C, and S. Due to the varied substrate preferences of cathepsins, functional overlap might obscure the activation-promoting effects of a specific cathepsin. Because cathepsins have diverse substrate preferences, functional redundancy may mask the activation-stimulating effects of a given cathepsin. Overall, active lysosomal enzyme leakage plays a significant role, although their lack can also be compensated by other mechanisms.

ACTIVATION PROCESS OF NLRP3 INFLAMMASOME *VIA* CANONICAL AND NON-CANONICAL PATHWAYS

Currently, canonical and non-canonical pathways of NLRP3 activation have been identified as two independent steps. Transcription (priming) and oligomerization (activation) are two separate and simultaneous stages required for canonical NLRP3 inflammasome stimulation [26]. A special protein in the body called nuclear factor-kappa B (NF-κB) helps to make NLRP3 and pro-IL-1 when our immune system is activated. This happens because of the signals from certain proteins like the tumor necrosis factor (TNF) receptor and toll-like receptors. Then, later on, NLRP3 and another protein called ASC come together and start a chain reaction that leads to the release of IL-18 and IL-1 [27]. NLRP3 inflammasome is activated by a diverse array of stimuli, such as by inhibiting glycolytic or mitochondrial metabolism, viral RNA, changes in the body's salt balance, and *via* the accumulation of amyloid (A) protein and synuclein (Syn) and also by post-translational modifications of NLRP3 (such as ubiquitination and phosphorylation).Thus, there are many ways our body can trigger NLRP3 to work. Research involving macrophages and animal models has revealed that the NLRP3 inflammasome can also be activated by oxidized low-density lipoprotein (oxLDL) and cholesterol crystals. Furthermore, monosodium urate crystals play a role in causing gout in both macrophages and animal models with an accumulation of uric acid, primarily by activating the NLRP3 inflammasome [28].

Additionally, as indicated by Hecker *et al.*, the activation of nicotinic acetylcholine receptors containing subunits 7, 9, and/or 10 resulted in the inhibition of ATP-mediated IL-1 production in both human and rat monocytes. This protective effect safeguards these cells from encountering unforeseen repercussions following an infarction. Notably, NLRP3 inflammasome-related proteins experience up-regulation in cardiac fibroblasts, a phenomenon that might play a role in determining the extent of the infarct during ischemia-reperfusion injury [29]. Caspase-1 maturation also contributes to pyroptosis, a vital defense mechanism against microbial infections independent of IL-1 activation. This process stops the facilitation of growing harmful microorganisms within the cell and allows the cell to engulf remaining bacteria through processes like phagocytosis. This also releases pro-inflammatory proteins, which are pivotal in the progression of various chronic inflammatory conditions. In humans, this alternative pathway relies on caspase-5 and caspase-4, while in mice, it hinges on caspase-11 [30].

Certain types of harmful bacteria like *Escherichia coli, Citrobacter rodentium, Legionella pneumophila, Vibrio cholerae,* and *Salmonella typhimurium* become active in our body through a couple of pathways called TRIF and TLR4-MyD88. These pathways also make a protein called interferon (IFN)-α. Later on, some unknown parts in our cells get activated by these bacteria, and this activates a protein called caspase-11. Caspase-11 starts a process called pyroptosis and releases IL-1, which causes inflammation. There is another way this can happen. Sometimes, certain molecules from damaged cells or the bacteria themselves can activate a protein called TLR4. This can trigger caspase-8 and its receptor to start a similar process. So, our body has different ways to protect itself from these harmful invaders [31].

Both the process of transcribing genetic information and the classical activation of the NLRP3 inflammasome can be triggered by the presence of receptor-interacting protein 1 (RIP1), fatty acid synthase (FAS), and the death domain associated with FADD protein. Endogenous damage-associated molecular patterns (DAMPs) that accumulate misfolded proteins and display an abnormal increase in various metabolites, characteristic of these illnesses, have been identified as direct factors that prime the NLRP3 inflammasome. The activation of a complex involving mucosa-associated lymphoid tissue lymphoma translocation protein 1 (MALT1), caspase-8, and ASC can also occur due to mycobacteria and fungal cell wall components such as glucans. This activation is facilitated by the stimulation of dectin-1, which subsequently enhances the production of interleukin-1 (IL-1). Notably, caspase-8 serves as a direct IL--converting enzyme, distinguishing it from caspase-1. The NLRP3 inflammasome is expressed in various cell types, predominantly macrophages, neutrophils, monocytes, and dendritic cells. Its expression extends to a wide array of non-immune cells, yet its role in endothelial cells, hepatocytes, and vascular smooth muscle cells remains uncertain and requires further elucidation [32]. If the NLRP3 and ASC genes are missing in bone marrow-derived dendritic cells (BMDCs), we do not see caspase-8 getting activated or IL-1 being processed. However, when there is a fungal infection, dendritic cells can make IL-1 because of a connection between caspase-8 and ASC. In simple terms, the NLRP3 inflammasome can be turned on or off by different things happening inside the cells, either separately or together [33 - 35].

ROLE OF NRLP3 INFLAMMASOME IN VARIOUS AILMENTS

Prognostic indicators for cardiovascular disorders like heart failure, diabetic cardiomyopathy, hypertension, diabetes, and atherosclerosis as well as the progression of these conditions after coronary obstruction, are significantly influenced by the NLRP3 inflammasome. During infection or inflammation, and also in stress situations, the NLRP3 inflammasome and the activity of IL-1β seem to regulate both pathogen-associated molecular patterns and damage-associated molecular patterns. Numerous inflammatory ailments are caused by excessive IL-1β activity, and inhibiting it appears to lessen cardiovascular pathology. In order to create safe medication for the management of cardiovascular disorders, it may be beneficial to comprehend the molecular pathways behind NLRP3 inflammasome formation and activation. Recent research has demonstrated that the development of cardiovascular disorders such as hypertension, ischemia damage, atherosclerosis, myocardial infarction, and cardiomyopathy is due to the NLRP3 stimulation in several ailments.

NLRP3 Inflammasome in Heart Failure

End-stage illness such as HF is defined as the incapacity to sustain regular blood output due to dysfunctioning in the diastolic or contractile mass, which results in increased CVD mortality. The underlying process of heart failure is now understood to involve myocardial remodeling, influenced by the modulatory actions of the NLRP3 inflammasome. Pyroptosis causing myocardial injury and cardiac fibroblast activation are the central steps in the remodeling process of physiological events. Another potential mechanism of apoptosis driven by inflammatory cytokines has been made feasible by the recent finding of NO physiological activities. By relaxing vascular smooth muscles or through other routes, low amounts of NO produced by constitutive NO synthase protect cardiomyocytes. However, excessive NO production from enzymes like inducible NO synthase (iNOS) causes cardiac damage and regulates leukocyte-endothelial interactions [33]. While IL-18 encourages iNOS overexpression, IL-1 is a powerful inducer of iNOS. Both require caspase-1 cleavage on the NLRP3 inflammasome to mature. A high iNOS level triggers the creation of tiny, uncharged NO molecules in addition to the overproduction of NO, apoptosis, and remodeling that follows. Reactive nitrogen species (RNS), which may change into NO molecules, have a similar function to ROS. TNF- α is not found in normal myocardium. TNF-α, on the other hand, is present in cardiomyocytes, reducing myocardial contractility in HF animal models *via* diminishing Ca^{2+} intracellular release. Among the downstream products of NLRP3 activation, TNF-α is generated due to the influence of IL-18. Meanwhile, the NF-κB pathway may activate the TNF- α, resulting in the transcription of NLRP3 and IL1β.

This interaction worsens the inflammatory damage to cardiac tissue. Previous research has thoroughly examined classic triggers such as ROS and oxLDL-C. Given that reactive oxygen species (ROS) and potassium ion (K^+) efflux from cardiac fibroblasts are recognized as crucial initiators of the NLRP3 inflammasome, their generation is promoted in the absence of oxygen. Following hypoxia, the NLRP3 inflammasome serves as the primary sensor for damage-associated molecular patterns (DAMPs). Fibroblasts promote and exacerbate inflammatory dysfunction following myocardial ischemia damage by activating the NLRP3 inflammasome. In addition to triggering the inflammatory response, hypoxia prompts the adoption of a fibrogenic phenotype in cardiac fibroblasts, leading to myofibroblast transdifferentiation and an increase in the production of collagen. Research findings reveal that NLRP3 influences mitochondrial ROS (mtROS) levels and enhances R-Smad signaling, ultimately culminating in the activation of pro-fibrotic genes. This establishes a novel route for myocardial fibrosis driven by NLRP3, ultimately contributing to remodeling and the development of heart failure (HF) [33].

NLRP3 Inflammasome in Dilated Cardiomyopathy

In epidemiological investigations, dilated cardiomyopathy (DCM) is the predominant contributor to both heart failure and the need for heart transplantation. This condition is characterized by the enlargement of the left ventricle and impaired contractile function, occurring independently of abnormal conditions, and is often associated with notable coronary artery disease. Cardiomyocyte pyroptosis is the critical factor where NLRP3 plays an essential role aside from other factors.

Caspase-1-dependent cardiomyocyte pyroptosis mediated by the NLRP3 inflammasome is important in dilated cardiomyopathy (DCM). TUNEL [Terminal deoxynucleotidyl transferase (TdT) dUTP Nick-End Labeling] and α –actinin and caspase-1triple-immunostaining were carried out on nine samples of human heart tissue. Increased pyroptotic cell death, as opposed to apoptotic cell death, was observed prominently among all patients diagnosed with dilated cardiomyopathy (DCM), while such an occurrence was absent in individuals with healthy cardiac function. The assessment of NF-κB expression or phosphorylation in the plasma of DCM patients revealed substantially elevated levels compared to those observed in the control group [34]. These results underscore the significance of the NLRP3 inflammasome in the advancement of DCM. NLRP3 might increase fibrosis and pro-fibrosis *via* a number of mechanisms, including cAMP signaling in fibroblasts and the Smad (R-Smad) pathway, according to other research. It has been proven that NLRP3 suppression by medication or genetics reduces myocardial fibrosis.

NLRP3 Inflammasome in Hypertension

Significant morbidity and death are caused by hypertension and its manifestations. High blood pressure and its associated outcomes, such as ischemic heart conditions, congestive heart failure (HF), strokes, peripheral vascular issues, impaired vision, and chronic kidney ailments, contribute significantly to global morbidity and mortality rates. Various researchers demonstrated that elevated levels of IL-1β are detected in individuals with hypertension, which indicate that enhanced levels of serum IL-1β can be considered as a marker or inducer of systemic hypertension.

The pathophysiology of hypertension is partially mediated by inflammation, which is effectively activated by NF-κB and NLRP3. Through the inhibition of NF-κB, high-salt-induced hypertension can be averted by reducing the activation of NLRP3 and caspase-1, as well as by diminishing oxidative stress and the presence of pro-inflammatory cytokines within the paraventricular nucleus of salt-sensitive hypertensive rats. The key pro-inflammatory cytokine IL-1β has pleiotropic effects and is produced by the activation of the NLRP3 inflammasome [36].

Evidence has shown that Ang II infusion increases the production of IL-1β and other proinflammatory cytokines as well as the NLRP3 initiation [33]. The role of the NLRP3 inflammasome in cardiac remodeling in Ang II-induced hypertensive rats is evident, as demonstrated by the substantial reduction in Ang II-induced cardiac fibrosis without impacting blood pressure when NLRP3 inflammasome activation is blocked [37].

NLRP3 Inflammasome in Diabetic Cardiomyopathy

Interstitial fibrosis, predominantly affecting the left ventricle, along with diastolic and systolic contractile dysfunction, are the defining features of diabetic cardiomyopathy. Cardiovascular diseases (CVDs) contribute to approximately half of the mortality associated with diabetes mellitus (DM). Pyroptosis is the primary cause of DCM pathogenesis, and as was already noted, the NLRP3 inflammasome is crucial to this process. Although it has been demonstrated that hyperglycemia is one of the factors that activates the NLRP3 inflammasome, the precise connection between the inflammatory response and hyperglycemia has not been thoroughly investigated. Hyperglycemia occurs from both T1D and T2D, while hyperlipidemia results from T2D [35]. In DCM, lipotoxicity and glucotoxicity are important signals in the NLRP3 inflammatory process, which encompasses both the priming and activation phases. Numerous studies have revealed that high fat, as well as blood glucose levels, can produce ROS upregulation, which initiates the NF-κB pathway and increases NLRP3 and pro-

IL-1 and pro-IL-18 transcription. The subsequent signal in NLRP3 activation is thioredoxin interacting/inhibiting protein (TXNIP), which binds to it directly to control its oligomerization.

The inflammatory response mediated by the innate immune system was shown to be more closely associated with the development of T2D in earlier investigations. The NLRP3 inflammasome, a pivotal component of the innate immune system, exerts a notable influence on the development of type 2 diabetes (T2D), where IL-1β assumes a central role as a critical mediator. The crucial part played by NLRP3 in the pathophysiology of T2D was reviewed by Liu *et al*. Research has demonstrated elevated IL-1β levels in individuals with type 2 diabetes (T2D), suggesting a potential link between IL-1β and the onset of T2D. According to Kim *et al*., NLRP3 inflammasome suppression by α- tocotrienol can alleviate and slow the course of T2D.

Diabetes serves as a prominent precursor of obesity, a chronic inflammatory state marked by the secretion of inflammatory cytokines such as IL-1β and TNF-α. Moreover, the roles of IL-1β and TNF-α extend to pancreatic islet cell deterioration and demise, inflammation induced by obesity, and subsequent development of insulin resistance. Targeted disruption of the NLRP3 inflammasome has been shown to enhance glucose tolerance in obese mice. The NLRP3 inflammasome is strongly linked to obesity-induced inflammation and insulin resistance [38, 39].

In addition to the conventional ROS-triggered activation pathway, cytosolic calcium ions (Ca^{2+}) also play a substantial role, effectively augmenting the activation process of the NLRP3 inflammasome. The facilitation of reticulum-t--cytoplasm transport is orchestrated by Sarcoplasmic/Endoplasmic Reticulum Calcium ATPase 2 (SERCA2a), an essential enzyme pivotal in the activation of NLRP3 and subsequent pyroptosis. In rats afflicted with type 1 diabetes (T1D), there was a concurrent decline in sarcoplasmic reticulum function alongside reduced levels of SERCA2a [36]. Information derived from mice with type 2 diabetes (T2D) indicated a similar decrease in SERCA2a expression levels. The elevated expression of SERCA2a in diabetic cardiomyocytes, on the other hand, substantially improved contractile function in contraction trials.

NLRP3 Inflammasome in Atherosclerosis

Given that both crystalline cholesterol and oxidized low-density lipoprotein trigger NLRP3 inflammasome activation, and these pathways exhibit significant shared characteristics such as oxidative stress, mitochondrial dysfunction, endoplasmic reticulum stress, and lysosome rupture, a conjecture has emerged suggesting a correlation between lipid metabolism and inflammatory processes.

An atherosclerotic plaque is regarded as an inflammatory lesion intertwined with the innate immune system, with sustained inflammation playing a pivotal role in its formation [15, 36]. Atherosclerotic lesions have advanced in a manner highly correlated with pathways driving pro-IL-1β release.

In addition to the heart's capacity to pump blood, myocardial infarction (heart failure) also causes electrical instability and deadly arrhythmias. Myocardial infarction is mostly caused by atherosclerotic plaque, constriction of the coronary arteries as well as instability and disruption of the plaque. A severe and complicated inflammatory response brought on by myocardial infarction is what causes cardiac remodeling and healing. Inflammation is crucial in determining the severity of tissue damage and healing following myocardial infarction, in addition to its function in the acute stage of myocardial infarction pathophysiology. The size of infarcts has been demonstrated to be reduced by interventions focused on inflammatory signals [40].

NLRP3 Inflammasome in Cardiac Remodelling

Cardiac fibroblasts, among the most abundant cell types within the human heart, are intricately linked to the NLRP3 inflammasome. Myocardial dysfunction results from improper NLRP3 activation in cardiac fibroblasts. Through the inhibition of NLRP3 inflammasome activation in cardiac fibroblasts, the introduction of exogenous carbon monoxide (CO) *via* CO-releasing molecule-3 exhibits an augmentative effect on myocardial function in rats affected by sepsis. The catalysis of heme degradation to CO by heme oxygenase-1 (HO-1) inhibits the activation of the NLRP3 inflammasome. Because the post-ischemic inflammatory response in mice is excessively vigorous and protracted, HO-1 deficiency causes late left ventricular remodeling [41]. It is widely recognized that a significant suppressor of NLRP3 inflammasome activation, inducible nitric oxide (NO) synthase (iNOS), governs the production of bioactive nitric oxide (NO).

MODULATION OF INFLAMMASOME

Various research studies have shown ways to reduce the damage to changes in the structure of the heart in heart failure caused by a heart attack or lack of blood flow to the heart. These include various genetic techniques, including genetic knockouts *via* blocking the effects of certain proteins in the blood (like IL-1 Trap), using medicines that block IL-1β receptors (such as anakinra), and using genetic tools to silence specific genes (siRNA silencing). All of these methods help improve the condition of the heart after a heart attack or in situations where the blood flow to the heart muscle is reduced. In the absence of an exercise intervention, a two-week therapy with anakinra can enhance peak VO2 in people with ST-segment elevation myocardial infarction. This suggests that reducing the activity of a protein called IL-1β can help the heart heal better. Evidence has shown that the IL-18 binding protein protects the heart against systolic dysfunction in certain mouse models. Also, treatment with IL-18 antibodies may be crucial in lowering harmful inflammatory processes brought on by inflammasome activation with reduced immunological suppression since IL-1β family cytokines are crucial in innate immune responses, such as fever [42].

CONCLUSION

Multiprotein signaling of NLRP3 attenuates HF disease by activating the IL-1β, IL-18, caspase-1, and pro-inflammatory cytokines by controlling the responses of inflammatory pathways. A large body of evidence supports that NLRP3 might be a target for drug development in cardiovascular diseases. NLRP3 inflammasome is an ongoing research area associated with cardiovascular disease with many promising interventions in the future. The pathogenesis of different diseases is ultimately linked to the activation of NLRP3 inflammasome. In HF patients, current insights into targeting the NLRP3 inflammasome-associated research are warranted for reducing deleterious responses.

REFERENCES

[1]   Shah A, Gandhi D, Srivastava S, Shah KJ, Mansukhani R. Heart failure: A class review of pharmacotherapy. P&T 2017; 42(7): 464-72.
        [PMID: 28674474]

[2]   Butts B, Gary RA, Dunbar SB, Butler J. The importance of NLRP3 inflammasome in heart failure. J Card Fail 2015; 21(7): 586-93.
        [http://dx.doi.org/10.1016/j.cardfail.2015.04.014] [PMID: 25982825]

[3]   Kanneganti TD. The inflammasome: Firing up innate immunity. Immunol Rev 2015; 265(1): 1-5.
        [http://dx.doi.org/10.1111/imr.12297] [PMID: 25879279]

[4]   Nógrádi B, Nyúl-Tóth Á, Kozma M, *et al.* Upregulation of nucleotide-binding oligomerization domain-, LRR-and pyrin domain-containing protein 3 in motoneurons following peripheral nerve injury in mice. Front Pharmacol 2020; 11: 584184.
        [http://dx.doi.org/10.3389/fphar.2020.584184] [PMID: 33328988]

[5]   Carriere J, Dorfleutner A, Stehlik C. NLRP7: From inflammasome regulation to human disease. Immunology 2021; 163(4): 363-76.
        [http://dx.doi.org/10.1111/imm.13372] [PMID: 34021586]

[6]   Ting JPY, Lovering RC, Alnemri ES, *et al.* The NLR gene family: A standard nomenclature. Immunity 2008; 28(3): 285-7.
        [http://dx.doi.org/10.1016/j.immuni.2008.02.005] [PMID: 18341998]

[7]   Srinivasula SM, Poyet JL, Razmara M, Datta P, Zhang Z, Alnemri ES. The PYRIN-CARD protein ASC is an activating adaptor for caspase-1. J Biol Chem 2002; 277(24): 21119-22.
        [http://dx.doi.org/10.1074/jbc.C200179200] [PMID: 11967258]

[8]   Zahid A, Li B, Kombe AJK, Jin T, Tao J. Pharmacological inhibitors of the NLRP3 inflammasome. Front Immunol 2019; 10: 2538.
        [http://dx.doi.org/10.3389/fimmu.2019.02538] [PMID: 31749805]

[9]   Jin Y, Fu J. Novel insights into the NLRP 3 inflammasome in atherosclerosis. J Am Heart Assoc 2019; 8(12): e012219.
        [http://dx.doi.org/10.1161/JAHA.119.012219] [PMID: 31184236]

[10]   Robinson AP, Harp CT, Noronha A, Miller SD. The experimental autoimmune encephalomyelitis (EAE) model of MS. Handb Clin Neurol 2014; 122: 173-89.
        [http://dx.doi.org/10.1016/B978-0-444-52001-2.00008-X] [PMID: 24507518]

[11]   Chen QL, Yin HR, He QY, Wang Y. Targeting the NLRP3 inflammasome as new therapeutic avenue for inflammatory bowel disease. Biomed Pharmacother 2021; 138: 111442.
        [http://dx.doi.org/10.1016/j.biopha.2021.111442] [PMID: 33667791]

[12]   Kolb R, Liu GH, Janowski AM, Sutterwala FS, Zhang W. Inflammasomes in cancer: A double-edged sword. Protein Cell 2014; 5(1): 12-20.
        [http://dx.doi.org/10.1007/s13238-013-0001-4] [PMID: 24474192]

[13]   Moltrasio C, Romagnuolo M, Marzano AV. NLRP3 inflammasome and NLRP3-related autoinflammatory diseases: From cryopyrin function to targeted therapies. Front Immunol 2022; 13: 1007705.
        [http://dx.doi.org/10.3389/fimmu.2022.1007705] [PMID: 36275641]

[14]   Sonnessa M, Cioffi A, Brunetti O, *et al.* NLRP3 inflammasome from bench to bedside: new perspectives for triple negative breast cancer. Front Oncol 2020; 10: 1587.
        [http://dx.doi.org/10.3389/fonc.2020.01587] [PMID: 33014808]

[15]   Kelley N, Jeltema D, Duan Y, He Y. The NLRP3 inflammasome: An overview of mechanisms of activation and regulation. Int J Mol Sci 2019; 20(13): 3328.
        [http://dx.doi.org/10.3390/ijms20133328] [PMID: 31284572]

[16]   Walev I, Klein J, Husmann M, *et al.* Potassium regulates IL-1 β processing *via* calcium-independent phospholipase A2. J Immunol 2000; 164(10): 5120-4.
        [http://dx.doi.org/10.4049/jimmunol.164.10.5120] [PMID: 10799869]

[17]   Muñoz-Planillo R, Kuffa P, Martínez-Colón G, Smith BL, Rajendiran TM, Núñez G. K⁻ efflux is the common trigger of NLRP3 inflammasome activation by bacterial toxins and particulate matter. Immunity 2013; 38(6): 1142-53.
        [http://dx.doi.org/10.1016/j.immuni.2013.05.016] [PMID: 23809161]

[18]   Muñoz-Planillo R, Kuffa P, Martínez-Colón G, Smith BL, Rajendiran TM, Núñez G. K⁻ efflux is the common trigger of NLRP3 inflammasome activation by bacterial toxins and particulate matter. Immunity 2013; 38(6): 1142-53.
        [http://dx.doi.org/10.1016/j.immuni.2013.05.016] [PMID: 23809161]

[19]   Rossol M, Pierer M, Raulien N, *et al.* Extracellular Ca2+ is a danger signal activating the NLRP3 inflammasome through G protein-coupled calcium sensing receptors. Nat Commun 2012; 3(1): 1329.
        [http://dx.doi.org/10.1038/ncomms2339] [PMID: 23271661]

[20]   Lee GS, Subramanian N, Kim AI, *et al.* The calcium-sensing receptor regulates the NLRP3 inflammasome through Ca2+ and cAMP. Nature 2012; 492(7427): 123-7.
        [http://dx.doi.org/10.1038/nature11588] [PMID: 23143333]

[21]   Murakami T, Ockinger J, Yu J, *et al.* Critical role for calcium mobilization in activation of the NLRP3 inflammasome. Proc Natl Acad Sci USA 2012; 109(28): 11282-7.
        [http://dx.doi.org/10.1073/pnas.1117765109] [PMID: 22733741]

[22]   Seok JK, Kang HC, Cho YY, Lee HS, Lee JY. Regulation of the NLRP3 inflammasome by post-translational modifications and small molecules. Front Immunol 2021; 11: 618231.
        [http://dx.doi.org/10.3389/fimmu.2020.618231] [PMID: 33603747]

[23]   Swanson KV, Deng M, Ting JPY. The NLRP3 inflammasome: Molecular activation and regulation to therapeutics. Nat Rev Immunol 2019; 19(8): 477-89.
        [http://dx.doi.org/10.1038/s41577-019-0165-0] [PMID: 31036962]

[24]   Verhoef PA, Kertesy SB, Lundberg K, Kahlenberg JM, Dubyak GR. Inhibitory effects of chloride on the activation of caspase-1, IL-1β secretion, and cytolysis by the P2X7 receptor. J Immunol 2005; 175(11): 7623-34.
[http://dx.doi.org/10.4049/jimmunol.175.11.7623] [PMID: 16301672]

[25]   Tang T, Lang X, Xu C, *et al.* CLICs-dependent chloride efflux is an essential and proximal upstream event for NLRP3 inflammasome activation. Nat Commun 2017; 8(1): 202.
[http://dx.doi.org/10.1038/s41467-017-00227-x] [PMID: 28779175]

[26]   Pellegrini C, Antonioli L, Lopez-Castejon G, Blandizzi C, Fornai M. Canonical and non-canonical activation of NLRP3 inflammasome at the crossroad between immune tolerance and intestinal inflammation. Front Immunol 2017; 8: 36.
[http://dx.doi.org/10.3389/fimmu.2017.00036] [PMID: 28179906]

[27]   Tran TAT, Grievink HW, Lipinska K, *et al.* Whole blood assay as a model for *in vitro* evaluation of inflammasome activation and subsequent caspase-mediated interleukin-1 beta release. PLoS One 2019; 14(4): e0214999.
[http://dx.doi.org/10.1371/journal.pone.0214999] [PMID: 30958862]

[28]   Kingsbury SR, Conaghan PG, McDermott MF. The role of the NLRP3 inflammasome in gout. J Inflamm Res 2011; 4: 39-49.
[PMID: 22096368]

[29]   Dani JA. Neuronal nicotinic acetylcholine receptor structure and function and response to nicotine. Int Rev Neurobiol 2015; 124: 3-19.
[http://dx.doi.org/10.1016/bs.irn.2015.07.001] [PMID: 26472524]

[30]   Viganò E, Diamond CE, Spreafico R, *et al.* Human caspase-4 and caspase-5 regulate the one-step non-canonical inflammasome activation in monocytes. Nat Commun 6: 8761.
[http://dx.doi.org/10.1038/ncomms9761]

[31]   Yang Y, Wang H, Kouadir M, Song H, Shi F. Recent advances in the mechanisms of NLRP3 inflammasome activation and its inhibitors. Cell Death Dis 2019; 10(2): 128.
[http://dx.doi.org/10.1038/s41419-019-1413-8] [PMID: 30755589]

[32]   Kany S, Vollrath JT, Relja B. Cytokines in inflammatory disease. Int J Mol Sci 2019; 20(23): 6008.
[http://dx.doi.org/10.3390/ijms20236008] [PMID: 31795299]

[33]   Latz E, Xiao TS, Stutz A. Activation and regulation of the inflammasomes. Nat Rev Immunol 2013; 13(6): 397-411.
[http://dx.doi.org/10.1038/nri3452] [PMID: 23702978]

[34]   Bauernfeind FG, Horvath G, Stutz A, *et al.* Cutting edge: NF-kappaB activating pattern recognition and cytokine receptors license NLRP3 inflammasome activation by regulating NLRP3 expression. J Immunol 2009; 183(2): 787-91.
[http://dx.doi.org/10.4049/jimmunol.0901363] [PMID: 19570822]

[35]   Faustin B, Lartigue L, Bruey JM, *et al.* Reconstituted NALP1 inflammasome reveals two-step mechanism of caspase-1 activation. Mol Cell 2007; 25(5): 713-24.
[http://dx.doi.org/10.1016/j.molcel.2007.01.032] [PMID: 17349957]

[36]   De Miguel C, Pelegrín P, Baroja-Mazo A, Cuevas S. Emerging role of the inflammasome and pyroptosis in hypertension. Int J Mol Sci 2021; 22(3): 1064.
[http://dx.doi.org/10.3390/ijms22031064] [PMID: 33494430]

[37]   Zheng Y, Xu L, Dong N, Li F. NLRP3 inflammasome: The rising star in cardiovascular diseases. Front Cardiovasc Med 2022; 9: 927061.
[http://dx.doi.org/10.3389/fcvm.2022.927061] [PMID: 36204568]

[38]   Galicia-Garcia U, Benito-Vicente A, Jebari S, *et al.* Pathophysiology of type 2 diabetes mellitus. Int J Mol Sci 2020; 21(17): 6275.
[http://dx.doi.org/10.3390/ijms21176275] [PMID: 32872570]

[39]   Masters SL, Dunne A, Subramanian SL, *et al.* Activation of the NLRP3 inflammasome by islet amyloid polypeptide provides a mechanism for enhanced IL-1β in type 2 diabetes. Nat Immunol 2010; 11(10): 897-904.
[http://dx.doi.org/10.1038/ni.1935] [PMID: 20835230]

[40]   Grebe A, Hoss F, Latz E. NLRP3 inflammasome and the IL-1 pathway in atherosclerosis. Circ Res 2018; 122(12): 1722-40.
[http://dx.doi.org/10.1161/CIRCRESAHA.118.311362] [PMID: 29880500]

[41]   Butts B, Gary RA, Dunbar SB, Butler J. The Importance of NLRP3 Inflammasome in Heart Failure. J Card Fail 2015; 21(7): 586-93.
[http://dx.doi.org/10.1016/j.cardfail.2015.04.014] [PMID: 25982825]

[42]   Chauhan D, Vande Walle L, Lamkanfi M. Therapeutic modulation of inflammasome pathways. Immunol Rev 2020; 297(1): 123-38.
[http://dx.doi.org/10.1111/imr.12908] [PMID: 32770571]

CHAPTER 4

TB and Inflammasome: A Complex Relationship

Monika Joon[1] and **Manisha Yadav**[2,*]

¹ Government College Bahadurgarh, Affiliated to MDU, Rohtak, Haryana, India

² Dr. B. R. Ambedkar Centre for Biomedical Research (ACBR), University of Delhi, Delhi-110007, India

Abstract: The reputation of *Mycobacterium tuberculosis* (*Mtb*) as one of the most successful human pathogens has been corroborated bysignificant experimental and clinical evidence. It infects the human host for long enough to co-evolve with the host, developing a robust repertoire of effectors to evade the immune response of the host. It has the capability to survive and multiply inside the very tools of the host immune system that are employed to eradicate it. Granuloma is a classical structure formed as a compensatory step in which both the host and the pathogen benefit partially. While a lot of mycobacterial virulence factors like cell wall envelope components, secreted proteins and dormancy regulon have been researched extensively, the comparatively newer concepts of inflammasomes need much attention. This chapter is an attempt to understand the complex relationship between the inflammasomes and *Mtb* in light of recent studies. With the emerging problems of drug resistance in the treatment of Tb, understanding the relationship between inflammasome and *Mtb* may present newer avenues in the development of host-directed therapy (HDT) strategies for combating Tb .

Keywords: Caspase-1, Interleukin-1beta, Innate immunity, Inflammasome, *Mtb*, Pattern recognition receptors, Pyroptosis, Virulence.

INTRODUCTION

Tuberculosis (TB) is a communicable disease that has been prevalent for thousands of years, as evidenced by scientific studies on skeletons of humans as well as literature. Scientific investigations of the archaeological pieces of evidence by various groups across the world have shown ancient TB prevalence. An important evidence in this contextis Pott's disease, as demonstrated in Peruvian mummies and *Mycobacterium tuberculosis (Mtb)* DNA recovered from Egyptian mummified tissues [1]. TB is known by several other names in historical literature such as phthisis and consumption. Notably, despite its considerable

* **Corresponding author Manisha Yadav:** Dr. B. R. Ambedkar Centre for Biomedical Research (ACBR), University of Delhi, Delhi-110007, India; E-mail: manisha.dhanda@gmail.com

Puneetpal Singh (Ed.)
All rights reserved-© 2024 Bentham Science Publishers

prevalence in human history, the disease was romanticized in European literature. The infectious nature of TB was demonstrated by a French military surgeon Jean-Antoine Villemin in 1865 [2]. However, the pathbreaking discovery and elucidation of the causative agent bacillus were done by Dr Robert Koch in 1882 for which he was awarded the Noble Prize in Medicine or Physiology in 1905. His elucidation of the aetiology of tuberculosis changed the course of events and its subsequent nomenclature as *Mycobacterium tuberculosis*. On the basis of the tissues affected, TB is described as pulmonary (lungs) and extrapulmonary (tissues other than lungs). Though TB is a contagious disease that spreads *via* the respiratory route and typically affects lungs (Pulmonary TB), it can also affect other sites (extrapulmonary TB). *Mtb* has co-evolved with its human host for millennia and has consequently adapted itself exquisitely to navigate the host immune system. It has developed a repertoire of effectors to not only evade the innate immune response but also to exploit it for survival and persistence. A remarkable feature of the pathogen is its ability to survive in different diverse intracellular microenvironments of different cell types of the host [3]. In the tug-of-war like situation between the pathogen and the host during infection, the outcome is determined by the genetic determinants of the host as well as the pathogen, co-morbidities, environmental factors and others.

Understanding the advancements in the innate host response to *Mtb* has promising potential in the developmentof host-directed therapy to counter TB. The concept of inflammasome activation is one such area that requires special attention [4].

The Causative Organism, *Mycobacterium Tuberculosis* (Mtb)

Mtb is a Gram-positive, facultative intracellular bacterium that has a doubling time of 12-24 hours under optimal conditions. It infects the mammalian host cells and not only can survive but also replicates within the host macrophages. Its capability to avoid macrophage-killing repertoire makes it a major reason for causing infectious diseases and a malady for mankind. Some of the main effectors that play a fundamental role in its virulence are as follows [5].

Peculiar Cell Wall Structure

The cell wall of *Mtb* is a strong, impermeable barrier consisting of outer membrane, periplasmic space and inner membrane. The outer membrane is further composed of peptidoglycan and arabinogalactan and is rich in mycolic acids that form an exceptionally thick, waxy, impermeable barrier and significantly contribute to drug resistance. It is also known as the mycolyl-arabinogalacta--peptidoglycan (mAGP) complex and represents the core cell wall structure of *Mycobacterium*.

Protein Secretion Systems

These are complex secretion systems that are used to secrete proteins across the cell envelope of Mycobacteria. *Mtb* has five secretion systems: ESX-1 [early secreted antigen 6 kilodaltons (ESAT-6) system 1] to ESX-5. These systems have been reported to have various functions in *Mtb* virulence. To describe briefly, ESX-1 secretes antigens that cause phagosomal membrane rupture. ESX-2 has an important role in survivability in slow-growing mycobacterial species within immune cells. ESX-3 is considered to be essential in regulating the metal ion homeostasis. It is reported to have a role in Fe^{2+} and Zn^{2+} ion uptake as well as in hindering phagosome maturation. ESX-4 is phylogenetically ancient in origin and is required in conjugation. ESX-5 releases proline-glutamate (PE) /proline-proline-glutamate (PPE) and PE- polymorphic GC-rich repetitive sequences (PGRS) proteins, which play a role in immunomodulation.

The Dormancy Survival Eegulon (Dos)

Mtb has the ability to sense unfavourable hypoxic, nutrient-depleted microenvironmental conditions inside macrophages and granulomas. In such conditions, it undergoes dormancy by activating its Dormancy Survival Regulator (DosR) regulon that regulates a myriad of genes, ultimately resulting in a dormant state of the bacillus wherein it stops multiplying, metabolises anaerobically and stays latent until the host becomes immunocompromised.

TB Pathogenesis

Typically, *Mtb* enters the human host through aerosol inhalation and reaches the alveoli in the lungs. The pathogen encounters the mucosa and alveolar epithelial cells, macrophages, dendritic cells and neutrophils as the first line of defence [5 - 7]. These cells have various receptors to recognize the pathogen as a threat and phagocytose it for elimination and to mount an immune response *via* antigen presentation. If the bacilli are all killed, the pathogen is cleared. However, if the pathogen manages to survive within the phagocytes, it replicates exponentially and results in a high bacterial burden. After the initial uptake, primarily by the alveolar resident macrophages, other cells like dendritic cells and monocyte-derived macrophages also take part in phagocytic processes. These phagocytic cells play a crucial role in mounting and directing adaptive T-cell immunity of the host by mycobacterial antigen presentation and expression of costimulatory signals and cytokines. Also, *Mtb* can diffuse to other sites *via* hematogenous and lymphatic routes. This leads to the mounting of immune response and initiation of the adaptive immune response to tackle the infection. Neutrophils, lymphocytes and other immune cells infiltrate the site of infection that culminates in granuloma formation, representing a stalemate between the bacterium and the host. It is a strategy of the host to check the spread of pathogens to surrounding healthy tissue as well as to prevent the total eradication of bacteria. With the onset of cell-mediated immunity, the bacterial multiplication is reduced considerably, and the disease enters the latent stage until the time the host becomes immunocompromised. It is then that the disease goes into active TB state [8 - 10].

Host Innate Immune Components

The host innate immune response employs cells, signalling molecules and the associated cellular functions (Fig. **1**). Airway epithelial cells (AECs) form a barrier and prevent invasion. However, they are also equipped to recognize Pathogen-associated molecular pattern molecules (PAMPs) [9]. The layer of surfactant above it acts like a trap for the pathogen and causes agglutination. Alveolar Macrophages are the battleground of the *Mtb,* and the outcome depends on the intrinsic microbicidal capacity of the host cell and the virulence factors of the ingested *Mtb*. Dendritic cells act as middlemen between innate and adaptive immunity. They carry out the function of antigen presentation. Neutrophils are professional phagocytes that have a complex role to play in *Mtb* pathogenesis. After stimulation with *Mtb*, neutrophils secrete chemokines and pro-inflammatory cytokines. Natural killer cells are recruited to the site of infection early and contribute to the antimicrobial defence of the host cells. These can lyse infected macrophages [5]. (Fig. **1**) summarises some of the important elements of host innate immunity.

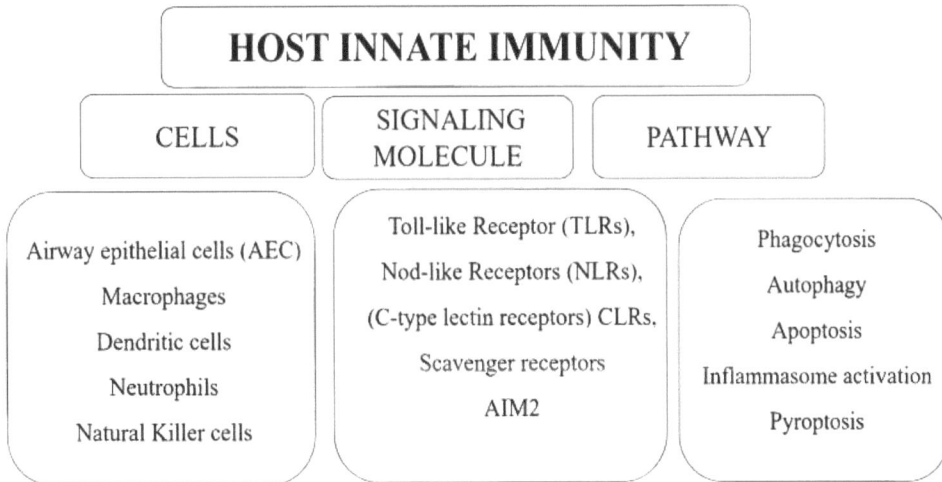

HOST INNATE IMMUNITY

CELLS	SIGNALING MOLECULE	PATHWAY
Airway epithelial cells (AEC) Macrophages Dendritic cells Neutrophils Natural Killer cells	Toll-like Receptor (TLRs), Nod-like Receptors (NLRs), (C-type lectin receptors) CLRs, Scavenger receptors AIM2	Phagocytosis Autophagy Apoptosis Inflammasome activation Pyroptosis

Fig. (1). Some of the main elements of the host innate immune response towards *Mtb* infection.

Inflammasomes are a comparatively new concept in host innate immunity and have contributed immensely to understanding microbial pathogenesis and metabolic or autoimmune diseases of the host [11].

Inflammasome

Inflammasomes are evolutionarily conserved cytosolic multimeric, macromolecular signaling complexes that are formed as an essential component of the innate immune response of the host cells in response to a variety of physiological and pathogenic stimuli. It is a design of nature to get rid of the invading pathogen or diseased host cells so as to maintain homeostasis. The activation of inflammasome requires the detection of foreign or host-derived insults of the host cells. This happens due to the recognition of certain components of the pathogen or the altered host cell type by the host immune cells. Interestingly, it has been observed that several pathogens have evolved to adopt ways to evade inflammasome activation and, hence survival within the host [11 - 14].

The detection of the "danger" signal takes place *via* Germline-encoded pattern recognition receptors (PRRs), which are sensors on or in host immune cells and are responsible for sensing the presence of threat. These molecular sensors are expressed by host cells that are at the front line of defence (*e.g.*, macrophages, monocytes, dendritic cells, neutrophils, and epithelial cells) and also the cells of the adaptive immune system. PRRs detect infection or tissue damage signals, such as conserved antigenic structures called danger-associated molecular patterns (DAMPs), such as host DNA/RNA, ATP, Uric acid and PAMPs *e.g.*, Lipoproteins, pathogen DNA/RNA, toxins *etc* [15, 16]. Based on their subcellular localization, PRRs are of two types.

Membrane-bound PRR

These scan the extracellular microenvironment and endosomal compartments for the presence of PAMPs. Typical examples of these PRRs are Toll-like receptors (TLRs) and C-type lectins (CTLs).

Intracellular PRRs

These provide cytosolic surveillance. Examples are RNA-sensing RIG-like helicases (RLHs) and NOD-like receptors.

Through their cooperation with PRRs, the inflammasomes activate host defence pathways to get rid of the pathogen or the diseased cells. The activation of PRRs due to molecular recognition of the external threat or host-derived insult signals triggers a cascade of signal transduction that finally results in the secretion of proinflammatory cytokines, such as IL-1β and IL-18, which in turn lead to the production of oxygen and nitrogen radicals that are crucial for intracellular killing of pathogens. Inflammasomes are basically high-molecular weight, caspase-activating molecular platforms that regulate the maturation and secretion of proinflammatory cytokines [11, 14, 16]. (Fig. **2**) depicts a unit of inflammasome. Typically, they are composed of three components.

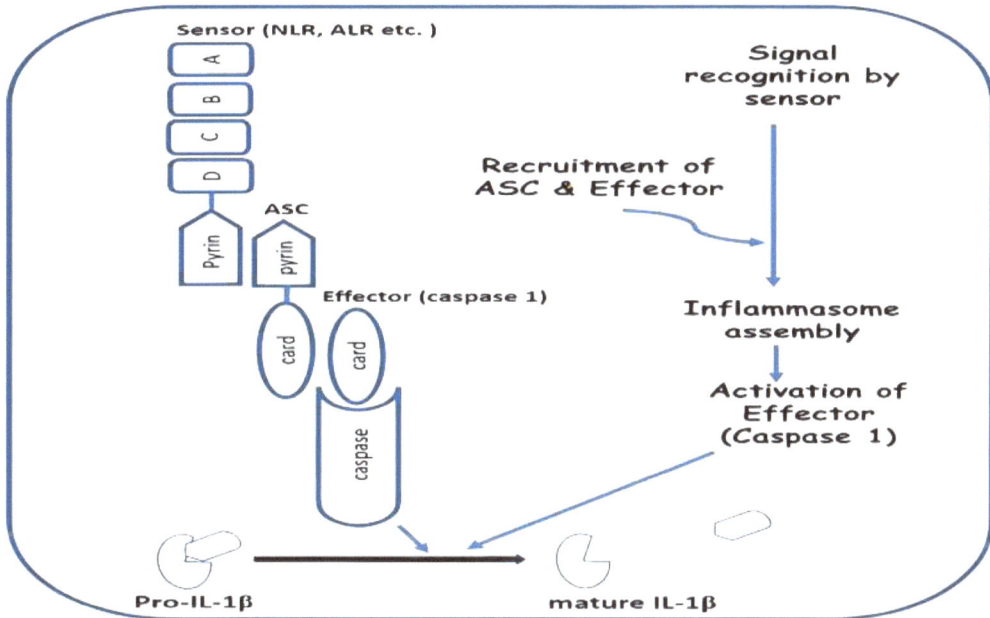

Fig. (2). The basic structural unit of the classical inflammasome and the dynamics of its activation culminating in the production of inflammasome-dependent IL-1β during innate immune response.

Sensor

It recognizes microbial components and cell injury *e.g.*, Nucleotide-binding domain–like (NLR) proteins, absent in melanoma 2–like (AIM2) proteins and PYRIN.

Adaptor

It serves as a bridge between the sensor and the effector. Apoptosis-associated speck-like (ASC) protein has a crucial role in the formation of an effective inflammasome. It is a bipartite molecule that contains an N-terminal pyrin domain

(PYD) and a C-terminal caspase activation and recruitment domain (CARD) that enable it to act like a bridge between the sensor and the effector (pro-caspase-1).

Effector (Caspase-1 or 11)

(Caspases belong to a family of Cysteine proteases that are aspartate-specific and are conserved through evolution. Caspase 1 is a heterodimeric cysteine protease composed of two subunits and also called interleukin-1β-converting enzyme (ICE). On interaction with the sensor *via* adaptor, it undergoes autocatalysis from inactive procaspase-1 to active caspase-1. Active caspase-1 mediates the conversion of pro-IL-1β (inactive) into an active form of interleukin-1beta (IL-1β) as well as the processing of pro-IL-18 into IL-18. Caspases 1 and 11 both have large domains that mediate interactions with other proteins.

On initiation of this complex formation, caspase-1 is activated, which proteolytically processes pro-inflammatory cytokines, pro-IL-1β and pro-IL-18 into their respective active forms. These interleukins, in turn, initiate a type of cell death called pyroptosis. Due to its cytotoxic end result, inflammasome activation is a tightly regulated phenomenon with the aim to provide defence against invading pathogens and avoid damage to the host. An insufficient inflammatory response may lead to recurrent infections, whereas excessive activation may result in chronic systemic inflammatory and autoimmune disorders. A variety of molecular and cellular events are therefore involved in maintaining the balance between inflammatory response and resolution.

Pyroptosis

Pyroptosis is a distinct form of cell death that requires the enzymatic activity of caspase-1 or 11. It is a lytic mode of cell death that is characterized by cytoplasmic swelling and rupture of the plasma membrane. Pyroptosis occurs to get rid of the infection and to mount further inflammation to combat the infection or disease. Though pyroptosis is a protective response of the host, it can be detrimental if it is in exuberance or inappropriately high levels [14, 17].

Based on whether caspase 1 or 11 is activated, the inflammasomes are of two types: canonical or noncanonical [13]. Canonical or classical inflammasome brings about the conversion of procaspase-1 into the catalytically active enzyme caspase-1. Several subtypes have been assigned to this type of inflammasome and named after its NLR or ALR protein scaffold. Noncanonical inflammasome involves the activation of procaspase-11. It has been found that caspase 11 is activated by most Gram-negative bacteria but does not respond to Gram-positive bacteria. The activation of caspase 11 has been found to be triggered by intracellular lipopolysaccharide (LPS) or acylated lipid A (a component found in many Gram-negative bacteria) [14, 18].

There are different inflammasomes named according to their sensor (receptor) components, namely nucleotide-binding domain-like receptors (NLRs), absent in melanoma 2–like receptors (ALRs), and pyrin. These receptors detect a variety of effectors and have the ability to assemble the inflammasome. (Fig. **2**) highlights the basic structural variations of different inflammasomes.

Role of IL-1β in Host Immunity against *Mtb*: Goldilocks Principle

It has been established that IL-1β plays a crucial role in modulating host immunity towards *Mtb*. The processing of pro-IL-1β into active IL-1β depends on cleavage by proteases. An eminent enzyme is caspase-1, which in turn is activated by the macromolecular platform called inflammasome. However, it is known that inflammasome activation varies across different cell types. Alternative mechanisms of processing and activation of IL-1β have been reported, for example, neutrophil-derived serine proteases or proteases that are released from certain microbial pathogens. A study on a mouse model revealed that IL-1β production is found to be inflammasome-independent during *Mtb* infections [19, 20]. Hence, IL-1β generation can happen *via* both inflammasome-dependent and inflammasome-independent pathways. Also, IL-1β is found to have a complex role in host immunity during the *Mtb* infection, with some studies indicating a host protective role while some other data support its role in increasing the host susceptibility to the pathogen. These are briefly described as follows.

Protective Role

The protective effect of IL-1β *in vivo* has been linked to its ability to suppress interferon-beta (IFN-β), a cytokine produced by host cells (both immune as well as non-immune) and has immunomodulatory functions. Increased IFN-β has been found to increase host susceptibility. Mouse studies have demonstrated the hypersusceptibility of mice deficient in the expression of either IL-1a/-b or the IL-1β receptor. *In vivo*, IL-1β suppresses necrosis of lung cells [19 - 22].

Detrimental Role

The main evidence in favour of a positive correlation between the severity of the Tb disease and increased levels of IL-1β is found in studies based on genetic variability and clinical outcomes. Single nucleotide polymorphism analysis of the human IL-1β gene revealed that SNPs in the promoter region causing enhanced IL-1β expression are found to be associated with severe Tb cases [19, 23].

Another clinical study reported that polymorphism in the IL-1 receptor agonist (IL1RA) gene, resulting in decreased IL1RA expression and increased IL-1β expression, is correlated with tuberculoid pleurisy patients [24]. Additionally, some studies also indicated the suppression of inflammasome activation during *Mtb* infection, hence, indicating the detrimental role of IL-1β to host defense [25]. MCC950, a small molecule inhibitor of NLRP3 inflammasome activation, reduces IL-1β processing in *Mtb*-infected Murine bone marrow-derived macrophages (BMDMs) and also results in decreased survival of *Mtb* [26].

Hence, it can be concluded that the Goldilocks principle applies to the production of IL-1β, implying that the right amount of the cytokine IL-1β at the right time during the infection results in a host-protective outcome.

Inflammasomes and Tb: A Complex Relationship

Mtb has been reported to have a complex relationship with inflammasome activation. While some studies show prevention of inflammasome activation as well as IL-1β, others provide evidence of inflammasome activation. The gene *zmp1* encoding a putative Zn^{2+} metalloprotease has been found to be essential for the inhibition of inflammasome activation and IL-1β production as well as required for the survival of *Mtb* in macrophages [27]. Two main types of inflammasomes have been found to be associated with *Mtb* pathogenesis, namely NLRP3 and AIM2 [7, 18].

NLRP3-inflammasome and *Mtb*

In this type of inflammasome, the cytosolic immune sensor NLRP3 mediates inflammasome activation by binding to a variety of intracellular ligands that serve as danger signals. Scientific literature shows that there is both a positive as well as negative correlation of *Mtb* infection on NLRP3- inflammasome activation.

It has been found that *Mtb* is capable of activating the NLRP3 inflammasome *via* its several constituents such as ESX-1 secretion system, Rv1579c (or EST12), Rv0878c (or PPE13), mannosylated lipoarabinomannan and dsRNA. Additionally, the Tb bacillus physically damages the plasma membrane and phagosomal membrane during the process of its phagocytosis by the host cell, leading to K+ efflux and the subsequent activation of NLRP3-dependent IL-1β release and eventually pyroptosis [27]. The activation of NLRP3 inflammasome by *Mtb* infection has been reported in several cell types by several studies based on *ex vivo* analysis of macrophages, dendritic cells, polymorphonuclear neutrophils (PMN) cells, BMDMs, Bone marrow-derived dendritic cells (BMDCs), primary murine microglial cells, *etc.* [7, 28, 29]. Also, a drop in the cytosolic K+ brought about by bacterial toxins like LPS, phagocytosis or any other cellular insult is found to activate caspase-1 *via* NLRP3 [30]. In macrophages and dendritic cells, the host cell inflammasome is crucial for the generation of secreted IL-1β in response to *Mtb* infections. In these cell types, *Mtb* infection activates the NLRP3-inflammasome. *Mtb* ESAT-6 has been well known to activate NLRP3 [31]. The involvement of NLRP3 in *Mtb* ESAT-6-promoted necrosis in macrophages has also been shown experimentally by researchers using two independent inhibitors of NLRP3, along with siRNA treatment against NLRP3 [32].

The negative regulators of NLRP3-inflammasomes have been identified as IFN-β, Nitric oxide (NO) and mega-3 fatty acids. NO brings about direct S-nitrosylation of NLRP3. The inhibition or negative regulation of NLRP3-inflammasome is a mechanism to check excessive inflammatory response and to prevent host tissue damage caused thereby [19, 33]. Interferon IFN-β, which is induced in the host by *Mtb* infection, can have an inhibitory impact on NLRP3-inflammasome activation.

Absent in Melanoma 2-Inflammasome and *Mtb*

Absent in Melanoma 2 (AIM2) Inflammasome was first identified as a gene that was lacking in melanoma cell lines using subtractive cDNA hybridization. Since its discovery by several research groups independently in 2009, the understanding of AIM2 inflammasome has been of critical significance in understanding host response to not only microbial pathogenesis but also to metabolic as well as autoimmune diseases. AIM2 inflammasome is responsible for sensing dsDNA in the host cell cytosol. In eukaryotic cells, under a homeostatic state, the nuclear as well as mitochondrial DNA is confined to compartmentalization, and its presence in cytosol is indicative of active infection or host derived pathological DNA damage. Naked DNA has been known to be recognized by host innate immune system components, such as Toll-like receptor 9 (TLR9). Structurally, the AIM2 inflammasome has an N-terminal PYD (pyrin) domain and one C-terminal hematopoietic interferon-inducible nuclear localization (HIN) domain. The PYD domain is responsible for recruiting the ASC adapter, while the HIN domain is responsible for binding to dsDNA in the host cell cytosol [34, 35]. AIM2 sensor recognizes not only microbial but also the host dsDNA, such as the mitochondrial DNA released during mitochondrial stress. As per current knowledge, AIM2 inflammasomes are activated by both "canonical" and "non-canonical" pathways. However, the downstream events are the same, *i.e.*, inflammasome assembly, activation of caspase-1 and the maturation of IL-1β/IL-18.

The role of AIM2- inflammasome in mycobacterial infection still remains unknown, and extensive research needs to be conducted to understand the underlying molecular mechanisms in the host immunity. AIM2 is found to be indispensable for host defense against *Mtb* infection. *In vivo* studies on the murine model showed that AIM$^{2-/-}$ deficient mice were found to be highly sensitive to intratracheal infection with *Mtb* H37Rv virulent strain and died within 7 weeks, whereas the wild-type mice survived for at least 8 weeks. The study also showed that AIM2 mediated the induction of caspase-1 activation in a *Mtb* DNA-dependent manner and the subsequent IL-1β/IL-18 secretion. Also, AIM2 inflammasomes are reported to be inhibited by the pathogen *Mtb*. During *Mtb* infection, the mycobacterial DNA in the extracellular microenvironment enters the host cell cytosol *via* the ESX-1 secretion system-dependent pathway. The process is found to be dependent on the ESX-1 secretion system of the pathogen, as reflected by the studies on the esxA mutant. EsxA deficient strain of *Mtb* fails to inhibit IL-1β secretion induced by *M. smegmatis* [18, 19]. A study elucidated the significant role of AIM2 in *Mtb* infection *via Mtb* DNA recognition [36].

Hence, there is a modulatory relationship between these two inflammasomes and the Tb pathogen. The mechanism still needs to be researched to completely understand the correlations.

It has been reported that clinical isolates from severe TB patients exhibit lower cytokine production. This is proposed as the pathogen has evolved the mechanisms to escape the cytosolic recognition by host cells [37]. Also, studies have shown that mitofusin 2 (MFN2) has a significant role in modulating the host response during *Mtb* infection [38]. Therefore, it can be inferred that *Mtb* modulates host immunity to its benefit in terms of survival and adaptation (Table **1**).

Table 1. Some studies that highlight the immunomodulatory role of *Mtb via* its interaction with inflammasomes.

Pathogen Strain/Effector/Mediator	Target Inflammasome	Observations/Results of the Study	Year of Publication	Refs.
ESAT-6	NLRP3/ASC	ESAT-6 is involved in the recognition of *Mtb* infection by the NLRP3 inflammasome.	2010	[31]
H37Rv strain of *M. tuberculosis*	Caspase 1 dependent	The study reports that inflammasomes are dispensable for IL-1β production *in vivo* in mice infected with the TB pathogen.	2010	[20]
ESAT-6	NLRP3	The study reveals that in macrophages, NLRP3 functions in *M. tuberculosis* ESAT-6-promoted necrosis.	2011	[32]

(Table 1) cont.....

Pathogen Strain/Effector/Mediator	Target Inflammasome	Observations/Results of the Study	Year of Publication	Refs.
M.tuberculosis strain H37Rv	AIM2	AIM2 plays a significant role in *Mtb* infection *via Mtb* DNA recognition.	2012	[36]
LPS	NLRP3	A drop in cytosolic K⁻ is necessary and sufficient for caspase-1 activation of the NLRP3 inflammasome.	2013	[30]
Clinical *Mtb* strains	NLRP3	Mitochondrial MFN2 interacts and activates NLRP3 inflammasome.	2020	[38]
Clinical *Mtb* strains	NLRP3	*Mtb* strains from severe tuberculosis show evasion of cytosolic surveillance systems.	2020	[37]
Clinical *Mtb* strains	AIM2 and NLRP3	Different clinical isolates of *Mtb* lead to differential inflammasome activation and IL-1β processing.	2020	[26]

CONCLUSION

In view of the significant problem of drug resistance and genetic diversity having implications in virulence in clinical isolates, it is indeed the need of the hour that anti-TB therapy based on non-conventional targets in the pathogen as well as the host be explored. Inflammasomes present one such avenue for host-directed therapeutic intervention. They can play a significant role as an adjunctive antimicrobial drug treatment by modulating the host immune response in a suitable way to promote pathogen clearance. Since studies have shown differences in inflammasome activation by different clinical isolates, adjunctive therapy may help mitigate the problem on an individual level in patients. Studies like these highlight the potential of inflammasomes in host-directed therapy (HDT) against M. *tuberculosis*. HDT. In the present context, inflammasomes offer a good scope of investigation and have applications in medicine.

REFERENCES

[1]   Daniel TM. The history of tuberculosis. Respir Med 2006; 100(11): 1862-70.
      [http://dx.doi.org/10.1016/j.rmed.2006.08.006] [PMID: 16949809]

[2]   Major RH III, Ed. Classic descriptions of disease. Springfield, IL: Charles C. Thomas 1945.

[3]   van Crevel R, Ottenhoff THM, van der Meer JWM. Innate immunity to *mycobacterium tuberculosis*. Clin Microbiol Rev 2002; 15(2): 294-309.
      [http://dx.doi.org/10.1128/CMR.15.2.294-309.2002] [PMID: 11932234]

[4]   Rastogi S, Briken V. Interaction of mycobacteria with host cell inflammasomes. Front Immunol 2022; 13: 791136.
      [http://dx.doi.org/10.3389/fimmu.2022.791136] [PMID: 35237260]

[5]   Liu CH, Liu H, Ge B. Innate immunity in tuberculosis: Host defense vs pathogen evasion. Cell Mol
        Immunol 2017; 14(12): 963-75.
        [http://dx.doi.org/10.1038/cmi.2017.88] [PMID: 28890547]

[6]   Roy S, Ghatak D, Das P, BoseDasgupta S. ESX secretion system: The gatekeepers of mycobacterial
        survivability and pathogenesis. Eur J Microbiol Immunol 2020; 10(4): 202-9.
        [http://dx.doi.org/10.1556/1886.2020.00028] [PMID: 33174865]

[7]   Ma J, Zhao S, Gao X, *et al.* The roles of inflammasomes in host defense against *mycobacterium
        tuberculosis.* Pathogens 2021; 10(2): 120.
        [http://dx.doi.org/10.3390/pathogens10020120] [PMID: 33503864]

[8]   Delogu G, Sali M, Fadda G. The biology of mycobacterium tuberculosis infection. Mediterr J Hematol
        Infect Dis 2013; 5(1): e2013070.
        [http://dx.doi.org/10.4084/mjhid.2013.070] [PMID: 24363885]

[9]   Lerner TR, Borel S, Gutierrez MG. The innate immune response in human tuberculosis. Cell
        Microbiol 2015; 17(9): 1277-85.
        [http://dx.doi.org/10.1111/cmi.12480] [PMID: 26135005]

[10]   Chandra P, Grigsby SJ, Philips JA. Immune evasion and provocation by *Mycobacterium tuberculosis.*
        Nat Rev Microbiol 2022; 20(12): 750-66.
        [http://dx.doi.org/10.1038/s41579-022-00763-4] [PMID: 35879556]

[11]   Schroder K, Tschopp J. The inflammasomes. Cell 2010; 140(6): 821-32.
        [http://dx.doi.org/10.1016/j.cell.2010.01.040] [PMID: 20303873]

[12]   Sharma D, Kanneganti TD. The cell biology of inflammasomes: Mechanisms of inflammasome
        activation and regulation. J Cell Biol 2016; 213(6): 617-29.
        [http://dx.doi.org/10.1083/jcb.201602089] [PMID: 27325789]

[13]   Lee KH, Kang TB. The molecular links between cell death and inflammasome. Cells 2019; 8(9): 1057.
        [http://dx.doi.org/10.3390/cells8091057] [PMID: 31509938]

[14]   Lamkanfi M, Dixit VM. Mechanisms and functions of inflammasomes. Cell 2014; 157(5): 1013-22.
        [http://dx.doi.org/10.1016/j.cell.2014.04.007] [PMID: 24855941]

[15]   Takeuchi O, Akira S. Pattern recognition receptors and inflammation. Cell 2010; 140(6): 805-20.
        [http://dx.doi.org/10.1016/j.cell.2010.01.022] [PMID: 20303872]

[16]   Wawrocki S, Druszczynska M. Inflammasomes in *mycobacterium tuberculosis* -driven immunity. Can
        J Infect Dis Med Microbiol 2017; 2017: 1-9.
        [http://dx.doi.org/10.1155/2017/2309478] [PMID: 29348763]

[17]   Bergsbaken T, Fink SL, Cookson BT. Pyroptosis: Host cell death and inflammation. Nat Rev
        Microbiol 2009; 7(2): 99-109.
        [http://dx.doi.org/10.1038/nrmicro2070] [PMID: 19148178]

[18]   Briken V, Ahlbrand SE, Shah S. Mycobacterium tuberculosis and the host cell inflammasome: a
        complex relationship. Front Cell Infect Microbiol 2013; 3: 62.
        [http://dx.doi.org/10.3389/fcimb.2013.00062] [PMID: 24130966]

[19]   Rastogi S, Briken V. Interaction of mycobacteria with host cell inflammasomes. Front Immunol 2022;
        13: 791136.
        [http://dx.doi.org/10.3389/fimmu.2022.791136] [PMID: 35237260]

[20]   Mayer-Barber KD, Barber DL, Shenderov K, *et al.* Caspase-1 independent IL-1beta production is
        critical for host resistance to mycobacterium tuberculosis and does not require TLR signaling *in vivo.* J
        Immunol 2010; 184(7): 3326-30.
        [http://dx.doi.org/10.4049/jimmunol.0904189] [PMID: 20200276]

[21]   Mayer-Barber KD, Sassetti CM. Type I interferon and interleukin-1 driven inflammatory pathways as
        targets for HDT in tuberculosis. In: Karakousis PC, Hafner R, Gennaro ML, Eds. Advances in Host-

Directed Therapies Against Tuberculosis. Springer International Publishing 2021; pp. 219-32.
[http://dx.doi.org/10.1007/978-3-030-56905-1_14]

[22]   Sugawara I, Yamada H, Hua S, Mizuno S. Role of interleukin (IL)-1 type 1 receptor in mycobacterial infection. Microbiol Immunol 2001; 45(11): 743-50.
[http://dx.doi.org/10.1111/j.1348-0421.2001.tb01310.x] [PMID: 11791667]

[23]   Zhang G, Zhou B, Li S, *et al.* Allele-specific induction of IL-1β expression by C/EBPβ and PU.1 contributes to increased tuberculosis susceptibility. PLoS Pathog 2014; 10(10): e1004426.
[http://dx.doi.org/10.1371/journal.ppat.1004426] [PMID: 25329476]

[24]   Wilkinson RJ, Patel P, Llewelyn M, *et al.* Influence of polymorphism in the genes for the interleukin (IL)-1 receptor antagonist and IL-1beta on tuberculosis. J Exp Med 1999; 189(12): 1863-74.
[http://dx.doi.org/10.1084/jem.189.12.1863] [PMID: 10377182]

[25]   Mishra BB, Rathinam VAK, Martens GW, *et al.* Nitric oxide controls the immunopathology of tuberculosis by inhibiting NLRP3 inflammasome–dependent processing of IL-1β. Nat Immunol 2013; 14(1): 52-60.
[http://dx.doi.org/10.1038/ni.2474] [PMID: 23160153]

[26]   Subbarao S, Sanchez-Garrido J, Krishnan N, Shenoy AR, Robertson BD. Genetic and pharmacological inhibition of inflammasomes reduces the survival of Mycobacterium tuberculosis strains in macrophages. Sci Rep 2020; 10(1): 3709.
[http://dx.doi.org/10.1038/s41598-020-60560-y] [PMID: 32111888]

[27]   Master SS, Rampini SK, Davis AS, *et al.* Mycobacterium tuberculosis prevents inflammasome activation. Cell Host Microbe 2008; 3(4): 224-32.
[http://dx.doi.org/10.1016/j.chom.2008.03.003] [PMID: 18407066]

[28]   Dorhoi A, Nouailles G, Jörg S, *et al.* Activation of the NLRP3 inflammasome by *Mycobacterium tuberculosis* is uncoupled from susceptibility to active tuberculosis. Eur J Immunol 2012; 42(2): 374-84.
[http://dx.doi.org/10.1002/eji.201141548] [PMID: 22101787]

[29]   Eklund D, Welin A, Andersson H, *et al.* Human gene variants linked to enhanced NLRP3 activity limit intramacrophage growth of Mycobacterium tuberculosis. J Infect Dis 2014; 209(5): 749-53.
[http://dx.doi.org/10.1093/infdis/jit572] [PMID: 24158955]

[30]   Muñoz-Planillo R, Kuffa P, Martínez-Colón G, Smith BL, Rajendiran TM, Núñez G. K⁻ efflux is the common trigger of NLRP3 inflammasome activation by bacterial toxins and particulate matter. Immunity 2013; 38(6): 1142-53.
[http://dx.doi.org/10.1016/j.immuni.2013.05.016] [PMID: 23809161]

[31]   Mishra BB, Moura-Alves P, Sonawane A, *et al.* Mycobacterium tuberculosis protein ESAT-6 is a potent activator of the NLRP3/ASC inflammasome. Cell Microbiol 2010; 12(8): 1046-63.
[http://dx.doi.org/10.1111/j.1462-5822.2010.01450.x] [PMID: 20148899]

[32]   Wong KW, Jacobs WR Jr. Critical role for NLRP3 in necrotic death triggered by *Mycobacterium tuberculosis.* Cell Microbiol 2011; 13(9): 1371-84.
[http://dx.doi.org/10.1111/j.1462-5822.2011.01625.x] [PMID: 21740493]

[33]   Yan Y, Jiang W, Spinetti T, *et al.* Omega-3 fatty acids prevent inflammation and metabolic disorder through inhibition of NLRP3 inflammasome activation. Immunity 2013; 38(6): 1154-63.
[http://dx.doi.org/10.1016/j.immuni.2013.05.015] [PMID: 23809162]

[34]   Wang L, Sun L, Byrd KM, Ko CC, Zhao Z, Fang J. AIM2 inflammasome's first decade of discovery: Focus on oral diseases. Front Immunol 2020; 11: 1487.
[http://dx.doi.org/10.3389/fimmu.2020.01487] [PMID: 32903550]

[35]   Kumari P, Russo AJ, Shivcharan S, Rathinam VA. AIM2 in health and disease: Inflammasome and beyond. Immunol Rev 2020; 297(1): 83-95.
[http://dx.doi.org/10.1111/imr.12903] [PMID: 32713036]

[36]   Saiga H, Kitada S, Shimada Y, *et al.* Critical role of AIM2 in mycobacterium tuberculosis infection. Int Immunol 2012; 24(10): 637-44.
[http://dx.doi.org/10.1093/intimm/dxs062] [PMID: 22695634]

[37]   Sousa J, Cá B, Maceiras AR, *et al.* Mycobacterium tuberculosis associated with severe tuberculosis evades cytosolic surveillance systems and modulates IL-1β production. Nat Commun 2020; 11(1): 1949.
[http://dx.doi.org/10.1038/s41467-020-15832-6] [PMID: 32327653]

[38]   Xu F, Qi H, Li J, *et al.* Mycobacterium tuberculosis infection up-regulates MFN2 expression to promote NLRP3 inflammasome formation. J Biol Chem 2020; 295(51): 17684-97.
[http://dx.doi.org/10.1074/jbc.RA120.014077] [PMID: 33454007]

CHAPTER 5

Mechanism of NLRP3 Activation, Associated Cardiovascular Complications and Update on its Inhibitors Acting as Cardioprotective Agents

Syed Ehtaishamul Haque[1],*, Aamir Khan[1] and Ashif Iqubal[1]

[1] *Department of Pharmacology, School of Pharmaceutical Education and Research, Jamia Hamdard, New Delhi-110062, India*

Abstract: Cardiovascular disorders (CVDs) are a major healthcare issue worldwide and are accountable for significant mortality and morbidity. Despite advancements in cellular, molecular, physiological and pathological understanding, a comprehensive understanding of CVDs is still lacking. Hence, a better understanding of pathological changes is needed to develop a potential cardioprotective agent. In recent times, NLRP3 inflammasome has been extensively studied in various disease conditions, including CVDs. The activation of NLRP3 inflammasome has been found to be positively correlated with various CVDs, such as hypertension, angina, arrhythmia, cardiac fibrosis, myocardial infarction, heart failure, *etc*. Moreover, a number of NLRP3 inflammasome activators have been explored for their role in CVDs, and the outcomes of these studies are found to be promising. Therefore, in the present manuscript, we have discussed the structural component of NLRP3 inflammasome, its molecular mechanism of activation, and the outcome of various NLRP3 inflammasome inhibitors in CVDs. We found that NLRP3 inflammasome is an indispensable player of pathogenesis in CVDs, and thus, targeting this inflammasome can be an effective approach for managing and treating these diseases.

Keywords: Myocardial infarction and MCC950, NLRP3 Inflammasome, Nuclear factor kappa B (NF-kB), Oxidative stress.

INTRODUCTION

Cardiovascular disorders (CVDs) are one of the major causes of mortality and morbidity globally and significantly affect patients' quality of life [1]. Moreover, the management and treatment of CVDs have an enormous socioeconomic impact. As per the published evidence, more than 130 million cases of CVDs will be reported by the end of 2035 [2]. Undoubtedly, there has been a significant

---
* **Corresponding author Syed Ehtaishamul Haque:** Department of Pharmacology, School of Pharmaceutical Education and Research, Jamia Hamdard, New Delhi-110062, India; E-mail: sehaq@jamiahamdard.ac.in

Puneetpal Singh (Ed.)
All rights reserved-© 2024 Bentham Science Publishers

increase in the understanding of CVDs; still, there is a lack of information on molecular pathogenesis and precise target-based therapeutic approach. The inflammasome is considered a macromolecular and multiprotein complex that plays a pivotal role in the production and maturation of various proinflammatory cytokines, such as interleukin-1beta (IL-1β). The produced cytokines play a vital role in generating systemic inflammation and various other conditions, including CVDs [3]. NOD-, LRR- and Pyrin domain-containing protein 3 (NLRP3) is an extensively studied inflammasome having a potential pathogenic role in various CVDs, such as hypertension, angina pectoris, arrhythmia, myocardial fibrosis, heart failure, *etc*. Initially, under normal physiological conditions, NLRP3 inflammasome remains inactivated, but in response to pathogen-associated molecular patterns (PAMPs) and damage-associated molecular patterns (DAMPs), it becomes activated and releases IL-1β and IL-18, which play a crucial role in CVD pathogenesis [4]. NLRP3 inflammasomes have been reported to promote atherosclerosis, coronary heart disease, hypertensive disorders, and other CVDs [5]. No doubt, the role of NLRP3 and IL-1β is well established in CVDs, but the molecular mechanism of pathogenesis is unclear. Moreover, clinical findings have also shown that IL-1β inhibitors are effective cardioprotective agents. Hence, a more detailed cellular and molecular mechanism of NLRP3 activation in CVDs is needed to design and develop potent NLRP3 inhibitors for managing and treating cardiovascular disorders.

Structure of NLRP3 Inflammasome

Inflammation is the body's physiological reaction to the incursion of external microorganisms [6]. Inflammasome plays a crucial role in this process [7, 8]. There are five primary Nucleotide-binding oligomerization domain, Leucine-rich Repeat, and Pyrin domain containing inflammasomes (NLRP) known as NLRP10, NLRP1, NLRP3, ice protease-activating factor (IPAF) and absent in melanoma 2 (AIM2). Among them, NLRP3 has received the utmost attention [9]. Inflammasomes are complexes of multi proteins of the Nucleotide-binding oligomerization domain (NOD)-like receptors (NLR) family. The complex of proteins (NLRP3, ASC, and pro-caspase-1 effector) forms the NLRP3 inflammasome. Cytosolic protein NLRP3, previously identified as a novel inflammatory gene, is now considered the primary component of the NLRP3 inflammasome and has C-terminal and N-terminal function structural domains [10]. The N-terminal contains the protein pyrin domain (PYD), the nucleotide-binding oligomerization domain (NOD), and the caspase-associated recruitment domain (CARD), whereas the C-terminal contains the leucine-rich repeat (LRR), which serves as a cap to recognize different patterns associated with the pathogen and other ligands. Rearrangement of the NOD structure domain occurs after the recognition of ligands by LRR, triggering the biological effects [11]. NOD is centrally located and surrounded by the N-terminal protein PYD, CARD, and C-terminal protein LLR. NLRP3 activation and processing of IL-1β are mediated by the NOD domain having an ATP-binding site. NLRP3 detects pathogen and body's signals, attaches to pro-caspase-1 and converts it to caspase-1 *via* ASC protein, followed by caspase-1 autocatalytic activation. Consequently, caspase-1 processes pro-IL-1β and pro-IL-18 into its active forms, thereby arbitrating the consequent responses [12].

Activation of NLRP3 Inflammasome

Pattern recognition receptors (PRRs) are genetically coded receptors present in the innate immune system. Agonists with binding properties to the same PRR are identified as PAMPs. PAMPs are associated with NLRP3 inflammasome activation. PRRs with membrane-bound toll-like receptors (TLRs) and C-type lectins (CTLs) are used by the body's innate immune system to recognize PAMPs. DAMPs are referred to as self-molecules generated by injured cells. These may trigger PRR activation in the absence of an active contagion and are accountable for the activation of NLRP3 inflammasome [13, 14]. PAMPs and DAMPs are both recognized by NLRs and thus play a pivotal role in activating NLRP3 inflammasome [15]. Specifically, the NLRP3 inflammasome is activated in two phases. One is through PAMPs and DAMPs, which form the NLRP3 inflammasome protein complex of NLRP3, ASC, and pro-caspase-1 [16]. The second is *via* TLR and Nuclear factor kappa B (NF-kB) signaling pathways, which cause the synthesis of pro-cytokine, such as pro-IL-1β, leading to pyroptosis, as shown in Fig. (**1**) [17].

The Lysosomal Damage Mediating NLRP3 Activation

When macrophage cells swallow up the PAMPs, they damage lysosomes by destabilizing phagocytes and activating caspase-1 for processing pro-cytokines like pro-IL-1β and pro-IL-18 [18]. Particulate matters like urea, calcium, cholesterol crystals, and silica are engulfed by the macrophages that damage the integrity of the lysosomal membrane. Furthermore, cathepsin B is released in the cytosol after rupturing the lysosome and is accountable for triggering the NLRP3 inflammasome activation [4, 18]. The mechanistic understanding of lysosome destabilization-mediated NLRP3 activation is unknown. However, based on previous studies, it is found that monosodium urate releases an enormous amount of sodium ions that reduce the concentration of intracellular K^+ efflux [19]. Lysosome destruction causes K^+ outflow *via* pore formation and is responsible for activating the NLRP3 inflammasome [20]. Lysosomal damage can also be due to oxidative stress induced by intracellular Ca^{2+} ion, macrophage, and dysfunctional mitochondria, which causes NLRP3 inflammasome activation leading to cardiovascular complications [21].

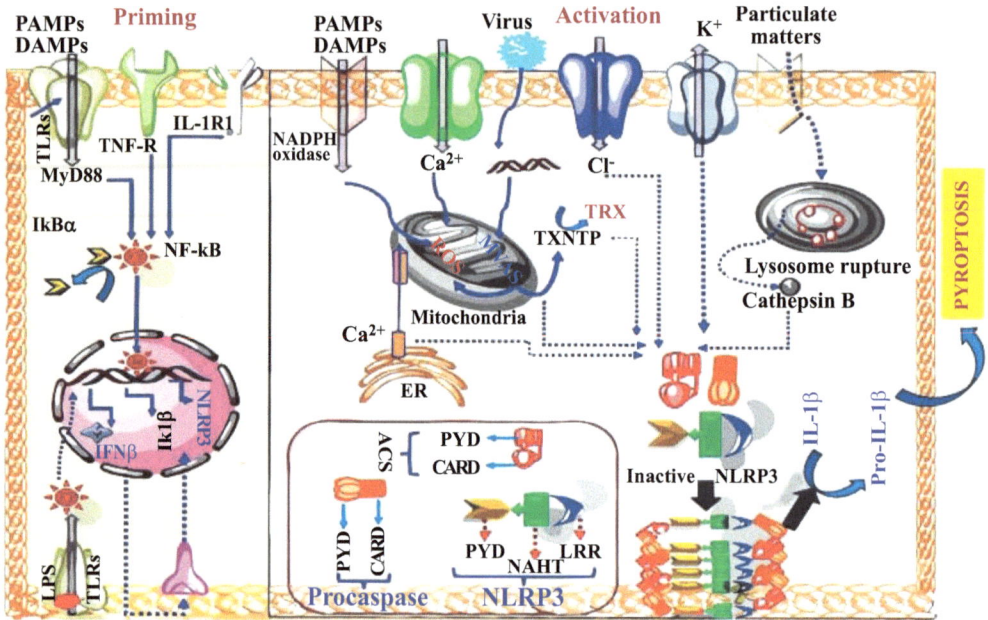

Fig. (1). Mechanism of NLRP3 activation. The figure is permitted for use under Creative Commons open licenses.

K^+ Efflux Mobilization-Mediated Activation Pathway

The efflux of K^+ ions can trigger the stimulation of the NLRP3 inflammasome. Different activators of NLRP3, such as nigericin and ATP, induce the efflux of K^+ ion, which regulates the secretion of IL-1β from monocytes and promotes the transformation of pro-IL-1β into IL-1β [22, 23]. Previous research has shown that the K^+ efflux-mediated NLRP3 inflammasome activation pathway involves a P2X7 ATP-gated ion channel. The purinergic 2X7 receptor (P2X7R) activates the NLRP3 inflammasome. Extracellular ATP activates the P2X7 ATP-gated ion channel to initiate the quick K^+ ion expulsion [20]. The outflow of K^+ ions results in its low concentration, leading to the formation of reactive oxygen species (ROS), apoptosis and mitochondrial damage, which activates the NLRP3 inflammasome. Various published research has also shown that K^+ efflux could also be initiated by asbestos and aluminum hydroxide silica to activate the inflammasome [21]. Consequently, the efflux of K^+ may not be a significant and self-reliant factor for the activation of NLRP3 inflammasome.

Ca^{2+} Mobilization Mediated NLRP3 Activation

Many signaling pathways use calcium mobilization. Numerous studies have demonstrated that Ca^{2+} plays a pathogenic role in NLRP3 activation. The phospholipase C enzyme catalyzes phosphatidylinositol4,5-bisphosphate (PIP2) to inositol 1,4,5-triphosphate (IP3), which, in the presence of ATP, causes Ca^{2+} efflux from the endoplasmic reticulum (ER) and increases the concentration of intracellular Ca^{2+} [24]. Opening of voltage-gated Ca^{2+} channels also increases the concentration of Ca^{2+} ions inside the cell. Previous research has shown a link between intracellular Ca^{2+} levels and NLRP3 activation [25]. Systematically, ATP and other stimuli increase the Ca^{2+} efflux from ER and elevate the Ca^{2+} concentration, which triggers mitochondrial dysfunction and ROS elevation and increases NF-kB expression, thereby triggering the NLRP3 inflammasome activation [26]. The study in which a Ca^{2+} blocker and IP3 inhibitor were used to confirm the pathogenic role of Ca^{2+} in NLRP3 activation showed a reduction in Ca^{2+}efflux and thus reduced the activation of NLRP3 [27]. Thus, the probable role of increased calcium concentration was positively correlated with NLRP3 activation and CVDs.

Na$^+$ And Cl$^-$ Efflux Mediated NLRP3 Activation

Various published research have described the importance of Na$^+$ and Cl$^-$ efflux in the NLRP3 activation. Blocking the Na$^+$ influx by lowering extracellular Na$^+$ ion concentration reduces the activation of the NLRP3 inflammasome complex [19]. Increased Na+ ions inside the cell result in swelling and water inflow, reduction of intracellular K$^+$ ions and triggering the NLRP3 inflammasome activation [19]. Previous studies stated that elevation in intracellular Cl$^-$ ion level increases the pro-IL-1β secretion followed by its activation in IL-1β, whereas increased extracellular Cl$^-$ ion concentration decreases the secretion and activation of IL-1β [28]. The importance of chloride ions in triggering inflammasome is well accounted in a previous study where fenamate, a Cl-channel inhibitor, prevents the activation of NLRP3 inflammasome [29]. However, a thorough study is further required to comprehend the role of Na$^+$ and Cl$^-$ ions efflux in NLRP3 inflammasome activation.

ROS-Mediated Activation Pathway

Excessive production of ROS through the NADPH oxidase and mitochondria is responsible for oxidative stress and causes the NLRP3 inflammasome activation [30]. In the presence of elevated ROS levels, the complex of thioredoxin and thioredoxin-interacting protein (TXNIP) get dissociated, and TXNIP then attaches to NLRP3 and activates it by forming TXNIP-NLRP3 inflammasome complex [31]. DAMPs, PAMPs, and ATP promote the production of ROS [21].

Mitochondrial production of ROS induced by NLRP3 agonists shows that ROS are also accountable for NLRP3 inflammasome activation [32]. Previous studies have reported that mitochondrial damage by autophagy decreases ROS generation and inhibits the induction of NLRP3 inflammasome [33]. Mitochondrial damage upregulates the activation of NLRP3 by producing ROS to start NLRP3 oligomerization [33]. Furthermore, ROS inhibitors inhibit the early activation phase of NLRP3, but they have no direct effect on the activation of NLRP3 [34, 35].

Mechanisms and Role of NLRP3 Activation in Cardiovascular Diseases

Despite significant improvements in CVD prevention and treatment, the lack of extensive knowledge of the mechanisms underlying CVD expansion remains a major contributor to mortality and morbidity worldwide [36]. Coronary heart disease, the most common type of CVD, accounts for roughly half of all CVD cases in America. More than 130 million individuals are expected to suffer from various forms of CVD by 2035, increasing the financial burden due to raised medical costs [37]. Thus, understanding the pathological process of CVDs and looking for new treatments by targeting signalling pathways are required. NLRP3 inflammasome has been the most thoroughly described inflammasome, which is involved in the progression of diseases because it can be activated by various mechanisms [15]. Exploring the inhibitory pathway of NLRP3 could be a novel perspective for CVD treatment and prevention [15].

Different types of DAMPs mediate the priming phase. Following myocardial ischemia, infarction (MI) and post-ischemic damage produce DAMPs and release intracellular and extracellular alarmins. Furthermore, metabolites and neurohormonal activation promote priming in cardiovascular diseases, such as hypertension and myocardial infarction or chronic diseases, such as obesity or diabetes [38 - 41]. Diabetes-related priming causes an elevation in the manifestation of NLRP3 inflammasome complex and substrates, which perpetuates the body's reaction to acute experimental MI [42]. As previously stated, some stimuli, such as PAMPs and DAMPs, contribute to the activation of NLRP3. Potassium ions efflux, which is mediated by different intracellular and extracellular proteins, is one of the main causes of the activation of NLRP3. When ATP binds to the P2X7 receptor outside the cell, it opens a K^+ channel that causes potassium efflux [43, 44]. Following an acute MI, P2X7 inhibition or gene silencing reduces cardiac damage. Other factors like lysosomal content leakage into the cytoplasm may be responsible for K^+ ions efflux [45]. PAMPs monosodium urate, silica, calcium pyrophosphate, and cholesterol cause phagocytosis, lysosome weakening, and swelling, ultimately leading to lysosome rupture and leakage of cathepsin B, which cause K$^+$ ions efflux and activation of NLRP3 leading to manifestations of CVDs [45, 46].

Moreover, autophagy causes the breakdown of proteins and organelles present in the cytoplasm, such as mitochondria. Autophagy modulates the inflammasome pathway in experimental settings. Mitophagy dysfunction increases ROS and cytosolic accumulation of mitochondrial DAMPS in the cytoplasmic matrix, such as mitochondrial DNA (mtDNA) and cardiolipin [47 - 50]. ROS and redox balance in the cells are key factors that activate NLRP3. The TXNIP is an oxidative stress-sensitive protein that binds with the thioredoxin oxidoreductase (TRX). The detachment of TXNIP from TRX initiates the activation of NLRP3 in response to oxidative stress (Fig. **2**) [51 - 53].

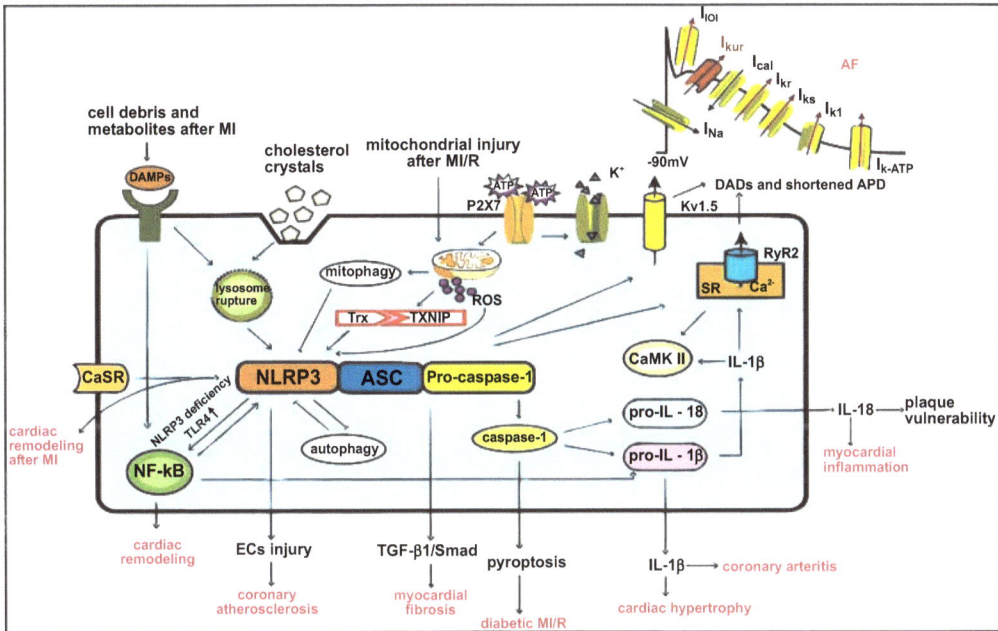

Fig. (2). Pathogenic role of NLRP3 activation in various cardiovascular diseases. The figure is permitted for use under Creative Commons open licenses.

Association Between NLRP3 Inflammasomes and Coronary Heart Diseases

NLRP3 plays a key role in the initial stages of coronary heart disease . The elevated level of low-density lipoprotein increases the deposition of cholesterol in the coronary vessels. After this, phagocytosis of lipoprotein occurs by the macrophages, and then macrophages transform into foam cells. Activated foam cells trigger the inflammatory cycle reaction by different mechanisms: (a) lysosomal damage in which lysosome loses its integrity after phagocytosis by the macrophages and produces ROS. The excessive production of ROS activates NLRP3 [54, 55]. (b) The capsular TLR-4 recognizes LDL and free fatty acids that have undergone limited oxidation.It increases the interferon TIR domain-containing adapter-inducing interferon-beta (TRIF) and myeloid differentiation primary response gene 88 to activate NF-κB. NF-κB stimulates the expression of the NLRP3 gene and IL-lβ to encourage inflammation [56]. (c) IL-lβ activates the platelets by stimulating mononuclear cells and promotes their release [57]. (d) The production of IL-18 by the activated macrophages causes vascular smooth muscle cell necrosis and liberating metalloprotease, which reduces plaque stability [58].

Association Between NLRP3 Inflammasome and Myocardial Ischemia

Inflammation is a major part of the pathophysiology of myocardial ischemia. However, the exact mechanism of cardiac ischemia that causes inflammation is unknown. Different studies have suggested that NLRP3 inflammasome regulates a sterile inflammatory response induced by cell damage. The detection of DAMPs and PAMPs through extracellular and intracellular pattern recognition receptors initiates the inflammatory response [59]. In myocardial ischemia, the inflammasome acts as early detection for danger signals. In 2011, it was discovered that the activation of NLRP3 in heart fibroblasts is critical in the early inflammatory response following ischemia [60]. TXNIP may be involved in the mechanism of NLRP3 action in myocardial ischemia. *In vitro* study suggests that TXNIP causes NLRP3 inflammasome to activate in cardiac microvascular endothelial cells *via* ROS [61]. This complex dissociates as the intracellular ROS concentration increases and activates the NLRP3 inflammasome by binding TXNIP to the leucine-rich repeat domain of NLRP3 [62].

The Association Between NLRP3 Inflammasome, Heart Failure and Arrhythmia

NLRP3 inflammasome activation induces inflammatory gene expression in myocytes. These responses may signal cardiac fibrosis, phagocytosis, and myocardial dysfunction. Previous findings suggest that heart failure can be prevented by inhibiting primary inflammatory responses persuaded by NLRP3 inflammasome-associated pathways [63, 64]. An *in vivo* study also revealed that elevated IL-1β signaling in response to Tet methylcytosine dioxygenase 2 (TET2) deficiency in hematopoietic cells has been linked to increased heart dysfunction in the cardiac failure rodent model [65]. TET2-mediated clonal hematopoiesis may increase the risk of cardiac failure and improve response to NLRP3-IL-1β inhibition [65]. Arrhythmia is common in patients with heart failure due to changes in electrical remodeling [66]. Mice with diabetes mellitus produce IL-1β after activating the NLRP3 inflammasome in cardiac macrophages [67]. IL-1β then reduces the density of calcium ions, upregulating ROS signaling and protein kinase C activation, leading to arrhythmia and cardiac failure [68]. Chronic inflammation in the case of heart failure causes collagen accumulation and cardiac fibrosis and exacerbates the condition [68]. Treatment of cardiac fibroblasts with anti-fibrotic medications inhibits the NLRP3 expression, inflammasome complex, and NLRP3-transforming growth factor 1 (TGF1)-Smad pathway [69].

The Association Between NLRP3 Inflammasome and Cardiac Fibrosis

Cardiac fibrosis is a clinical situation in many CVDs and is characterized by an extreme build-up of extracellular matrix, which causes organ dysfunction and tissue damage. The NLRP3 inflammasome is associated with the development of cardiac fibrosis [70]. Previous research has shown that the stimulation of TGF-β modulates the activation of NLRP3 inflammasome [71]. Recent studies have also shown that NLRP3 regulates TGF-β signaling pathways rather than TGF regulating NLRP3. It has been found that serelaxin inhibits the NLRP3 inflammasome and TLR-4 and decreases IL-1β and TGF-β1 levels in myofibroblasts [72]. This research is still in its early stages, and more evidence is required to understand the mechanism of cardiac fibrosis. A study conducted on mice with MI showed that MCC950, a potent NLRP3 inflammasome inhibitor, ameliorated cardiac fibrosis and strengthened heart function by reducing the expression of NLRP3 inflammasome [73]. Another study demonstrated that the expression of NLRP3 inflammasome was increased by angiotensin II, causing cardiac fibrosis and inflammation, whereas MCC950 reversed these pathological changes [74].

Hyperglycemia has also been shown to cause inflammasome activation, significantly contributing to cardiac fibrosis, as seen in diabetic cardiomyopathy [75]. Hyperglycemia causes the extreme generation of mitochondrial ROS and leads to oxidative stress. Under normal circumstances, thioredoxin oxidoreductase (TRX) prevents the activity of the thioredoxin-binding protein (TXNIP) by binding to it. The generation of ROS dissociates the TXNIP-TRX complex, followed by the binding of TXNIP to NLRP3 to induce inflammasome activation [76]. It has also been found that the inhibition of NLRP3 inflammasome activation improves cardiac function in diabetic mice [77]. Autophagy has been linked to NLRP3-mediated cardiac fibrosis. Autophagy prevents inflammasome activation by reducing cell ROS generation [78]. In a rodent model of cardiotoxicity induced by isoproterenol administration and left anterior descending artery ligation, autophagy was found to be impaired, ameliorating myocardial fibrosis. Aspirin treatment considerably improves cardiac fibrosis, whereas an autophagy promoter rapamycin inhibits the cardiac fibroblast advancement, implying that autophagy has a significant role in the progression of cardiac fibrosis [79].

The Association Between NLRP3 Inflammasome and Cardiac Hypertrophy

IL-18 has proven to be a potential diagnostic marker of coronary artery disease in cohort studies. IL-18 has a significant role in cardiac hypertrophy, as evidenced by the downregulation of hypertrophy-related genes in IL-18-deficient mice [80]. The NLRP3 inflammasome expression is significantly elevated in transverse aortic constricted mice. It plays a vital role in the upregulation of inflammatory markers and profibrotic factor production, leading to hypertrophy, cardiac fibrosis and heart dysfunction [81]. Under oxidative stress, due to excessive ROS, cardiac cells are activated, and calcium ions are liberated into the cytoplasm, which leads to changes in the mitochondrial membrane's potential, resulting in the apoptosis of the myocardium [82]. An *in-vitro* study on H9C2 cells showed that Receptor for Advanced Glycation End products (RAGE) induced myocardial hypertrophy was linked to NF-κB and NLRP3, which was induced by the NF-κB-NLRP3-IL- 1β signaling pathway [83]. Transverse aortic constriction-induced cardiac hypertrophy in mice is ameliorated by pirfenidone *via* inhibiting the NLRP3-I--1β signaling pathway [84]. These outcomes suggest that NLRP3 inflammasome signaling pathways have a significant role in the pathogenesis and progression of cardiac hypertrophy.

NLRP3 Inhibitors: New Therapies Related to the NLRP3 Inflammasome

A large number of inflammatory diseases, such as stroke in diabetic patients, hypertension, small vessel disease, kidney damage, CVDs, and autoimmune and genetic syndromes, are associated with the NLRP3 inflammasome pathway [85]. For this purpose, scientists have focused in recent years on developing molecules that could proficiently hinder the NLRP3 inflammasome Table **1**. Selective NLRP3 inhibitors have their own advantage like the inhibition of NLRP3 inflammasome prevents pyroptosis, which is unaffected by inhibiting the IL-1β or IL-18 cytokines [85] (Fig. **3**). Most of the compounds discussed in this article have been studied in different rodent models of CVDs.

Table 1. Showing the various NLRP3 inhibitors against cardiovascular disorders.

S. No.	NLRP3 Inhibitors	Mechanism of NLRP3 Inhibitors	Refs.
1.	MCC950	Inhibits NLRP3-ATPase activity and blocks ASC oligomerization	[87]
2.	JC-124	Suppresses NLRP3 complex, Trop-I and Caspase-1	[95, 98]
3.	Bay 11-7082	Inhibits NLRP3 activation and reduction in expression of caspase-1 and IL-1β	[42]

(Table 1) cont.....

S. No.	NLRP3 Inhibitors	Mechanism of NLRP3 Inhibitors	Refs.
4.	INF4E	Inhibits caspase-1 and NLRP3 ATPase activities and activates RISK pathway	[101, 102]
5.	OLT1177	Limits NLRP3-ASC interaction and oligomerization of NLRP3 through inhibition of ATPase activity	[104]
6.	CY-09	Prevents NLRP3 complex activation and ATPase activity through the bond formation with the ATP-binding motif NACHT domain	[108]
7.	Tranilast	Binds to the NACHT domain of NLRP3 and prevents NLRP3 oligomerization	[111]
8.	Colchicine	Inhibits P2X7-mediated pore formation and ASC expression	[115, 119]
9.	Glyburide	Inhibits K^+ efflux and prevents ACS oligomerization	[95]
10.	VX-765	Directly inhibits Caspase-1 and NLRP3 inflammasome activation	[120]
11.	HQQR	Inhibits NLRP3, IL-1β and caspase-1 pathway and ameliorates cardiac fibrosis	[121]
12.	Allopurinol	Inhibits cardiac fibrosis and inflammation by suppressing NLRP3 and TGF-β/Smads signaling pathway	[122]
13.	Empagliflozin	Inhibits calcium ion efflux and NLRP3, reduces inflammation	[123]
14.	Triptolide	NLRP3-ASC interaction and decreases IL-1β	[69]
15.	Emodin	Alleviates inflammatory cytokines and inhibits NLRP3 inflammasome to reduce pyroptosis	[124]
16.	Anakinra	Suppresses IL-1β processing and inhibits NLRP3 inflammasome	[125]

ASC; apoptosis-associated speck-like protein containing a CARD, Trop-I; Troponin-I, RISK; reperfusion injury salvage kinase.

MCC950

MCC950 is a potent NLRP3 inhibitor, but it cannot inhibit NLRP1, NLRC4, or AIM2 [86]. It is a small molecule that forms a noncovalent bond with NLRP3, blocking NLRP3-ATPase activity and thus preventing ASC oligomerization and subsequent IL-1 release [87]. MCC950 is also recognized by other names, such as CP-456,773 and CRID3. It was first discussed in 2001 for its ability to prevent the processing of IL-1β along with other compounds containing diarylsulfonylurea [88]. NLRP3 in cryopyrin-associated periodic syndrome (CAPS) is a molecular target of diarylsulfonylurea inhibitors, and as a result, MCC950 cannot effectively inhibit these forms of NLRP3 [89].

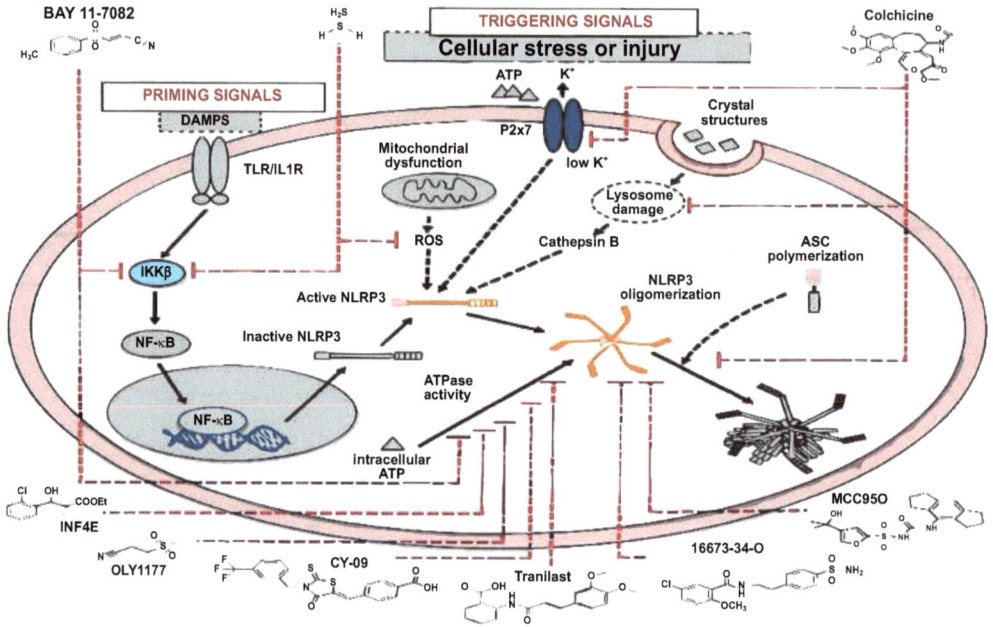

Fig. (3). Showing details and target of NLRP3 inflammasome inhibitor in managing and treating CVDs.

A study has shown that the administration of MCC950 (10 mg/kg dose) in angiotensin II infusion-challenged hypertensive mice decreases IL-1β levels and cardiac fibrosis [90]. The administration of MCC950 in hypertensive mice for 25 days reduced renal inflammation and controlled elevated blood pressure [91]. Additionally, MCC950 considerably decreases the manifestation of NLRP3 inflammasome, leading to reduced aortic dilation and disintegration in thoracic aortic sections in a high-fat diet and angiotensin II-challenged mice [91]. Both mouse and pig models of acute myocardial infarction have demonstrated the beneficial effects of MCC950. In the pig model of MI, the administration of MCC950 (6 mg/kg) improved the cardiac function and decreased the infarct size and IL-1β level [92]. The treatment of postmenopausal heart disease in mice with MCC950 (10 mg/kg) for eight weeks ameliorated cardiac remodeling and improved cardiac functions [93].

Glyburide, JC-124 and 16673-34-0

Glyburide, known as glibenclamide, was first used for the management of type II diabetes [94]. It was the first NLRP3 inflammasome inhibitor discovered in bone marrow-derived macrophages. Glyburide is a selective NLRP3 inhibitor as it does not affect NLRC4, AIM2, and NLRP1 activity [95]. However, the required dose of glyburide to prevent the NLRP3 inflammasome activation causes hypoglycemia, thus limiting its use as an anti-inflammatory drug [96]. 16673-34-0 is an orally active compound with inhibition properties of NLRP3 inflammasome without influencing glucose metabolism. In a mice model of myocardial ischemia, a 100 mg/kg dose of 16673-34-0 decreases the infarct size by inhibiting caspase-1 [97]. Based on 16673-34-0 activity, a new compound was developed, *i.e.*, JC-124. It was found that intraperitoneal administration of JC-124 (30 mg/kg) decreased the level of Troponin I and infarct size in mice with ischemia [98].

Bay 11-7082 and INF4E

Bay 11-7082, a phenyl vinyl sulfone, was discovered as an NF- κB pathway inhibitor. Bay 11-7082 effectively inhibits the NLRP3 inflammasome while not impacting NLRP1 and NLRC4 [53]. Intraperitoneal administration of Bay 11-7082, 10 minutes before reperfusion, decreased the infarct size, inflammation, and apoptosis in a murine model of ischemia/reperfusion [99]. In a diabetic model of rats, it was found to inhibit the activation of NLRP3 inflammasome with a reduction in the expression of IL-1β and caspase-1 to reduce cardiac injury following ischemia-reperfusion [42]. However, it is challenging to distinguish the effects of Bay 11-7082, which are reliant on the down-regulation of the NF- κB pathway, from those that are dependent on NLRP3 inhibition *in vivo*.

INF4E is an electrophilic moiety that shows nucleophile reactivity and can inhibit the activation of NLRP3, NLRP3-dependent pyroptosis, and IL-1β processing [100]. INF4E is an effective inhibitor of NLRP3 and inhibits the activities of NLRP3 ATPase and caspase-1. INF4E protects the myocardium from IR-induced injury and dysfunction [101]. In a rat ischemia model, administration of INF4E improved cardiac function and decreased infarct size. Additionally, INF4E-treated hearts decreased the NLRP3 inflammasome expression, activated the RISK pathway to prevent reperfusion injury and enhanced mitochondrial function [102]. Other compounds have also been developed that have the Michael acceptor moiety of INF4E in response to the compound's potential cytotoxicity [103]. INF58, the most promising of these chemicals, has not yet been proven to be a cardio-protective agent.

OLT1177 and CY-09

OLT1177 is a potent NLRP3 inflammasome inhibitor with beta-sulfonyl nitrile moiety. OLT1177 directly binds with NLRP3 and prevents NLRP3-ASC interaction and NLRP3 oligomerization by blocking of ATPase activity of NLRP3 [104]. OLT1177 has been evaluated in several animal models of inflammation and has consistently displayed the prevention of NLRP3 activation. Isolated mononuclear cells from CAPS patients continuously released IL-18 and IL-1β, and OLT1177 inhibited cytokine release in these mononuclear cells [104]. An animal study found that treatment with OLT1177 decreased the infarct area of the heart and retained the cardiac functions in ischemic mice [105]. OLT1177 is currently in clinical trials. In gout patients, it was found to be safe and effective in decreasing target joint pain [106]. Patients suffering from heart failure were taken for a pilot phase 1B-double blind study, in which OLT1177 was given to patients, and itwas found that OLT1177 was safe at a high dose and linked to an increment in left ventricular ejection fraction and treadmill exercise period [107]. CY-09 is a newly developed inhibitor of NLRP3 that inhibits NLRP3 complex activation and ATPase activity by binding to the NACHT domain's ATP-binding motif. Various animal models of CAPS and type-2 diabetes have been used to evaluate its therapeutic effectiveness [108]. The administration of CY-09 in mice with diabetic ischemic stroke prevents myocardial dysfunction [109].

Tranilast and Colchicine

Tranilast is a newly identified potent inhibitor of NLRP3 inflammasome and has no influence on NLRC4 and AIM2. Tranilast is primarily used for the treatment of a number of allergic disorders [110]. Tranilast has been shown to bind to the NACHT domain of NLRP3, preventing it from oligomerizing independently of NLRP3 ATPase activity. The inhibitory mechanism of tranilast is also unaffected by excessive ROS generation, Na^+- K^+ efflux, and mitochondrial damage [111]. It has been studied on various rodent models of gout, type-2 diabetes, and CAPS. It was used for its pharmacological effects in MI, hypertension, cardiac fibrosis, and cardiomyopathy [111 - 113]. Several clinical trials showed that a high dose of tranilast is safe in patients [114].

Colchicine is orally taken to cure gout, Behçet's disease and other inflammatory diseases. Besides this, colchicine is now also used as an NLRP3 inflammasome inhibitor. Colchicine produces its inhibitory effects by inhibiting the pore formation mediated by P2X7 and intracellular transportation [115]. In a rodent model of AMI, colchicine attenuated the cardiac functions at a daily dose of 0.1 mg/kg for seven days and decreased neutrophil infiltration and NLRP3 inflammasome expression [116]. Clinical trials have shown that colchicine is safe and pharmacologically effective at 0.5 mg/kg. The administration of 0.5 mg/kg colchicine in patients with AMI decreases the ischemic events [117]. A clinical study on patients with post-acute coronary syndrome found that colchicine administration alters the coronary plaque and high-sensitivity C-reactive protein [118]. Moreover, colchicine decreases pericardial inflammation and ASC expression in mice with pericarditis [119].

DISCUSSION AND CONCLUSION

Based on the aforementioned incidence and prevalence of CVDs and the potential pathogenic role of NLRP3 inflammasome, it can be inferred that the design and development of selective NLRP3 inhibitors could be one of the novel and future therapeutic implications in the management and treatment of various cardiovascular disorders. NLRP3 also effectively interacts with the viruses, bacteria, and other intracellular components such as endotoxins, ROS, MDA, *etc.*, and causes the activation of caspase-1 from pro-caspase-1. Activated caspase-1 then regulates the production of pro-IL-1β to IL-1β and IL-18. Hence, selective targeting of NLRP3 assembly and its activation is a pivotal and novel therapeutic approach for NLRP3-mediated cardiac inflammation and associated pathogenic attributes. Studies have shown that when S194 phosphorylation is inhibited, NLRP3 inflammasome activation gets prevented, exhibiting cardiovascular effects. Moreover, the selective targeting of the NLRP3-NACHT domain and hydrolysis of ATP also appear to be promising approaches in the inhibition of NLRP3-mediated CVDs.

Considering the existing NLRP3 inhibitors, such as MCC950, JC-124, Bay 11-7082, INF4E, CY-09, tranilast, and glyburide, their study on preclinical models has shown significant cardioprotection with the utmost safety profile. However, a more detailed cellular and molecular mechanism of cardioprotection is needed. We further conclude that well-designed clinical trials should be conducted to bring NLRP3 inhibitors from the bench to the bedside.

ACKNOWLEDGEMENT

The authors are thankful to the School of Pharmaceutical Education and Research, Jamia Hamdard, New Delhi, for providing the necessary facilities.

REFERENCES

[1]   Ezzati M, Obermeyer Z, Tzoulaki I, Mayosi BM, Elliott P, Leon DA. Contributions of risk factors and medical care to cardiovascular mortality trends. Nat Rev Cardiol 2015; 12(9): 508-30.
      [http://dx.doi.org/10.1038/nrcardio.2015.82] [PMID: 26076950]

[2]   Benjamin EJ, Virani SS, Callaway CW, *et al.* Heart disease and stroke statistics-2018 update: A reportfrom the American Heart Association. Circulation 2018; 137(12): e67-e492.
      [http://dx.doi.org/10.1161/CIR.0000000000000558] [PMID: 29386200]

[3]   An N, Gao Y, Si Z, *et al.* Regulatory mechanisms of the NLRP3 inflammasome, a novel immune-inflammatory marker in cardiovascular diseases. Front Immunol 2019; 10: 1592.
      [http://dx.doi.org/10.3389/fimmu.2019.01592] [PMID: 31354731]

[4]   Schroder K, Tschopp J. The inflammasomes. Cell 2010; 140(6): 821-32.
      [http://dx.doi.org/10.1016/j.cell.2010.01.040] [PMID: 20303873]

[5]   Su Q, Li L, Sun Y, Yang H, Ye Z, Zhao J. Effects of theTLR4/Myd88/NF-κB signaling pathway on NLRP3 inflammasomein coronary microembolization-induced myocardialinjury. Cell Physiol

Biochem 2018; 47(4): 1497-508.
[http://dx.doi.org/10.1159/000490866] [PMID: 29940584]

[6] Yang CS, Shin DM, Jo EK. The Role of NLR-related Protein 3 Inflammasome in Host Defense and Inflammatory Diseases. Int Neurourol J 2012; 16(1): 2-12.
[http://dx.doi.org/10.5213/inj.2012.16.1.2] [PMID: 22500248]

[7] Broz P, Dixit VM. Inflammasomes: Mechanism of assembly, regulation and signalling. Nat Rev Immunol 2016; 16(7): 407-20.
[http://dx.doi.org/10.1038/nri.2016.58] [PMID: 27291964]

[8] Kanneganti TD, Lamkanfi M, Núñez G. Intracellular NOD-like receptors in host defense and disease. Immunity 2007; 27(4): 549-59.
[http://dx.doi.org/10.1016/j.immuni.2007.10.002] [PMID: 17967410]

[9] Fidler TP, Xue C, Yalcinkaya M, *et al*. The AIM2 inflammasome exacerbates atherosclerosis in clonal haematopoiesis. Nature 2021; 592(7853): 296-301.
[http://dx.doi.org/10.1038/s41586-021-03341-5] [PMID: 33731931]

[10] Compan V, Martín-Sánchez F, Baroja-Mazo A, *et al*. Apoptosis-associated speck-like protein containing a CARD forms specks but does not activate caspase-1 in the absence of NLRP3 during macrophage swelling. J Immunol 2015; 194(3): 1261-73.
[http://dx.doi.org/10.4049/jimmunol.1301676] [PMID: 25552542]

[11] Zhang Q, Yu W, Lee S, Xu Q, Naji A, Le AD. Bisphosphonate induces osteonecrosis of the jaw in diabetic mice *via* NLRP3/caspase-1-dependent IL-1β mechanism. J Bone Miner Res 2015; 30(12): 2300-12.
[http://dx.doi.org/10.1002/jbmr.2577] [PMID: 26081624]

[12] Madouri F, Guillou N, Fauconnier L, *et al*. Caspase-1 activation by NLRP3 inflammasome dampens IL-33-dependent house dust mite-induced allergic lung inflammation. J Mol Cell Biol 2015; 7(4): 351-65.
[http://dx.doi.org/10.1093/jmcb/mjv012] [PMID: 25714839]

[13] Mogensen TH. Pathogen recognition and inflammatory signaling in innate immune defenses. Clin Microbiol Rev 2009; 22(2): 240-73.
[http://dx.doi.org/10.1128/CMR.00046-08] [PMID: 19366914]

[14] Takeuchi O, Akira S. Pattern recognition receptors and inflammation. Cell 2010; 140(6): 805-20.
[http://dx.doi.org/10.1016/j.cell.2010.01.022] [PMID: 20303872]

[15] Guarda G, Zenger M, Yazdi AS, *et al*. Differential expression of NLRP3 among hematopoietic cells. J Immunol 2011; 186(4): 2529-34.
[http://dx.doi.org/10.4049/jimmunol.1002720] [PMID: 21257968]

[16] Hornung V, Latz E. Critical functions of priming and lysosomal damage for NLRP3 activation. Eur J Immunol 2010; 40(3): 620-3.
[http://dx.doi.org/10.1002/eji.200940185] [PMID: 20201015]

[17] Katsnelson MA, Lozada-Soto KM, Russo HM, Miller BA, Dubyak GR. NLRP3 inflammasome signaling is activated by low-level lysosome disruption but inhibited by extensive lysosome disruption: Roles for K^+ efflux and Ca^{2+} influx. Am J Physiol Cell Physiol 2016; 311(1): C83-C100.
[http://dx.doi.org/10.1152/ajpcell.00298.2015] [PMID: 27170638]

[18] Martinon F, Pétrilli V, Mayor A, Tardivel A, Tschopp J. Gout-associated uric acid crystals activate the NALP3 inflammasome. Nature 2006; 440(7081): 237-41.
[http://dx.doi.org/10.1038/nature04516] [PMID: 16407889]

[19] Muñoz-Planillo R, Kuffa P, Martínez-Colón G, Smith BL, Rajendiran TM, Núñez G. K^+ efflux is the common trigger of NLRP3 inflammasome activation by bacterial toxins and particulate matter. Immunity 2013; 38(6): 1142-53.
[http://dx.doi.org/10.1016/j.immuni.2013.05.016] [PMID: 23809161]

[20]   Nakanishi A, Kaneko N, Takeda H, *et al.* Amyloid β directly interacts with NLRP3 to initiate inflammasome activation: identification of an intrinsic NLRP3 ligand in a cell-free system. Inflamm Regen 2018; 38(1): 27.
[http://dx.doi.org/10.1186/s41232-018-0085-6] [PMID: 30459926]

[21]   Fulp J, He L, Toldo S, *et al.* Structural insights of benzenesulfonamide analogues as NLRP3 inflammasome inhibitors: Design, synthesis, and biological characterization. J Med Chem 2018; 61(12): 5412-23.
[http://dx.doi.org/10.1021/acs.jmedchem.8b00733] [PMID: 29877709]

[22]   Marchetti C, Toldo S, Chojnacki J, *et al.* Pharmacologic inhibition of the NLRP3 inflammasome preserves cardiac function after ischemic and nonischemic injury in the mouse. J Cardiovasc Pharmacol 2015; 66(1): 1-8.
[http://dx.doi.org/10.1097/FJC.0000000000000247] [PMID: 25915511]

[23]   Walev I, Klein J, Husmann M, *et al.* Potassium regulates IL-1 beta processing *via* calcium-independent phospholipase A2. J Immunol 2000; 164(10): 5120-4.
[http://dx.doi.org/10.4049/jimmunol.164.10.5120] [PMID: 10799869]

[24]   Murakami T, Ockinger J, Yu J, *et al.* Critical role for calcium mobilization in activation of the NLRP3 inflammasome. Proc Natl Acad Sci 2012; 109(28): 11282-7.
[http://dx.doi.org/10.1073/pnas.1117765109] [PMID: 22733741]

[25]   Lee GS, Subramanian N, Kim AI, *et al.* The calcium-sensing receptor regulates the NLRP3 inflammasome through Ca2+ and cAMP. Nature 2012; 492(7427): 123-7.
[http://dx.doi.org/10.1038/nature11588] [PMID: 23143333]

[26]   Lacroix-Lamandé S, Fanton d'Andon M, Michel E, *et al.* Downregulation of the Na/K-ATPase pump by leptospiral glycolipoprotein activates the NLRP3 inflammasome. J Immunol 2012; 188(6): 2805-14.
[http://dx.doi.org/10.4049/jimmunol.1101987] [PMID: 22323544]

[27]   Chu J, Thomas LM, Watkins SC, Franchi L, Núñez G, Salter RD. Cholesterol-dependent cytolysins induce rapid release of mature IL-1β from murine macrophages in a NLRP3 inflammasome and cathepsin B-dependent manner. J Leukoc Biol 2009; 86(5): 1227-38.
[http://dx.doi.org/10.1189/jlb.0309164] [PMID: 19675207]

[28]   Schorn C, Frey B, Lauber K, *et al.* Sodium overload and water influx activate the NALP3 inflammasome. J Biol Chem 2011; 286(1): 35-41.
[http://dx.doi.org/10.1074/jbc.M110.139048] [PMID: 21051542]

[29]   Daniels MJD, Rivers-Auty J, Schilling T, *et al.* Fenamate NSAIDs inhibit the NLRP3 inflammasome and protect against Alzheimer's disease in rodent models. Nat Commun 2016; 7(1): 12504.
[http://dx.doi.org/10.1038/ncomms12504] [PMID: 27509875]

[30]   Wu J, Li X, Zhu G, Zhang Y, He M, Zhang J. The role of Resveratrol-induced mitophagy/autophagy in peritoneal mesothelial cells inflammatory injury *via* NLRP3 inflammasome activation triggered by mitochondrial ROS. Exp Cell Res 2016; 341(1): 42-53.
[http://dx.doi.org/10.1016/j.yexcr.2016.01.014] [PMID: 26825654]

[31]   Shi H, Zhang Z, Wang X, *et al.* Inhibition of autophagy induces IL-1β release from ARPE-19 cells *via* ROS mediated NLRP3 inflammasome activation under high glucose stress. Biochem Biophys Res Commun 2015; 463(4): 1071-6.
[http://dx.doi.org/10.1016/j.bbrc.2015.06.060] [PMID: 26102024]

[32]   Coll RC, Hill JR, Day CJ, *et al.* MCC950 directly targets the NLRP3 ATP-hydrolysis motif for inflammasome inhibition. Nat Chem Biol 2019; 15(6): 556-9.
[http://dx.doi.org/10.1038/s41589-019-0277-7] [PMID: 31086327]

[33]   Yang S, Xia C, Li S, Du L, Zhang L, Zhou R. Defective mitophagy driven by dysregulation of rheb and KIF5B contributes to mitochondrial reactive oxygen species (ROS)-induced nod-like receptor 3

(NLRP3) dependent proinflammatory response and aggravates lipotoxicity. Redox Biol 2014; 3: 63-71.
[http://dx.doi.org/10.1016/j.redox.2014.04.001] [PMID: 25462067]

[34] MacKenzie SH, Schipper JL, Clark AC. The potential for caspases in drug discovery. Curr Opin Drug Discov Devel 2010; 13(5): 568-76.
[PMID: 20812148]

[35] Lamkanfi M, Kanneganti TD, Franchi L, Núñez G. Caspase-1 inflammasomes in infection and inflammation. J Leukoc Biol 2007; 82(2): 220-5.
[http://dx.doi.org/10.1189/jlb.1206756] [PMID: 17442855]

[36] Ezzati M, Obermeyer Z, Tzoulaki I, Mayosi BM, Elliott P, Leon DA. Contributions of risk factors and medical care to cardiovascular mortality trends. Nat Rev Cardiol 2015; 12(9): 508-30.
[http://dx.doi.org/10.1038/nrcardio.2015.82] [PMID: 26076950]

[37] Benjamin EJ, Virani SS, Callaway CW, *et al.* Heart disease and stroke statistics-2018 update: A reportfrom the american heart association. Circulation 2018; 137(12): e67-e492.
[http://dx.doi.org/10.1161/CIR.0000000000000558] [PMID: 29386200]

[38] Pasqua T, Pagliaro P, Rocca C, Angelone T, Penna C. Role of NLRP-3 inflammasome in hypertension: A potential therapeutic target. Curr Pharm Biotechnol 2018; 19(9): 708-14.
[http://dx.doi.org/10.2174/1389201019666180808162011] [PMID: 30091406]

[39] Pavillard LE, Marín-Aguilar F, Bullon P, Cordero MD. Cardiovascular diseases, NLRP3 inflammasome, and western dietary patterns. Pharmacol Res 2018; 131: 44-50.
[http://dx.doi.org/10.1016/j.phrs.2018.03.018] [PMID: 29588192]

[40] Rong L, Sun S, Zhu F, *et al.* Effects of irbesartan on myocardial injury in diabetic rats: The role of NLRP3/ASC/Caspase-1 pathway. J Renin Angiotensin Aldosterone Syst 2020; 21: 2.
[http://dx.doi.org/10.1177/1470320320926049] [PMID: 32466695]

[41] Gao J, Xie Q, Wei T, Huang C, Zhou W, Shen W. Nebivolol improves obesity-induced vascular remodeling by suppressing NLRP3 activation. J Cardiovasc Pharmacol 2019; 73(5): 326-33.
[http://dx.doi.org/10.1097/FJC.0000000000000667] [PMID: 31082961]

[42] Qiu Z, Lei S, Zhao B, *et al.* NLRP3 inflammasome activation-mediated pyroptosis aggravates myocardial ischemia/reperfusion injury in diabetic rats. Oxid Med Cell Longev 2017; 2017: 1-17.
[http://dx.doi.org/10.1155/2017/9743280] [PMID: 29062465]

[43] Mariathasan S, Weiss DS, Newton K, *et al.* Cryopyrin activates the inflammasome in response to toxins and ATP. Nature 2006; 440(7081): 228-32.
[http://dx.doi.org/10.1038/nature04515] [PMID: 16407890]

[44] Pétrilli V, Papin S, Dostert C, Mayor A, Martinon F, Tschopp J. Activation of the NALP3 inflammasome is triggered by low intracellular potassium concentration. Cell Death Differ 2007; 14(9): 1583-9.
[http://dx.doi.org/10.1038/sj.cdd.4402195] [PMID: 17599094]

[45] Lima H Jr, Jacobson L, Goldberg M, *et al.* Role of lysosome rupture in controlling Nlrp3 signaling and necrotic cell death. Cell Cycle 2013; 12(12): 1868-78.
[http://dx.doi.org/10.4161/cc.24903] [PMID: 23708522]

[46] Gold M, El Khoury J. β-amyloid, microglia, and the inflammasome in Alzheimer's disease. Semin Immunopathol 2015; 37(6): 607-11.
[http://dx.doi.org/10.1007/s00281-015-0518-0] [PMID: 26251237]

[47] Klionsky DJ, Abdelmohsen K, Abe A, *et al.* Guidelines for the use and interpretation of assays for monitoring autophagy (3rd edition). Autophagy 2016; 12(1): 1-222.
[http://dx.doi.org/10.4161/auto.19496]

[48] Schofield JH, Schafer ZT. Mitochondrial Reactive Oxygen Species and Mitophagy: A Complex and Nuanced Relationship. Antioxid Redox Signal 2021; 34(7): 517-30.

[http://dx.doi.org/10.1089/ars.2020.8058] [PMID: 32079408]

[49] Zhong Z, Liang S, Sanchez-Lopez E, *et al.* New mitochondrial DNA synthesis enables NLRP3 inflammasome activation. Nature 2018; 560(7717): 198-203.
[http://dx.doi.org/10.1038/s41586-018-0372-z] [PMID: 30046112]

[50] Iyer SS, He Q, Janczy JR, *et al.* Mitochondrial cardiolipin is required for Nlrp3 inflammasome activation. Immunity 2013; 39(2): 311-23.
[http://dx.doi.org/10.1016/j.immuni.2013.08.001] [PMID: 23954133]

[51] Alhawiti NM, Al Mahri S, Aziz MA, Malik SS, Mohammad S. TXNIP in metabolic regulation: Physiological role and therapeutic outlook. Curr Drug Targets 2017; 18(9): 1095-103.
[PMID: 28137209]

[52] Gao P, He FF, Tang H, *et al.* NADPH oxidase-induced NALP3 inflammasome activation is driven by thioredoxin-interacting protein which contributes to podocyte injury in hyperglycemia. J Diabetes Res 2015; 2015: 1-12.
[http://dx.doi.org/10.1155/2015/504761] [PMID: 25834832]

[53] Liu Y, Lian K, Zhang L, *et al.* TXNIP mediates NLRP3 inflammasome activation in cardiac microvascular endothelial cells as a novel mechanism in myocardial ischemia/reperfusion injury. Basic Res Cardiol 2014; 109(5): 415.
[http://dx.doi.org/10.1007/s00395-014-0415-z] [PMID: 25015733]

[54] He J, Yang Y, Peng DQ. Monosodium urate (MSU) crystals increase gout associated coronary heart disease (CHD) risk through the activation of NLRP3 inflammasome. Int J Cardiol 2012; 160(1): 72-3.
[http://dx.doi.org/10.1016/j.ijcard.2012.05.083] [PMID: 22726397]

[55] Heid ME, Keyel PA, Kamga C, Shiva S, Watkins SC, Salter RD. Mitochondrial reactive oxygen species induces NLRP3-dependent lysosomal damage and inflammasome activation. J Immunol 2013; 191(10): 5230-8.
[http://dx.doi.org/10.4049/jimmunol.1301490] [PMID: 24089192]

[56] Chuang SY, Yang CH, Chou CC, Chiang YP, Chuang TH, Hsu LC. TLR-induced PAI-2 expression suppresses IL-1β processing *via* increasing autophagy and NLRP3 degradation. Proc Natl Acad Sci 2013; 110(40): 16079-84.
[http://dx.doi.org/10.1073/pnas.1306556110] [PMID: 24043792]

[57] Aloi M, Tromba L, Di Nardo G, *et al.* Premature subclinical atherosclerosis in pediatric inflammatory bowel disease. J Pediatr 2012; 161(4): 589-594.e1.
[http://dx.doi.org/10.1016/j.jpeds.2012.03.043] [PMID: 22579000]

[58] Zheng F, Xing S, Gong Z, Mu W, Xing Q. Silence ofNLRP3 suppresses atherosclerosis and stabilizes plaques inapolipoprotein E-deficient mice. Mediators Inflam 2014; 2014: 507208.

[59] Liu Y, Lian K, Zhang L, *et al.* TXNIP mediates NLRP3 inflammasome activation in cardiac microvascular endothelial cells as a novel mechanism in myocardial ischemia/reperfusion injury. Basic Res Cardiol 2014; 109(5): 415.
[http://dx.doi.org/10.1007/s00395-014-0415-z] [PMID: 25015733]

[60] Kawaguchi M, Takahashi M, Hata T, *et al.* Inflammasome activation of cardiac fibroblasts is essential for myocardial ischemia/reperfusion injury. Circulation 2011; 123(6): 594-604.
[http://dx.doi.org/10.1161/CIRCULATIONAHA.110.982777] [PMID: 21282498]

[61] Liu Y, Lian K, Zhang L, *et al.* TXNIP mediates NLRP3 inflammasome activation in cardiac microvascular endothelial cells as a novel mechanism in myocardial ischemia/reperfusion injury. Basic Res Cardiol 2014; 109(5): 415.
[http://dx.doi.org/10.1007/s00395-014-0415-z] [PMID: 25015733]

[62] Zhou J, Chng WJ. Roles of thioredoxin binding protein (TXNIP) in oxidative stress, apoptosis and cancer. Mitochondrion 2013; 13(3): 163-9.
[http://dx.doi.org/10.1016/j.mito.2012.06.004] [PMID: 22750447]

[63]   Byrne NJ, Matsumura N, Maayah ZH, *et al.* Empagliflozinblunts worsening cardiac dysfunction associated with reducedNLRP3 (nucleotide-binding domain-like receptor protein 3)inflammasome activation in heart failure. Circ Heart Fail 2020; 13(1): e006277.
[http://dx.doi.org/10.1161/CIRCHEARTFAILURE.119.006277] [PMID: 31957470]

[64]   Suetomi T, Willeford A, Brand CS, *et al.* Inflammation andNLRP3 inflammasome activation initiated in response to pressureoverload by Ca2+/calmodulin-dependent protein kinase IIδ signaling in cardiomyocytes are essential for adverse cardiacremodeling. Circulation 2018; 138(22): 2530-44.
[http://dx.doi.org/10.1161/CIRCULATIONAHA.118.034621] [PMID: 30571348]

[65]   Sano S, Oshima K, Wang Y, *et al.* Tet2-mediated clonalhematopoiesis accelerates heart failure through a mechanism involving the IL-1β/NLRP3 inflammasome. J Am Coll Cardiol 2018; 71(8): 875-86.
[http://dx.doi.org/10.1016/j.jacc.2017.12.037] [PMID: 29471939]

[66]   Long VP III, Bonilla IM, Vargas-Pinto P, *et al.* Heart failure duration progressively modulates the arrhythmia substrate through structural and electrical remodeling. Life Sci 2015; 123: 61-71.
[http://dx.doi.org/10.1016/j.lfs.2014.12.024] [PMID: 25596015]

[67]   Monnerat G, Alarcón ML, Vasconcellos LR, *et al.* Macrophage-dependent IL-1β production induces cardiac arrhythmias in diabetic mice. Nat Commun 2016; 7(1): 13344.
[http://dx.doi.org/10.1038/ncomms13344] [PMID: 27882934]

[68]   Westermann D, Lindner D, Kasner M, *et al.* Cardiac inflammation contributes to changes in the extracellular matrix in patients with heart failure and normal ejection fraction. Circ Heart Fail 2011; 4(1): 44-52.
[http://dx.doi.org/10.1161/CIRCHEARTFAILURE.109.931451] [PMID: 21075869]

[69]   Pan XC, Liu Y, Cen YY, *et al.* Dual role oftriptolide in interrupting the NLRP3 inflammasome pathway to attenuatecardiac fibrosis. Int J Mol Sci 2019; 20(2): 360.
[http://dx.doi.org/10.3390/ijms20020360]

[70]   Wang Y, Liu X, Shi H, *et al.* NLRP3 inflammasome, an immune-inflammatory target in pathogenesis and treatment of cardiovascular diseases. Clin Transl Med 2020; 10(1): 91-106.
[http://dx.doi.org/10.1002/ctm2.13] [PMID: 32508013]

[71]   Díaz-Araya G, Vivar R, Humeres C, Boza P, Bolivar S, Muñoz C. Cardiac fibroblasts as sentinel cells in cardiac tissue: Receptors, signaling pathways and cellular functions. Pharmacol Res 2015; 101: 30-40.
[http://dx.doi.org/10.1016/j.phrs.2015.07.001] [PMID: 26151416]

[72]   Cáceres FT, Gaspari TA, Samuel CS, Pinar AA. Serelaxin inhibits the profibrotic TGF-β1/IL-1β axis by targeting TLR-4 and the NLRP3 inflammasome in cardiac myofibroblasts. FASEB J 2019; 33(12): 14717-33.
[http://dx.doi.org/10.1096/fj.201901079RR] [PMID: 31689135]

[73]   Gao R, Shi H, Chang S, *et al.* The selective NLRP3-inflammasome inhibitor MCC950 reduces myocardial fibrosis and improves cardiac remodeling in a mouse model of myocardial infarction. Int Immunopharmacol 2019; 74: 105575.
[http://dx.doi.org/10.1016/j.intimp.2019.04.022] [PMID: 31299609]

[74]   Gan W, Ren J, Li T, *et al.* The SGK1 inhibitor EMD638683, prevents Angiotensin II–induced cardiac inflammation and fibrosis by blocking NLRP3 inflammasome activation. Biochim Biophys Acta Mol Basis Dis 2018; 1864(1): 1-10.
[http://dx.doi.org/10.1016/j.bbadis.2017.10.001] [PMID: 28986310]

[75]   Luo B, Li B, Wang W, *et al.* Rosuvastatin alleviates diabetic cardiomyopathy by inhibiting NLRP3 inflammasome and MAPK pathways in a type 2 diabetes rat model. Cardiovasc Drugs Ther 2014; 28(1): 33-43.
[http://dx.doi.org/10.1007/s10557-013-6498-1] [PMID: 24254031]

[76]   Zhang H, Chen X, Zong B, *et al.* Gypenosides improve diabetic cardiomyopathy by inhibiting ROS -
        mediated NLRP 3 inflammasome activation. J Cell Mol Med 2018; 22(9): 4437-48.
        [http://dx.doi.org/10.1111/jcmm.13743] [PMID: 29993180]

[77]   Che H, Wang Y, Li H, *et al.* Melatonin alleviates cardiac fibrosis *via* inhibiting lncRNA
        MALAT1/miR-141-mediated NLRP3 inflammasome and TGF-β1/Smads signaling in diabetic
        cardiomyopathy. FASEB J 2020; 34(4): 5282-98.
        [http://dx.doi.org/10.1096/fj.201902692R] [PMID: 32067273]

[78]   Li L, Tan J, Miao Y, Lei P, Zhang Q. ROS and autophagy: Interactions and molecular regulatory
        mechanisms. Cell Mol Neurobiol 2015; 35(5): 615-21.
        [http://dx.doi.org/10.1007/s10571-015-0166-x] [PMID: 25722131]

[79]   Liu P, Liu H, Sun S, *et al.* Aspirin alleviates cardiac fibrosis in mice by inhibiting autophagy. Acta
        Pharmacol Sin 2017; 38(4): 488-97.
        [http://dx.doi.org/10.1038/aps.2016.143] [PMID: 28216620]

[80]   Talman V, Ruskoaho H. Cardiac fibrosis in myocardial infarction-from repair and remodeling to
        regeneration. Cell Tissue Res 2016; 365(3): 563-81.
        [http://dx.doi.org/10.1007/s00441-016-2431-9] [PMID: 27324127]

[81]   Mastrocola R, Penna C, Tullio F, *et al.* Pharmacological inhibition of NLRP3 inflammasome
        attenuates myocardial ischemia/reperfusion injury by activation of RISK and mitochondrial pathways.
        Oxid Med Cell Longev 2016; 2016: 1-11.
        [http://dx.doi.org/10.1155/2016/5271251] [PMID: 28053692]

[82]   Yang X, Li X, Yuan M, *et al.* Anticancer therapyinducedatrial fibrillation: Electrophysiology and
        related mechanisms. Front Pharmacol 2018; 9: 1058.
        [http://dx.doi.org/10.3389/fphar.2018.01058] [PMID: 30386232]

[83]   Lim S, Lee ME, Jeong J, *et al.* sRAGE attenuates angiotensin II-induced cardiomyocyte hypertrophy
        by inhibiting RAGE-NFκB-NLRP3 activation. Inflamm Res 2018; 67(8): 691-701.
        [http://dx.doi.org/10.1007/s00011-018-1160-9] [PMID: 29796842]

[84]   Wang Y, Wu Y, Chen J, Zhao S, Li H. Pirfenidone attenuates cardiac fibrosis in a mouse model of
        TAC-induced left ventricular remodeling by suppressing NLRP3 inflammasome formation.
        Cardiology 2013; 126(1): 1-11.
        [http://dx.doi.org/10.1159/000351179] [PMID: 23839341]

[85]   An N, Gao Y, Si Z, *et al.* Regulatory mechanisms of the NLRP3 inflammasome, a novel immune-
        inflammatory marker in cardiovascular diseases. Front Immunol 2019; 10: 1592.
        [http://dx.doi.org/10.3389/fimmu.2019.01592] [PMID: 31354731]

[86]   Coll RC, Robertson AAB, Chae JJ, *et al.* A small-molecule inhibitor of the NLRP3 inflammasome for
        the treatment of inflammatory diseases. Nat Med 2015; 21(3): 248-55.
        [http://dx.doi.org/10.1038/nm.3806] [PMID: 25686105]

[87]   Coll RC, Hill JR, Day CJ, *et al.* MCC950 directly targets the NLRP3 ATP-hydrolysis motif for
        inflammasome inhibition. Nat Chem Biol 2019; 15(6): 556-9.
        [http://dx.doi.org/10.1038/s41589-019-0277-7] [PMID: 31086327]

[88]   Perregaux DG, McNiff P, Laliberte R, *et al.* Identification and characterization of a novel class of
        interleukin-1 post-translational processing inhibitors. J Pharmacol Exp Ther 2001; 299(1): 187-97.
        [PMID: 11561079]

[89]   van der Heijden T, Kritikou E, Venema W, *et al.* NLRP3Inflammasome inhibition by MCC950
        reduces atherosclerotic lesion development in apolipoprotein E-deficient mice-Brief Report.
        Arterioscler Thromb Vasc Biol 2017; 37(8): 1457-61.
        [http://dx.doi.org/10.1161/ATVBAHA.117.309575] [PMID: 28596375]

[90]   Willeford A, Suetomi T, Nickle A, Hoffman HM, Miyamoto S, Heller Brown J. CaMKIIδ-mediated
        inflammatory gene expression and inflammasome activation in cardiomyocytes initiate inflammation

and induce fibrosis. JCI Insight 2018; 3(12): e97054.
[http://dx.doi.org/10.1172/jci.insight.97054] [PMID: 29925681]

[91]   Wang H, Sun X, Hodge HS, Ferrario CM, Groban L. NLRP3 inhibition improves heart function in GPER knockout mice. Biochem Biophys Res Commun 2019; 514(3): 998-1003.
[http://dx.doi.org/10.1016/j.bbrc.2019.05.045] [PMID: 31092335]

[92]   Gao R, Shi H, Chang S, *et al.* The selective NLRP3-inflammasome inhibitor MCC950 reduces myocardial fibrosis and improves cardiac remodeling in a mouse model of myocardial infarction. Int Immunopharmacol 2019; 74: 105575.
[http://dx.doi.org/10.1016/j.intimp.2019.04.022] [PMID: 31299609]

[93]   Yao C, Veleva T, Scott L Jr, *et al.* EnhancedCardiomyocyte NLRP3 inflammasome signaling promotes atrial fibrillation. Circulation 2018; 138(20): 2227-42.
[http://dx.doi.org/10.1161/CIRCULATIONAHA.118.035202] [PMID: 29802206]

[94]   Luzi L, Pozza G. Glibenclamide: An old drug with a novel mechanism of action? Acta Diabetol 1997; 34(4): 239-44.
[http://dx.doi.org/10.1007/s005920050081] [PMID: 9451465]

[95]   Marchetti C, Chojnacki J, Toldo S, *et al.* A novel pharmacologic inhibitor of the NLRP3 inflammasome limits myocardial injury after ischemia-reperfusion in the mouse. J Cardiovasc Pharmacol 2014; 63(4): 316-22.
[http://dx.doi.org/10.1097/FJC.0000000000000053] [PMID: 24336017]

[96]   Marchetti C, Toldo S, Chojnacki J, *et al.* Pharmacologic inhibition of the NLRP3 inflammasome preserves cardiac function after ischemic and nonischemic injury in theMouse. J Cardiovasc Pharmacol 2015; 66(1): 1-8.
[http://dx.doi.org/10.1097/FJC.0000000000000247] [PMID: 25915511]

[97]   Toldo S, Marchetti C, Mauro AG, *et al.* Inhibition of the NLRP3 inflammasome limits the inflammatory injury following myocardial ischemia-reperfusion in the mouse. Int J Cardiol 2016; 209: 215-20.
[http://dx.doi.org/10.1016/j.ijcard.2016.02.043] [PMID: 26896627]

[98]   Fulp J, He L, Toldo S, *et al.* Structural insights ofBenzenesulfonamide analogues as NLRP3 inflammasome inhibitors: design, synthesis, and biological characterization. J Med Chem 2018; 61(12): 5412-23.
[http://dx.doi.org/10.1021/acs.jmedchem.8b00733] [PMID: 29877709]

[99]   Kim YS, Kim JS, Kwon JS, *et al.* BAY 11-7082, a nuclear factor-κB inhibitor, reduces inflammation and apoptosis in a rat cardiac ischemia-reperfusion injury model. Int Heart J 2010; 51(5): 348-53.
[http://dx.doi.org/10.1536/ihj.51.348] [PMID: 20966608]

[100]   Gastaldi S, Boscaro V, Gianquinto E, *et al.* Chemical Modulation of the 1-(piperidin-4-yl)-1,3-dihydro-2 H-benzo [d] imidazole-2-one Scaffold as a Novel NLRP3 Inhibitor. Molecules 2021; 26(13): 3975.
[http://dx.doi.org/10.3390/molecules26133975] [PMID: 34209843]

[101]   Mezzaroma E, Abbate A, Toldo S. NLRP3 inflammasome inhibitors in cardiovascular diseases. Molecules 2021; 26(4): 976.
[http://dx.doi.org/10.3390/molecules26040976] [PMID: 33673188]

[102]   Cocco M, Miglio G, Giorgis M, *et al.* Design, synthesis, and evaluation of acrylamide derivatives as direct NLRP3 inflammasome inhibitors. ChemMedChem 2016; 11(16): 1790-803.
[http://dx.doi.org/10.1002/cmdc.201600055] [PMID: 26990578]

[103]   Darakhshan S, Pour AB. Tranilast: A review of its therapeutic applications. Pharmacol Res 2015; 91: 15-28.
[http://dx.doi.org/10.1016/j.phrs.2014.10.009] [PMID: 25447595]

[104]   Sánchez-Fernández A, Skouras DB, Dinarello CA, López-Vales R. OLT1177 (dapansutrile), a

selective NLRP3 inflammasome inhibitor, ameliorates experimental autoimmune encephalomyelitis pathogenesis. Front Immunol 2019; 10: 2578.
[http://dx.doi.org/10.3389/fimmu.2019.02578] [PMID: 31736980]

[105] Toldo S, Mauro AG, Cutter Z, *et al.* The NLRP3 inflammasome inhibitor, OLT1177 (dapansutrile), reduces infarct size and preserves contractile function AfterIschemia reperfusion injury in the mouse. J Cardiovasc Pharmacol 2019; 73(4): 215-22.
[http://dx.doi.org/10.1097/FJC.0000000000000658] [PMID: 30747785]

[106] Klück V, Jansen TLTA, Janssen M, *et al.* Dapansutrile, an oral selective NLRP3 inflammasome inhibitor, for treatment of gout flares: an open-label, dose-adaptive, proof-of-concept, phase 2a trial. Lancet Rheumatol 2020; 2(5): e270-80.
[http://dx.doi.org/10.1016/S2665-9913(20)30065-5] [PMID: 33005902]

[107] Wohlford GF, Van Tassell BW, Billingsley HE, *et al.* A phase IB, randomized, double-blinded, dose escalation, Single Center, repeat dose Safetyand pharmacodynamics study of the oral NLRP3 inhibitor dapansutrile in subjects with NYHA II-III systolic heart failure. J Cardiovasc Pharmacol 2021; 77(1): 49-60.
[http://dx.doi.org/10.1097/FJC.0000000000000931] [PMID: 33235030]

[108] Jiang H, He H, Chen Y, *et al.* Identification of a selective and direct NLRP3 inhibitor to treat inflammatory disorders. J Exp Med 2017; 214(11): 3219-38.
[http://dx.doi.org/10.1084/jem.20171419] [PMID: 29021150]

[109] Lin HB, Wei GS, Li FX, *et al.* Macrophage-NLRP3 inflammasome activation exacerbates cardiac dysfunction after ischemic stroke in a mouse model of diabetes. Neurosci Bull 2020; 36(9): 1035-45.
[http://dx.doi.org/10.1007/s12264-020-00544-0] [PMID: 32683554]

[110] Huang Y, Jiang H, Chen Y, *et al.* Tranilast directly targets NLRP 3 to treat inflammasome-driven diseases. EMBO Mol Med 2018; 10(4): e8689.
[http://dx.doi.org/10.15252/emmm.201708689] [PMID: 29531021]

[111] Chen S, Wang Y, Pan Y, *et al.* Novel role for tranilast inRegulating NLRP3 ubiquitination, vascular inflammation, and atherosclerosis. J Am Heart Assoc 2020; 9(12): e015513.
[http://dx.doi.org/10.1161/JAHA.119.015513] [PMID: 32476536]

[112] Kazuo U, Shinji K, Yasuhiro S, Mitsuyoshi N. Inhibitory effect of tranilast on hypertrophic collagen production in the spontaneously hypertensive rat heart. Jpn J Pharmacol 1998; 78(2): 161-7.
[http://dx.doi.org/10.1254/jjp.78.161] [PMID: 9829619]

[113] Watanabe M. Early and delayed tranilast treatment reduces pathological fibrosis following myocardial infarction. Heart Lung Circ 2013; 22: 122-32.
[http://dx.doi.org/10.1016/j.hlc.2012.08.054]

[114] Konneh M. Tranilast kissei pharmaceutical. IDrugs 1998; 1(1): 141-6.
[PMID: 18465519]

[115] Leung YY, Yao Hui LL, Kraus VB. Colchicine-Update on mechanisms of action and therapeutic uses. Semin Arthritis Rheum 2015; 45(3): 341-50.
[http://dx.doi.org/10.1016/j.semarthrit.2015.06.013] [PMID: 26228647]

[116] Fujisue K, Sugamura K, Kurokawa H, *et al.* Colchicine improves survival, left ventricular remodeling, and chronic cardiac function after acute myocardial infarction. Circ J 2017; 81(8): 1174-82.
[http://dx.doi.org/10.1253/circj.CJ-16-0949]

[117] Tardif JC, Kouz S, Waters DD, *et al.* Efficacy and safety of low-dose colchicine after myocardial infarction. N Engl J Med 2019; 381(26): 2497-505.
[http://dx.doi.org/10.1056/NEJMoa1912388] [PMID: 31733140]

[118] Vaidya K, Arnott C, Martínez GJ, *et al.* Colchicine therapy andPlaque stabilization in patients with acute coronary syndrome: a CT coronary angiography study. J Am Coll Cardiol Imaging 2018; 11(2 Pt 2): 305-16.

[http://dx.doi.org/10.1016/j.jcmg.2017.08.013] [PMID: 29055633]

[119] Mauro AG, Bonaventura A, Vecchie A. The role of NLRP3 inflammasome in pericarditis: Potential for therapeutic approaches. JACC BTS 2021; 6(2): 137-50.

[120] Audia JP, Yang XM, Crockett ES, *et al.* Caspase-1 inhibition by VX-765 administered at reperfusion in P2Y$_{12}$ receptor antagonist-treated rats provides long-term reduction in myocardial infarct size and preservation of ventricular function. Basic Res Cardiol 2018; 113(5): 32.
[http://dx.doi.org/10.1007/s00395-018-0692-z] [PMID: 29992382]

[121] Lu B, Xie J, Fu D, *et al.* Huoxue Qianyang Qutan recipe attenuates cardiac fibrosis by inhibiting the NLRP3 inflammasome signalling pathway in obese hypertensive rats. Pharm Biol 2021; 59(1): 1043-55.
[http://dx.doi.org/10.1080/13880209.2021.1953541] [PMID: 34362291]

[122] Kang LL, Zhang DM, Ma CH, *et al.* Cinnamaldehyde and allopurinol reduce fructose-induced cardiac inflammation and fibrosis by attenuating CD36-mediated TLR4/6-IRAK4/1 signaling to suppress NLRP3 inflammasome activation. Sci Rep 2016; 6(1): 27460.
[http://dx.doi.org/10.1038/srep27460] [PMID: 27270216]

[123] Byrne NJ, Matsumura N, Maayah ZH, *et al.* Empagliflozin blunts worsening cardiac dysfunction associated with reduced NLRP3(nucleotide-binding domain-like receptor Protein 3) inflammasome activation in heart failure. Circ Heart Fail 2020; 13(1): e006277.
[http://dx.doi.org/10.1161/CIRCHEARTFAILURE.119.006277] [PMID: 31957470]

[124] Dai S, Ye B, Chen L, Hong G, Zhao G, Lu Z. Emodin alleviates LPS -induced myocardial injury through inhibition of NLRP3 inflammasome activation. Phytother Res 2021; 35(9): 5203-13.
[http://dx.doi.org/10.1002/ptr.7191] [PMID: 34131970]

[125] Potere N, Del Buono MG, Caricchio R, *et al.* Interleukin-1 and the NLRP3 inflammasome in COVID-19: Pathogenetic and therapeutic implications. EBioMedicine 2022; 85: 104299.
[http://dx.doi.org/10.1016/j.ebiom.2022.104299] [PMID: 36209522]

CHAPTER 6

Role of NLRP3 in Protozoan Parasitic Infections

Sonal Yadav[1], **Harpreet Kaur**[2], **Rakesh Singh Dhanda**[3] and **Manisha Yadav**[1,*]

[1] *Dr. B. R. Ambedkar Centre for Biomedical Research (ACBR), University of Delhi, Delhi-110007, India*

[2] *Department of Medical Parasitology (PGIMER), Chandigarh, India*

[3] *Celluleris AB, VentureLab, Scheelevägen 15, 223 70 Lund, Sweden*

Abstract: Nod-like receptors (NLRs) and the inflammasome complex have significant roles in regulating the innate immune system against bacterial and viral pathogens and have attracted significant attention to their role in protozoan infections. Several parasitic protozoan pathogens are the most prevalent that cause severe morbidity and pose a significant health burden. In the present article, we discussed the most common protozoan parasites and the roles of NLRs and inflammasomes against these parasites. *G. duodenalis*, *E. histolytica*, *T. vaginalis*, Plasmodium parasite, *T. cruzi*, *Schistosomes* parasite, *T. gondii*, and *Leishmania spp.* activate the NLRP3 inflammasome. The NLRP3 inflammasome protects the host in *Giardia, T. cruzi*, and *E. histolytica* infections. Also, its protective role in the case of *Trichomonas* infection has been suggested, but more studies are needed. However, NLRP3 induces pathology during *Schistosomes* and *Malaria* parasite infection. In *T. gondii* infection, NLRP3 causes inflammation and limits the parasite load burden and propagation. This provides a new dimension in the research on the role and exact mechanism of NLRP3 during *T. gondii* infection. The NLRP3 inflammasome protects the host by clearing the parasitic load; NLRP3 provides resistance toward some *Leishmania spp.* It alleviates the host's parasitic burden of *L. amazonensis* and *L. major*. However, *L. major* or *L. donovani* induces chronic non-healing infection-promoting lesion development. These contrary reports warrant more research on *Leishmaniasis*. For developing new treatment strategies, studying the role of NLRP3 in the host defense and inflammatory pathology is crucial in parasitic protozoan infection.

Keywords: IL-1β, IL-18, NLRP3, Protozoan infection.

INTRODUCTION

Protozoa are free-living or parasitic single-cell microorganisms. They propagate in humans and animals, leading to serious infection development. Protozoa

---

* **Corresponding author Manisha Yadav:** Dr. B. R. Ambedkar Centre for Biomedical Research (ACBR), University of Delhi, Delhi-110007, India; E-mail: manisha.dhanda@gmail.com

Puneetpal Singh (Ed.)
All rights reserved-© 2024 Bentham Science Publishers

infecting humans are classified into four groups: Sarcodina, Mastigophora, Ciliophora, and Sporozoa. Many protozoa have been poorly studied and come under the neglected tropical disease category.

Pathogen recognition receptors (PRRs) of the host play a role in the recognition of pathogens, the first initiating step of the host immune response and subsequent generation of an adaptive immune response [1]. These receptors recognize specific pathogen-associated molecular patterns (PAMPs) like Lipopolyglycan, flagellin protein, and many other pathogens and danger/damage-associated molecular patterns (DAMPs) like extracellular ATP, hemozoin and many other molecules [2, 3]. The four classes of PRRs are Toll-like receptors (TLRs), the Nucleotide-binding oligomerization domain (NOD)-Leucine-rich repeats (LRR)-containing receptors (NLR), the retinoic acid-inducible gene 1 (RIG-I)-like receptors (RLR; RIG-I-like helicases—RLH) and the C-type lectin receptors (CLRs) [1]. NLRs are central regulators of inflammation and immunity; they recognize pathogens and regulate TLR-mediated immune system pathways, mainly expressed by non-hematopoietic cells and immune cells [4].

Structure and Function of NOD-like Receptor 3 (NLRP3)

The NLR family consists of 22 mammalian genes with diverse functions in innate immune response and inflammation. They share common structural motifs such as a variable N-terminal effector domain, either a caspase recruitment domain (CARD) or pyrin domain (PYD), a C-terminal leucine-rich repeat (LRR) domain for ligand recognition, and a central NOD (nucleotide-binding and oligomerization (NACHT) domain) required for self-oligomerization [5]. Based on phylogenetic relationships, NLRs are mainly divided into three subfamilies: NODs, NLRPs (also known as NALPs), and IPAF. NLRP3 is the best-characterized intracellular sensor, consisting of NOD-, LRR-, and a pyrin domain-containing protein 3. NLRP3 is known to form the assembly of an inflammasome complex. It plays the role of a scaffold with the adaptor protein ASC (apoptosis-associated speck-like protein containing a CARD), leading to the cleavage of pro-caspase-1 and activation and secretion of interleukin-1beta (IL-1β) and IL-18 [6]. Viral, parasitic, bacterial, and fungal pathogens lead to NLRP3 inflammasome activation, and their diverse functions depend on the infection type [7]. The NLRP3 may play an essential role in innate immunity and regulating inflammatory reactions during parasitic infection by killing the pathogen or initiating the destructive pathology. NLRP3 plays a varied role as it can identify mitochondrial DNA and ATP and regulates signaling cascades of TLRs and NOD. It is also involved in chronic immune diseases, tissue homeostasis, embryonic development, cancer, and autophagy [1].

Activation of NLRP3 and its Signaling Cascade

NLRP3 has a vast and varied number of agonists; many cause cation flux K^+ efflux and increased cytosolic Ca^{2+} concentration) or chloride ions ($Cl-$), causing mitochondrial disruption, lysosomal disruption, mitochondrial dysfunction, metabolic changes, and trans-Golgi, disassembly Pathogen-derived products, sterile crystalline molecules, and ATP [8]. NLRP3 activation is mediated *via* a canonical and non-canonical pathway. Canonical activation is a two-step process that requires priming/transcription and activation. Priming occurs by recognizing PAMPs and DAMPs *via* PRRs, resulting in Nuclear factor kappa B (NF-κB) activation and upregulation of NLRP3 and pro-IL-1β transcription. Activation is caused by a pathogen (PAMPs and DAMPs) causing conformational change (post-translational modifications), causing the maturation of caspase 1 to induce the cleavage of GSDMD leading to pyroptosis and IL-1β and IL-18 release [1]. The non-canonical pathway directly activates the inflammasome (*via* caspase 4/5/11). It induces cell death and cleavage of Gasdermin D (GSDMD), causing N-terminal release and its assembly at the plasma membrane, resulting in membrane damage, potassium efflux, pyroptosis, and increased activation of NLRP3 inflammasome [1]. Caspase 8 and Fas-associated death domain (FADD) regulate the activation of NLRP3 inflammasome and maturation of IL-1β [9, 10].

Inflammasome Activation and Pyroptosis

Upon activation, NLRP3 couples with ASC and procaspase-1(inactive) and cleaves to convert it into caspase-1 (active form) that further cleaves the proIL-1β and proIL-18 into mature IL-1β and IL-18 (secreted forms) [11]. These cytokines further initiate inflammatory processes in the host. Activated NLRP3 inflammasome also leads to pyroptosis, a rapid, inflammatory-lytic type, programmed cell death. GSDMD has an amino-terminal cell death domain (GSDMDN term), a central short linker region, and a carboxy-terminal autoinhibition domain. Caspase 1 cleaves GSDMD, removing its autoinhibitory carboxyl terminus and releasing the GSDMDN term (amino-terminal), which binds, oligomerizes, and inserts into the plasma membrane, forming a pore, thus killing the cell [12 - 14].

The role of NLRs and inflammasomes in the detection of PRRs of the pathogen and their involvement in the host response are well defined, but their role in parasitic infection has been poorly studied. However, recently some studies reported the role of NLRs and inflammasomes in protozoan parasites. In this chapter, we have tried to discuss the role of NLRP3 in the parasitic protozoan infections in humans.

NLRP3 AND PARASITIC PROTOZOAN INFECTION

Giardiasis

Giardiasis (diarrheal disease) is caused by the flagellated, anaerobic parasitic protozoan *Giardia duodenalis*. *Giardia* lives in the intestine of infected humans and passes through stool. More than 1.2 million *Giardia* cases are reported in the United States annually [15]. According to a 2018 report, 15,579 giardiasis cases were reported in the United States, of which 96.8% were positive [16].

The attenuation of disease severity caused by *Citrobacter rodentium*, an equivalent of A/E *E. coli*, in C57BL/6 male mice co-infected with *Giardia* was achieved by elevating the levels of antimicrobial peptides (AMP) Murine β defensin 3 and Trefoil Factor 3, and also by elevating the bactericidal activity modulated *via* NLRP3. Increased levels of IL18 mRNA were expressed in the human adenocarcinoma (Caco-2) cell line when co-incubated with *Giardia* and Enteropathogenic *Escherichia coli* (EPEC). However, in this study, *Giardia* alone cannot activate the NLRP3 inflammasome in both *in-vitro* and *in-vivo* experimental models [17]. Another study has reported similar findings, *i.e.*, AMP-mediated protective effect during co-infection with *Giardia,* which is partially NLRP3-dependent. *Giardia* cathepsin B-like proteases contributed to AMP-mediated protection in co-infection models [18].

In a recent study, it was observed that NLRP3 upregulation could be triggered in macrophages infected with *Giardia* It secreted peptidyl-prolyl *cis-trans* isomerase B (PPIB), which promoted the activation of CASP1, ultimately cleaving Gasdermin E (GSDME) [19]. According to a recent report, extracellular vesicles secreted by *Giardia* (EVs) activate NLRP3 inflammasome signaling, and the production of IL-1β is dependent on dose and time in primary murine peritoneal macrophages [20] (Table **1**, Fig. **1**).

Table 1. Involvement of NLRP3 in recognizing PAMPs and DAMPs and its regulatory mechanisms in various parasitic protozoan infections.

Organism	Ligands	Experimental Model	NLRP3 Inflammasome	Effect/Outcome	Comments	Refs.
Giardia duodenalis	Giardia cathepsin B-like proteases	-	Activated	Protective effect	AMP-mediated protection	[18]
	Giardia and its secreted peptidyl-prolylcis-trans isomerase B	Macrophages	Upregulation	Protective effect	Promotes the activation of CASP1,ultimately cleaving GSDME	[19]
	Extracellular vesicles secreted by *Giardia* (EVs)	Primary murine peritoneal macrophages	Activated	Protective effect	IL-1β production dependent on dose and time	[20]

(Table 1) cont.....

Organism	Ligands	Experimental Model	NLRP3 Inflammasome	Effect/Outcome	Comments	Refs.
Entamoeba histolytica	Lipopeptidophosphoglycan	-	Activated	Protective effect	TLR2/TLR4 signaling and induce IL-33 expression; Increase pathogenesis	[23, 24]
	-	THP-1 macrophages	Activated	Protective effect	Activated caspase-1 and IL-1β	[25]
	Gal-lectin equivalent to LPS	THP-1 macrophages	Upregulation	-	Upregulation of pro-IL-1β and NLRP3 expression; activate NF-kB.	[26]
	Gal-lectin and CP-A5	-	Inhibited	Detrimental effect	Activate caspase-4 like caspase-1 and release higher IL-1β levels	[27]
	Cysteine proteinase EhCP5	-	-	-	Cysteine proteinase EhCP5	[30]
Trichomonas vaginalis	Glycosylated-Lipophosphoglycan (LPG)	-	Activated	Protective effect	NF-κB mediated increased secretion of IL-1β	[36]
	Ecto-ATPases	Prostate epithelial cell line	Inhibited	Detrimental effect	Digesting extracellular ATP	[37]
Leishmania spp.	-	Murine macrophages	Activated	Protective effect	Decrease IL-1β release in the case of L. amazonensis	[44]
	Metalloprotease GP63	-	Inhibited	-	Decreased secretion of IL-1β through inhibition of ROS production	[45]
	-	Nlrp3, ASC, and caspase 1/11 knockout mice	-	Protective effect	*L. major* upregulated IL-1β mRNA, and IL-1β leads to neutrophils recruitment to the infected Skin. Cleared L. major load and promoted lesion healing	[46]
	-	NLRP3, ASC, or caspase 1 knockout BALB/c	-	Protective effect	Production of defective IL-1β and IL-18 at the infection site	[47]
	Leishmania spp. lipophosphoglycan (LPG)	-	Activated	-	Engage TLR2, glycoproteins and glycosphingophoshplipids engage TLR4 and DNA engage TLR9, RNA virus (LRV) engage TLR3	[43]
	LPG of Leishmania spp.	C57BL/6 knockouts of Nlrp3 and Casp11	Activated (caspase-11 dependent (non-canonical))	-	Significantly increased ear swelling compared to wild-type ones; Casp-11 protects BMDM against Leishmania.	[51]
	-	C57BL/6	-	-	*L. major* or/ *L. donovani* leads to chronic non-healing infection by releasing significantly more IL-1β; promotes lesion development	[46, 54]
Toxoplasma gondii	Rhoptry protein 7 (ROP7)	THP-1-Derived Macrophages	Activated (GSDMD-independent manner)	-	Persistent release of IL1-β independent of pyroptosis.	[62]
	-	Primary human monocytes	-	-	Produced IL-1β *via* a Syk-PK--CARD9/MALT-1-NF-B signaling pathway	[63]
	Virulence gene wx2	-	Inhibited	Detrimental effect	Stimulates the multiplication and survival of *T. gondii*; deters GSDMD and caspase-1and deters the classical pyroptotic pathway	[64]

(Table 1) cont.....

Organism	Ligands	Experimental Model	NLRP3 Inflammasome	Effect/Outcome	Comments	Refs.
Plasmodium spp.	Crystalline particulates	-	Activated	Detrimental effect	Trigger the release of the lysosomal contents in the cytosol; NLRP3 activation induces IL 1b-mediated fever	[67]
	sHZ	-	Activated	Detrimental effect	Activates NF-κB and induces neuroinflammation in BV2 microglia and oxidative stress and caspase-6-mediated neurotoxicity	[69]
	β-hematin primed with LPS	Macrophages	-	-	Induce the secretion of IL-1β	[70]
	P. berghei ANKA or P. f	Nlrp3-/- mice brain endothelial cells	-	Detrimental effect	Increased the survival days of mice	[70]
	Migration inhibitory factor (MIF) inhibition	Dendritic cells and macrophages *in vitro* and *in vivo*	Activated	-	Secretion of IL-1β and IL-18 inhibition	[75]
Trypanosoma cruzi	MMP2 and MMP9	Human	Inhibited	Detrimental effect	MMP2 showed a positive correlation with IL 1β and CASP1 and NLRP3, whereas MMP9 showed a positive correlation with IL 1β but a negative correlation with CASP1 and NLRP3, the caspase 1 molecules dependent IL 1β activation pathway.	[76]
Schistosoma spp.	*S. mansoni* -derived SEA	knockout animals	Activated	Detrimental effect	IL-1β production; activates Syk kinase and results in ROS production andK⁺ efflux; yields milder disease	{85, 86]

Amebiasis

Entamoeba histolytica (Eh), the etiological agent of Amebiasis in humans, is an extracellular parasitic protozoan which colonizes the intestine. About 100 million cases of Amebiasis are reported every year, which causes 100,000 deaths worldwide [21]. According to a meta-analysis of articles published between the year 2001–2020, data from 289,659 human subjects obtained from 12 states and 4 union territories showed amoebiasis prevalence to be 3-23% in asymptomatic patients and 0.64–11% in symptomatic patients. The highest prevalence was found in Tamil Nadu, Andaman Nicobar Island, and North East India [22]. Amoebiasis affects about 15% of the Indian population. About 90% of the cases remain asymptomatic.

Recently, studies showed that NLRP3 inflammasome activation through toll-like receptor 2 (TLR2)/TLR6 signaling, TLR2, and TLR4 recognizes amebic lipopeptidophosphoglycan. Thus, PAMPs of Eh could activate NLRP3 through TLR2/TLR4 signaling and induce IL-33 expression [23, 24].

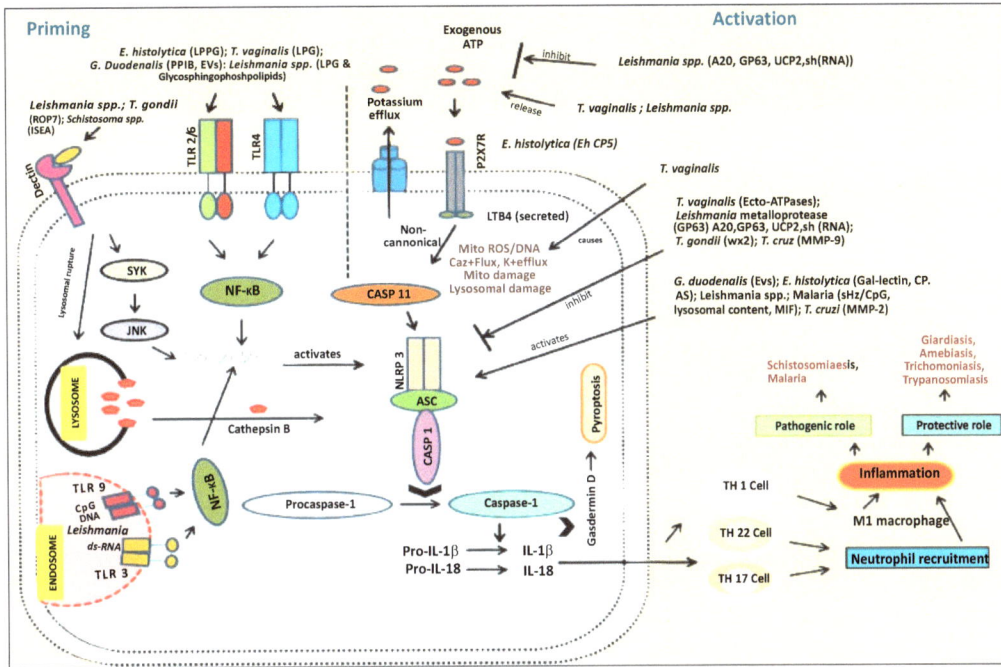

Fig. (1). NLR3 inflammasome activation and release of IL-1β and IL-18 cytokines during various parasitic protozoan infections.

An *In vitro* study showed that trophozoite-cultured THP-1 macrophages resulted in activated caspase-1 and IL-1β. The first study reported the activation of α5β1 integrin through direct contact with Eh for NLRP3 inflammasome activation. Integrin-binding cysteine protease (EhCP5) results in α5β1 integrin activation, which induces the release of ATP into the extracellular space through P2X7 receptors *via* opening pannexin-1 channels, which signal NLRP3 activation [25].

A previous study showed the upregulation of pro-IL-1β and NLRP3 expression *via* Gal-lectin, which is equivalent to LPS in THP-1 macrophages, inducing a priming step to activate NF-kB. Cross-linking of Gal-lectin to the host receptor could disrupt the movement of the plasma membrane/proteins, which could be sensed by the inflammasome [26]. Interestingly, Gal-lectin and CP-A5 of Eh also activate caspase-4 like caspase-1, leading to higher IL-1β levels. The IL-1β release is mediated by cleavage of GSDMD through both the caspases. Both the caspases can converge to regulate high proinflammatory responses in the pathogenesis of infection. NLRP3 CRISPR/Cas9 KO THP-1 macrophages exposed to Eh show that caspase-4 activation is independent of NLRP3 and ASC [27].

According to some studies, cysteine proteinase EhCP5 can cleave and inactivate recombinant IL-18 and IL-1β [28, 29]. Also reported is the down-regulation of IL-1β due to monocyte locomotion inhibitory factor produced by Eh [30]. Eh follows varied strategies to neutralize IL-1β and IL-18, suggesting their role in protection against Eh infection. More studies are required to directly determine the effects of NLRP3, inflammasomes, and cytokines in adaptive immune responses against Eh infection [31] (Table 1, Fig. 1).

CP, Cysteine proteases; EVs, extracellular vesicles; LPPG, lipopeptido-phosphoglycan; MMP, matrix metalloproteinases; MIF, migration inhibitory factor; UCP2, mitochondrial uncoupling protein2; PPIB, peptidyl-prolylcis-trans isomerase B; ROP7, rhoptry protein 7; (sh)RNA, short hairpin; SEA, soluble egg antigen, sHz/CpG, synthetic hemozoin.

Trichomoniasis

Trichomonas vaginalis (*Tv*) causes Trichomoniasis (a sexually transmitted infection (STI)). It is a pear-shaped flagellated parasite reported worldwide. The global prevalence of Tv is estimated to be 8.1% among women and 1% among men [32]. In India, its prevalace is estimated to be around 6-10% [33]. According to the CDC report, there were more than two million trichomoniasis infections reported in the United States in 2018 [34].

There is limited knowledge about the role of inflammasomes during *Tv* infection. Only a few studies have discussed the activation of NLRP3 during *Tv* infection in both *in-vitro* and *in-vivo* models, including human macrophages and human prostate epithelial cells.

Tv destroys cell membranes, releases adenosine triphosphate (ATP) and other DAMPs, sensed by NLRP3, and leads to inflammasome activation. Glycosylated-Lipophosphoglycan (LPG) of *Tv* activates NF-κB [35]. NF-κB mediates increased secretion of IL-1β, which initiates NLRP3 inflammasome complex. During *Tv* infection, reactive oxygen species (ROS) production, extracellular ATP sensing *via* purinoceptor 7 (P2X7) receptors, and potassium ion efflux induce NLRP3 inflammasomes in human macrophages, which contributes to the release of IL-1β, IL-18, and also causes pyroptosis process *via* cleavage of gasdermin D through caspase-1 which assembles in the host cell membrane to form pores [36]. *Tv*-mediated NLRP3 inflammasome activation pathways may be evoked in the vaginal and cervical cells. In the C57BL/6 model, IL-1β production is reported in the vaginal fluids in response to *Tv* infection [36]. Another study has reported NLRP3 inflammasome activation in the prostate epithelial cell line against *Tv* infection by sensing ROS, K^+ efflux, and extracellular ATP, resulting in IL-1β production. Interestingly, Ecto-ATPases expressed by *Tv* could attenuate NLRP3 inflammasome by digesting extracellular ATP [37].

Involvement of the endoplasmic reticulum (ER) in the apoptosis of human cervical cancer SiHa cells during *Tv* infection and its molecular mechanisms were investigated. The induction of apoptosis is caused *via* mitochondrial ROS production and ER stress responses. IRE1/ASK1/JNK/Bcl-2 pathways cause mitochondrial apoptosis, suggesting *Tv* mediated apoptosis [38].

A study showed a significant expression of *Nlrp3* in the vaginal tissue of BALB/c mice infected with Tv trophozoites obtained from the symptomatic patient on the 2nd day post-infection (dpi) and 14th dpi from the asymptomatic group. In the cervical tissue of the asymptomatic group, higher *Nlrp3* was expressed on the 14th dpi. It was concluded that early NLRP3 expression of *Nlrp3* was observed in the symptomatic group and late onset in the asymptomatic group [39].

These studies set a foundation for future studies in understanding the signaling pathway of NLRP3 inflammasome and its protective role against infection or in infection pathogenesis (Table **1**, Fig. **1**).

Leishmaniasis

Leishmania parasites cause leishmaniasis, which is a neglected tropical disease. Leishmaniasis is reported in about 89 countries and is endemic in Asia, Africa, America, and the Mediterranean [40]. Estimated new cases of cutaneous leishmaniasis ranged from 700,000 to 1.2 million per year, and that of visceral leishmaniasis decreased to <100,000 [41]. Three different clinical forms include Cutaneous Leishmaniasis (CL), Mucosal Leishmaniasis (MCL), and Visceral Leishmaniasis (VL). VL is the most deadly among others, also called kala-azar [42]. It is disseminated by the bite of an infected sand fly (*Phlebotomus* spp.), where it transfers metacyclic promastigotes into the host. Then they are phagocytosed by macrophages and transform into amastigotes and multiply [43].

In 2013, a report discussed the involvement of *L. amazonensis* in the activation of NLRP3 inflammasome in macrophages and *in vivo* models influencing cutaneous and visceral disease in mice. In this study, authors observed that NLRP3 inflammasome limited the intracellular growth of *L. amazonensis* in macrophages using knockout mice of NLRP3, ASC, and Caspase-1, showing increased lesion size and parasitic burden. They observed that it decreased IL-1β release in infected macrophages. *L. amazonensis, L. braziliensis,* and *L. mexicana* infected-macrophages expressed NLRP3, ASC, Caspase-1, and released IL-1β. *L. infantum* activated NLRP3 in the *in vivo* model [44]. *Leishmania* inhibits nitric oxide and pro-inflammatory cytokine to survive in macrophages. Also, the inhibition of IL-

1β production has been reported in several *in vitro* and *in vivo* studies. The exact mechanism is still unknown. Phorbol 12-myristate 13-acetate (PMA)-differentiated THP-1 cells infected with *Leishmania* effectively inhibit IL-1β production. Metalloprotease GP63 of *Leishmania* species mediates decreased secretion of IL-1β through the inhibition of ROS production [45]. Two possible elucidations of the mechanism have been proposed. Firstly, IL-1β production and TLR signal for inflammasome activation; secondly, significant tissue damage during chronic infection could result in DAMP release, leading to inflammasome activation. *Leishmania spp.*-induced ROS signals NLRP3 inflammasome activation [43]. Another study has reported that NLRP3 inflammasome is essential in providing resistance to *Leishmania* infection.

L. major upregulates IL-1β mRNA and IL-1β, leading to the recruitment of neutrophils to the infected skin. Nlrp3, ASC, and caspase-1/11 knockout mice, or mice lacking IL-1β receptor signaling, cleared *L. major* load and developed healing lesions. NLRP3 inflammasome recruited neutrophils are IL-1β dependent forms of cutaneous leishmaniasis [46]. In another study, NLRP3, ASC, or caspase 1 knockout BALB/c infected with *Leishmania* leads to the production of defective IL-1β and IL-18 at the infection site, which are resistant to cutaneous infection. NLRP3 inflammasome has detrimental effects during leishmaniasis. IL-18 neutralization reduced *L. major* titers, suggesting a potential therapeutic target to treat leishmaniasis [47].

Increased mRNA levels of IL-1ß, caspase-1, and NLRP3 have been reported in skin biopsies of patients suffering from localized cutaneous leishmaniasis (LCL) due to *L braziliensis*-infection [48]. *Leishmania spp.* lipophosphoglycan (LPG) can directly engage TLR2, glycoproteins and glycosphingophoshpolipids engage TLR4 and DNA engages TLR9, and dsRNA carried by *leishmania* RNA virus (LRV) engages TLR3, which could provide as a priming signal to activate NLRP3 inflammasome [43].

A recent article on *Leishmania* has discussed NLRP3's role during infection. It proposes two possible elucidations of the mechanism; firstly, IL-1β production and TLR signal for inflammasome activation, and secondly, significant tissue damage during chronic illness could result in DAMP release leading to inflammasome activation [43]. *L. amazonensis* infection during exogenous ATP-induced leukotriene B4 (LTB4) *via* P2X7 receptor activates the caspase-1--mediated non-canonical NLRP3 inflammasome in peritoneal macrophages. The generation and role of endogenous ATP or LTB4 during *L. amazonensis* infection and caspase11 and non-canonical NLRP3 activation are not studied [49].

During *Leishmania* infection, NLRP3 inflammasome activation takes place through Dectin-1/SYK/ROS signaling (canonical NLRP3 inflammasome) and LPG *via* the caspase-11 pathway (non-canonical NLRP3 inflammasome) [43]. *Leishmania* sensing promotes ROS production *in vitro* and *in vivo via* the Dectin-1/SYK pathway, which induces the NLRP3 inflammasome activation [50]. LPG of *Leishmania* spp. activates caspase-11 dependent (non-canonical) NLRP3 inflammasome. C57BL/6 knockouts of Nlrp3 and Casp11 show significantly increased ear swelling compared to wild-type ones [51]. Also, Casp-11 protects Bone-marrow-derived macrophage (BMDM) against *Leishmania*.

The indirect evidence of NLRP3 inflammasome protecting against *Leishmania* infection and evolved mechanisms to inhibit NLRP3 inflammasome *via* GP63 shows blockade of ROS production and cleavage of NLRP3. A20 or mitochondrial uncoupling protein2 (UCP2) short hairpin (sh)RNA [52], to inhibit ATP-induced NLRP3 inflammasome activation by modulating H3 histone modulation in macrophages [53], inhibits the activation of ATP-induced NLRP3 inflammasome [43]. NLRP3 inflammasome-induced IL-18 cytokines promote susceptibility to *L. major* infection in BALB/c mice, resulting in parasite persistence and lesion pathology. C57BL/6 infected with *L major* [46] or/ *L donovani* [54] induces chronic non-healing infection by releasing significantly more IL-1β accentuating neutrophil recruitment at the infection site to promote lesion development.

C57BL/6 mice are ameliorated by MCC950 or glyburide NLRP3 inflammasome inhibitors, showing a decrease in neutrophils [55]. *L. major* infected CD11b+ myeloid cells produce IL-1β through NLRP3 inflammasome activation *via* CD8+ T cells, which subsequently recruit neutrophils, resulting in immunopathology and lesion development [56].

High levels of IL-1β in biopsy samples of peripheral blood mononuclear cells from patients infected with *L. braziliensis* were observed, and this increase was NLRP3, caspase-1, and ASC dependent, which accords with the immunopathology during cutaneous leishmaniasis [57] (Table **1**, Fig. **1**).

Toxoplasmosis

Toxoplasma is an opportunistic intracellular parasite that infects humans and other warm-blooded animals and infects around 60% of the world's population. The mechanisms by which the parasite evades the host's immune response, and the host controls the parasite proliferation are still unclear. It is recently suggested that inflammasome activation plays a crucial role in the *Toxoplasma* pathogenesis in humans. NLRP1 and NLRP3 inflammasomes identify the parasite *Toxoplasma gondii*, leading to the generation of IL-1β and IL-18 *in vitro* and *in vivo* [58, 59].

NLRP3 activation induced by *T. gondii* involves different mechanisms depending upon the cell type [60, 61], as the responses are different in human monocytes from those in human macrophages. A recent study found that the interaction of *T. gondii* rhoptry protein 7 (ROP7) with NLRP3 induces the hyperactivation of inflammasomes in THP-1-derived macrophages [62] and results in a persistent release of IL1-β independent of pyroptosis. Primary human monocytes infected with *T. gondii* produce IL- 1β *via* a Syk-PKC-CARD9/MALT-1-NF-B signaling pathway and elicit the NLRP3 inflammasome in a GSDMD-independent manner for the production of IL-1β from the viable cells [63]. In another study, a virulence gene wx2 was shown to stimulate the multiplication and survival of *T. gondii* in the host by preventing the stimulation of the NLRP3 inflammasome, GSDMD, and caspase-1 and deterring the classical pyroptotic pathway [64] (Table **1**, Fig. **1**).

Malaria

Malaria is a mosquito-borne acute febrile illness caused by *Plasmodium* parasite that affects humans and other animals. Around 241 million cases were reported in 85 countries with endemic malaria, including the French Guiana territory in 2020, which accounted for 96% of malaria cases and deaths (WHO Report 2021). *Plasmodium* species proliferate inside the RBCs. A pro-inflammatory cytokine storm is induced with the rupture of infected RBCs that induces IL-1 β-mediated fever [65] in malaria patients [66] and is regulated by inflammasomes. NLRP3 inflammasomes are activated when the crystalline particulates trigger the release of the lysosomal contents in the cytosol [67]. Cytochalasin D inhibits the crystal engulfment that results in NLRP3 activity disruption in a dose-dependent manner as IL-1β production in macrophages is inhibited on exposure to synthetic hemozoin (sHz) complexed with CpG DNA. An H^+ ATPase inhibitor, bafilomycin A, blocks the sHz/CpG-mediated release of IL-1β by neutralizing the lysosomal pH and preventing the activation of lysosomal cathepsins. sHz does not seem to activate NLRP3 through the release of uric acid as monosodium urate stimulated cells, when treated with uricase, lowering IL-1β release in a dose-dependent manner. Thus, Hz delivers DNA to the cytosol, where cytosolic DNA receptors are activated by the DNA [68].

Recently, a study has shown that sHz activates NF-κB and NLRP3 inflammasome and induces neuroinflammation in BV 2 microglia, oxidative stress and caspase--mediated neurotoxicity [69]. β-hematin primed with LPS at high concentrations can induce the secretion of IL-1β when incubated with macrophages *in vitro*, whereas the *Plasmodium berghei* ANKA or *Plasmodium falciparum* cannot. NLRP3 but not inflammasome components participate in the experimental cerebral malaria pathogenesis as the NLRP3[-/-] mice succumbed to cerebral malaria after eight days compared to the median survival of 6 days in wild-type mice. Though the cytokine serum levels of IL-6, IL-10, Interferon-gamma (IFN-γ), and tumor necrosis factor (TNF) were produced similar to that in Nlrp3$^{-/-}$ and wild-type mice, IL-1β did not induce within five days of infection. *P. berghei* ANKA infection induces NLRP3 in the mouse brain endothelial cells [70]. Heme activates NLRP3 through NADPH-2, spleen tyrosine kinase, K$^+$ efflux, and mitochondrial reactive oxygen species but not through heme internalization, lysosomal damage, ATP release, the P2X7 receptor, and cell death. Macrophages, NLRP3 inflammasome components, IL-1R and IL-1β, participate in the sterile hemolysis that leads to lethality [71, 72]. A study has revealed that IL 33 is downregulated in the brain during cerebral malaria. IL 33 treatment further decreases the inflammasome activation and affects the IL 1β production in brain cells like microglia and intracerebral monocytes to suppress or regulate neuroinflammation and cerebral pathology. Moreover, co-treatment with NLRP3-inflammasome inhibitor MCC9950 alongside antiplasmodial drugs imitates the effects of IL 33 therapy [73]. Another study on placental malaria indicates the increased expression of AIM 2 and NLRP3 inflammasomes, which is paralleled with a reduction in birth weight of babies born to the malaria-infected mothers by activating caspase 1 and IL 1β production. A recombinant human IL-1 receptor antagonist (IL-1Ra), Anakinra, restored fetal growth and confirmed IL-1β signaling involvement in the molecular pathogenesis of placental malaria [74]. The inhibition of migration inhibitory factor (MIF) in dendritic cells and macrophages inhibits the secretion of IL-1β and IL-18 *via* NLRP3 activation *in vitro* and *in vivo*. Moreover, MIF is crucial in NLRP3–vimentin interaction and regulates inflammation [75] (Table **1**, Fig. **1**).

Trypanosomiasis

Trypanosomiasis, also known as Chagas disease or sleeping sickness, is caused by an obligate parasite, *Trypanosoma cruzi*. It causes cardiomyopathy in 30 to 50% of the population infected with *Trypanosoma.*

Matrix metalloproteinase 2 (MMP2) and MMP 9 interact antagonistically with IL1β mediated inflammation. MMP2 shows a positive correlation with IL 1β,CASP1 and NLRP3, whereas MMP9 shows a positive correlation with IL 1β but a negative correlation with CASP1 and NLRP3 in the caspase 1 molecules dependent IL 1β activation pathway. MMP9 induces IL 1 β activation in patients with cardiomyopathy, promoting fibrosis and inflammation. IL10 reduces the NLRP3 activation and regulates inflammation. High expression levels of IL 1β and IL 18 but not IL 33 were observed in the infected groups [76]. Patients with cardiomyopathy have reported increased TNF-α, IFN-γ, IL-1β, and nitric oxide (NO), leading to myocarditis, fibrosis, and myocardial hypertrophy. Moreover, the increased levels of TLR2 and NLRP3 induce the expression of IL-1β, IL-12, and TNF-α (a pro-inflammatory cytokine) and play a crucial role in the pathophysiology of Chronic Chagasic Cardiomyopathy [77]. Compared to control cells, a significant elevation in NLRP3 and mitochondrial ROS (mtROS) expression was observed in rapamycin-pretreated and infected macrophages. The inhibition of mTOR during *T. cruzi* infection activates NLRP3 inflammasome and production of mtROS that results in an inflammatory profile that regulates and controls *T. cruzi* replication in macrophages [78]. Macrophage galactose-C type lectin (MGL) 1 receptor (MGL1) in Mφ activates through the modulation of c-Jun, ERK1/2, NF-κB, and NLRP3 signaling pathways and develops protective innate immunity against experimental *T. cruzi* infection [79]. Parasitemia was similar in the infected *nlrp3-/-* and C57BL/6 wild-type (WT) mice, whereas it was higher in the livers of *nlrp3-/-* mice than in control mice, indicating that NLRP3 is required for combating *Trypanosoma* parasitemia [80]. High virulent strains can upregulate NLRP3, caspase 1, TNF α, IL 1β, and iNOS mRNA in heart muscle compared to low or medium virulent strains [81] (Table **1**; Fig.**1**).

Schistosomiasis

Schistosomiasis is a chronic and acute helminthic infectious disease that comes under the neglected tropical disease category caused by *S. mansoni, S. haematobium*, or *S. japonicum*. According to a WHO report, about 236.6 million people required preventive treatment in 2019, and more than 105.4 million people were treated [82]. Its transmission report includes around 78 countries. The cercariae (larval stage) penetrate the human skin. In the body, they transform into schistosomula, which migrate and reach the portal system. Then, they mature into adult form and lay eggs. These eggs induce granulomatous, fibrosing inflammation and tissue damage. Granulomatous and fibrosing inflammation is the primary pathological process of *S. japonicum* infection, when exposed to its soluble egg antigen (SEA). Targeting the granulomatous inflammation pathology might be a novel therapeutic approach to cure schistosomiasis-associated liver fibrosis (SSLF) [82]. Inflammasome activation in liver disease pathology has recently been reported in various studies. However, the role of NLRP3 inflammasome in schistosomiasis-associated liver fibrosis (SSLF) is yet to be extensively explored.

In a study, hepatic stellate cells (HSCs) of *S. japonicum*-infected mice showed NLRP3 activation in *in-vivo* and *in-vitro* experiments. In this study, researchers inhibited NLRP3 inflammasome in SEA-infected mouse HSCs, lowering inflammation and collagen deposition in the liver. They also found that the activation is dependent on spleen tyrosine kinase (Syk, an enzyme), Dectin-1, and JNK signaling, showing new details regarding the mechanism of NLRP3 activation during *S. japonicum* infection and in SSLF [83]. In a previous study, the authors reported higher levels of IL-1β and collagen deposition in mouse HSCs infected with *Schistosoma J.* for six weeks. Marked co-localization of IL-1β with Desmin was reported. They also explored SEA-induced NLRP3 inflammasome activation associated with redox regulation and lysosomal dysfunction without potassium channel activation [84].

S. mansoni-derived SEA activates NLRP3 inflammasomes, leading to IL-1β production. This activation depends on Dectin-2/FcRγ receptor complex, Card9 complex, mitochondrial ROS, spleen tyrosine kinase, and K^+ efflux. NLRP3 plays a critical role in TH-2 polarized immune responses [85]. In another study, knockout animals showed that NLRP3 complex activation was mediated by the binding of SEA component to Dectin-2, which associates with the FcRγchain; this binding activates Syk kinase and results in ROS production andK^+ efflux. *S. mansoni*-infected knockout mice (lacking NLRP3 or ASC) show a milder disease and low levels of Th1, Th2, and Th17 cytokine production [86]. *S. mansoni*-infected mouse livers showed significant levels of ROS and superoxides with increased NF-κB release. SEA stimulates HuH-7 hepatocellular carcinoma cells, resulting in NLRP3 inflammasome complex formation [87].

A study investigated whether the inhibition of NLRP3 can inhibit liver fibrosis and its molecular mechanism. BALB/c mice were infected with 15 cercariae, then injected with MCC950 (inflammasome inhibitor) on the same day and 22 days post-infection, followed by examining SSLF phenotype and the effect on liver fibrosis. Human hepatic stellate cell lines (human LX-2 cells) were treated with SEA and NLRP3 inflammasome and markers of liver fibrosis, granuloma, and ALT/AST were evaluated. MCC950 showed dual SSLF pathology and fibrosis in infected mice. Its treatment improved SSLF on infection day, but it exacerbated the pathological effects on 22 dpi; these effects were mediated *via* NF-κB [88].

Praziquantel is used as the current treatment option for liver fibrosis; it effectively kills the worm but cannot prevent re-infection and cannot resolve liver fibrosis. Also, a complete cure for liver fibrosis and splenic damage is not present. Growing resistance to praziquantel has compelled researchers to find new effective treatment options. Schisandrin B (Sch B) of *Schisandra chinensis* might have the potential to treat *S. mansoni*-induced liver fibrosis and splenic damage by inhibiting inflammasome activation and apoptosis [89]. In Schistosomiasis, inflammasome promotes pathology instead of curing or preventing it (Table **1**, Fig. **1**).

CONCLUSION

A large population is affected by infectious parasitic protozoans, causing significant morbidity and mortality globally. Still, it is less funded and studied than viral and bacterial pathogens, and many come under the list of neglected tropical diseases, including malaria, Chagas' disease, Trichomoniasis, Leishmaniasis, and Schistosomiasis. The NLRs play a crucial role in recognizing and responding to pathogens. Among NLRs, NLRP3 is the most widely studied, but in the case of protozoan infections, the effective signaling mechanism is not entirely understood. Its exact role in varied cell types, in immunity modulation, and in adaptive immunity remains unknown. Most of the available treatments for protozoan infections are non-specific and lead to severe side effects. The role of NLRP3 in host protection and inflammatory pathology is crucial in parasitic protozoan infection. It is the foundation for developing new treatment strategies and vaccines, which must be wisely balanced during inflammation in disease pathology and inflammation as protection against infection. Therefore, more research in this area is warranted to develop immunotherapies and vaccines. NLRP3 in some parasitic infections may be needed as a host response to parasite infection by initiating an inflammatory response, and in others, the inflammatory response results in the pathology of the infection.

In the case of *Giardia* infection, NLRP3 elevates bactericidal activity and IL-18 mRNA levels and reduces the severity of the infection. Also, the extracellular vesicles secreted by *Giardia* initiate NLRP3 inflammasome signaling and release of IL-1β. In the case of *Giardia* infection, NLRP3 plays a vital role in the protection or defense against infection. Amebic lipopeptidophosphoglycan (PAMP of *Eh*) induces NLRP3 activation *via* TLR2/6 and TLR4 signaling. Gal-lectin and CP-A5 of Eh are found to activate caspase-4, leading to the release of significant levels of IL-1β. *Eh*CP5 can cleave IL-18 and IL-1β. Also, the monocyte locomotion inhibitory factors produced by *Eh* can downregulate IL-1β and varied strategies to neutralize IL-1β and IL-18, suggesting their role in the defense against *Eh* infection. More studies are required to directly determine the effects of NLRP3, inflammasomes, and cytokines (IL-1β and IL-18) in adaptive immune responses against *Eh* infection.

Trichomonas's glycosylated- LPG activates NF-κB to release IL-1β, which further initiates the NLRP3 inflammasome complex. Ecto-ATPases expressed by *Tv* could attenuate the NLRP3 inflammasome by digesting extracellular ATP, thus used as an evasion strategy from the host's innate immune response. However, the exact outcome of NLRP3 inflammasome in pathogenesis or protection against infection is unclear. More research is warranted to understand the role and mechanism of NLRP3 in *Tv* infection.

NLRP3 inflammasome protects the host by clearing the parasitic load of *L. amazonensis* and *L. major* in macrophages using knockout mice of NLRP3, ASC, and Caspase-1. However, L. major or/ *L. donovani* induce chronic non-healing infection by releasing significantly more IL-1β to promote lesion development *via* neutrophil recruitment. These contrary reports provide grounds for more research. Also, IL-18 neutralization reduces *L. major* titers suggesting a potential therapeutic target to treat Leishmaniasis.

Schisandra chinensis has the potential to treat *S. mansoni*-induced liver fibrosis and splenic damage by inhibiting inflammasome activation. In schistosomiasis, inflammasome seems to promote pathology instead of curing or preventing it.

Parasite proteins are known to activate the inflammasomes, but how *T. gondii* activates the NLRP3 inflammasomes is still unclear. NLRP3 inflammasomes activation can lead to inflammation that limits the parasite burden and dissemination, thereby protecting the host. Similarly, in *T. cruzi* infection, the NLRP3 inflammasome takes part in the protective role in the host by mediating the parasite control and thus limiting the end organ damage. Although NLRP3 activation is protective in many diseases, it has detrimental effects on malaria pathogenesis. The NLRP3 and AIM2 inflammasome increase the malarial pathogenesis and decrease survival in the experimental model of cerebral malaria.

The NLRP3 inflammasome protects the host in *Giardia, T. cruzi, T. gondii,* and *Eh* infections. Also, its protective role in case of *Trichomonas* infection is suggested. NLRP3 inflammasome activation is the key mechanism to treat *Giardia, Eh,* and *Tv* using an agonist of NLRP3. *Leishmania* summons more research to understand NLRP3's role in developing the best strategy to treat the infection. NLRP3 promotes pathology in malaria, and schistosomiasis infection can be treated by neutralizing or downregulating NLRP3.

Therefore, more research on the role and mechanism of NLRs in parasitic protozoan infections using agonist or antagonist molecules is needed to design new immunotherapies.

REFERENCES

[1]   Babamale AO, Chen ST. Nod-like receptors: Critical intracellular sensors for host protection and cell death in microbial and parasitic infections. Int J Mol Sci 2021; 22(21): 11398.
      [http://dx.doi.org/10.3390/ijms222111398] [PMID: 34768828]

[2]   Gowda DC, Wu X. Parasite recognition and signaling mechanisms in innate immune responses to malaria. Front Immunol 2018; 9: 3006.
      [http://dx.doi.org/10.3389/fimmu.2018.03006] [PMID: 30619355]

[3]   Matzinger P. Tolerance, danger, and the extended family. Annu Rev Immunol 1994; 12(1): 991-1045.
      [http://dx.doi.org/10.1146/annurev.iy.12.040194.005015] [PMID: 8011301]

[4]   Liwinski T, Zheng D, Elinav E. The microbiome and cytosolic innate immune receptors. Immunol Rev 2020; 297(1): 207-24.
[http://dx.doi.org/10.1111/imr.12901] [PMID: 32658330]

[5]   Schroder K, Tschopp J. The inflammasomes. Cell 2010; 140(6): 821-32.
[http://dx.doi.org/10.1016/j.cell.2010.01.040] [PMID: 20303873]

[6]   Davis BK, Wen H, Ting JPY. The inflammasome NLRs in immunity, inflammation, and associated diseases. Annu Rev Immunol 2011; 29(1): 707-35.
[http://dx.doi.org/10.1146/annurev-immunol-031210-101405] [PMID: 21219188]

[7]   Franchi L, Muñoz-Planillo R, Núñez G. Sensing and reacting to microbes through the inflammasomes. Nat Immunol 2012; 13(4): 325-32.
[http://dx.doi.org/10.1038/ni.2231] [PMID: 22430785]

[8]   Swanson KV, Deng M, Ting JPY. The NLRP3 inflammasome: Molecular activation and regulation to therapeutics. Nat Rev Immunol 2019; 19(8): 477-89.
[http://dx.doi.org/10.1038/s41577-019-0165-0] [PMID: 31036962]

[9]   Antonopoulos C, Russo HM, El Sanadi C, *et al.* Caspase-8 as an effector and regulator of NLRP3 inflammasome signaling. J Biol Chem 2015; 290(33): 20167-84.
[http://dx.doi.org/10.1074/jbc.M115.652321] [PMID: 26100631]

[10]   Gurung P, Kanneganti TD. Novel roles for caspase-8 in IL-1β and inflammasome regulation. Am J Pathol 2015; 185(1): 17-25.
[http://dx.doi.org/10.1016/j.ajpath.2014.08.025] [PMID: 25451151]

[11]   Clay GM, Sutterwala FS, Wilson ME. NLR proteins and parasitic disease. Immunol Res 2014; 59(1-3): 142-52.
[http://dx.doi.org/10.1007/s12026-014-8544-x] [PMID: 24989828]

[12]   He W, Wan H, Hu L, *et al.* Gasdermin D is an executor of pyroptosis and required for interleukin-1β secretion. Cell Res 2015; 25(12): 1285-98.
[http://dx.doi.org/10.1038/cr.2015.139] [PMID: 26611636]

[13]   Ding J, Wang K, Liu W, *et al.* Pore-forming activity and structural autoinhibition of the gasdermin family. Nature 2016; 535(7610): 111-6.
[http://dx.doi.org/10.1038/nature18590] [PMID: 27281216]

[14]   Shi J, Zhao Y, Wang K, *et al.* Cleavage of GSDMD by inflammatory caspases determines pyroptotic cell death. Nature 2015; 526(7575): 660-5.
[http://dx.doi.org/10.1038/nature15514] [PMID: 26375003]

[15]   Scallan E, Hoekstra RM, Angulo FJ, *et al.* Foodborne illness acquired in the United States--major pathogens. Emerg Infect Dis 2011; 17(1): 7-15.
[http://dx.doi.org/10.3201/eid1701.P11101] [PMID: 21192848]

[16]   Prevention. Giardiasis NNDSS Summary Report for 2018. Retrieved July. Control CfD 2021; 12: 2021.

[17]   Manko-Prykhoda A, Allain T, Motta JP, *et al.* Giardia spp. promote the production of antimicrobial peptides and attenuate disease severity induced by attaching and effacing enteropathogens *via* the induction of the NLRP3 inflammasome. Int J Parasitol 2020; 50(4): 263-75.
[http://dx.doi.org/10.1016/j.ijpara.2019.12.011] [PMID: 32184085]

[18]   Manko A, Motta JP, Cotton JA, *et al.* Giardia co-infection promotes the secretion of antimicrobial peptides beta-defensin 2 and trefoil factor 3 and attenuates attaching and effacing bacteria-induced intestinal disease. PLoS One 2017; 12(6): e0178647.
[http://dx.doi.org/10.1371/journal.pone.0178647] [PMID: 28622393]

[19]   Liu L, Yang Y, Fang R, *et al.* Giardia duodenalis and its secreted PPIB trigger inflammasome activation and pyroptosis in macrophages through TLR4-induced ROS signaling and A20-mediated

NLRP3 deubiquitination. Cells 2021; 10(12): 3425.
[http://dx.doi.org/10.3390/cells10123425] [PMID: 34943932]

[20] Zhao P, Cao L, Wang X, *et al.* Extracellular vesicles secreted by *Giardia* duodenalis regulate host cell innate immunity *via* TLR2 and NLRP3 inflammasome signaling pathways. PLoS Negl Trop Dis 2021; 15(4): e0009304.
[http://dx.doi.org/10.1371/journal.pntd.0009304] [PMID: 33798196]

[21] Stanley SL Jr. Amoebiasis. Lancet 2003; 361(9362): 1025-34.
[http://dx.doi.org/10.1016/S0140-6736(03)12830-9] [PMID: 12660071]

[22] Gupta P, Singh KK, Balodhi A, Jain K, Deeba F, Salam N. Prevalence of amoebiasis and associated complications in India: A systematic review. Acta Parasitol 2022; 67(2): 947-61.
[http://dx.doi.org/10.1007/s11686-022-00547-z] [PMID: 35404011]

[23] Huang J, Gandini MA, Chen L, *et al.* Hyperactivity of innate immunity triggers pain *via* TLR2-IL-3-mediated neuroimmune crosstalk. Cell Rep 2020; 33(1): 108233.
[http://dx.doi.org/10.1016/j.celrep.2020.108233] [PMID: 33027646]

[24] Wong-Baeza I, Alcántara-Hernández M, Mancilla-Herrera I, *et al.* The role of lipopeptidophosphoglycan in the immune response to Entamoeba histolytica. J Biomed Biotechnol 2010; 2010: 1-12.
[http://dx.doi.org/10.1155/2010/254521] [PMID: 20145703]

[25] Mortimer L, Moreau F, Cornick S, Chadee K. The NLRP3 inflammasome is a pathogen sensor for invasive Entamoeba histolytica *via* activation of α5β1 integrin at the macrophage-amebae intercellular junction. PLoS Pathog 2015; 11(5): e1004887.
[http://dx.doi.org/10.1371/journal.ppat.1004887] [PMID: 25955828]

[26] Mortimer L, Moreau F, Cornick S, Chadee K. Gal-lectin-dependent contact activates the inflammasome by invasive Entamoeba histolytica. Mucosal Immunol 2014; 7(4): 829-41.
[http://dx.doi.org/10.1038/mi.2013.100] [PMID: 24253103]

[27] Quach J, Moreau F, Sandall C, Chadee K. Entamoeba histolytica-induced IL-1β secretion is dependent on caspase-4 and gasdermin D. Mucosal Immunol 2019; 12(2): 323-39.
[http://dx.doi.org/10.1038/s41385-018-0101-9] [PMID: 30361535]

[28] Que X, Kim SH, Sajid M, *et al.* A surface amebic cysteine proteinase inactivates interleukin-18. Infect Immun 2003; 71(3): 1274-80.
[http://dx.doi.org/10.1128/IAI.71.3.1274-1280.2003] [PMID: 12595442]

[29] Zhang Z, Wang L, Seydel KB, *et al. Entamoeba histolytica* cysteine proteinases with interleukin-1 beta converting enzyme (ICE) activity cause intestinal inflammation and tissue damage in amoebiasis. Mol Microbiol 2000; 37(3): 542-8.
[http://dx.doi.org/10.1046/j.1365-2958.2000.02037.x] [PMID: 10931347]

[30] Velázquez JR, Garibay-Martínez L, Martínez-Tejada P, Leal YA. An amebic anti-inflammatory peptide down-regulates ex vivo IL-1β expression in patients with rheumatoid arthritis. Reumatol Clin 2012; 8(6): 315-20.
[http://dx.doi.org/10.1016/j.reuma.2012.03.012] [PMID: 22749729]

[31] Gurung P, Kanneganti TD. Immune responses against protozoan parasites: A focus on the emerging role of Nod-like receptors. Cell Mol Life Sci 2016; 73(16): 3035-51.
[http://dx.doi.org/10.1007/s00018-016-2212-3] [PMID: 27032699]

[32] Global prevalence and incidence of selected curable sexually transmitted infections: overview and estimates. Geneva: World Health Organization 2001.

[33] Malla N, Kaur S, Khurana S, Bagga R, Wanchu A. Trichomoniasis among women in North India: A hospital based study. Indian J Sex Transm Dis 2008; 29(2): 76.
[http://dx.doi.org/10.4103/0253-7184.48729]

[34] CDC. Trichomoniasis – CDC basic fact sheet. Centers for Disease Control and Prevention 2022.

[35] Singh BN, Hayes GR, Lucas JJ, *et al.* Structural details and composition of Trichomonas vaginalis lipophosphoglycan in relevance to the epithelial immune function. Glycoconj J 2009; 26(1): 3-17.
[http://dx.doi.org/10.1007/s10719-008-9157-1] [PMID: 18604640]

[36] Riestra AM, Valderrama JA, Patras KA, *et al.* Trichomonas vaginalis induces NLRP3 inflammasome activation and pyroptotic cell death in human macrophages. J Innate Immun 2019; 11(1): 86-98.
[http://dx.doi.org/10.1159/000493585] [PMID: 30391945]

[37] De Jesus JB, Ferreira MA, Cuervo P, Britto C, Costa e Silva-Filho F, Roberto Meyer-Fernandes J. Iron modulates ecto-phosphohydrolase activities in pathogenic trichomonads. Parasitol Int 2006; 55(4): 285-90.
[http://dx.doi.org/10.1016/j.parint.2006.08.002] [PMID: 17010660]

[38] Gao FF, Quan JH, Lee MA, *et al.* Trichomonas vaginalis induces apoptosis *via* ROS and ER stress response through ER-mitochondria crosstalk in SiHa cells. Parasit Vectors 2021; 14(1): 603.
[http://dx.doi.org/10.1186/s13071-021-05098-2] [PMID: 34895315]

[39] Yadav S, Verma V, Dhanda RS, Khurana S, Yadav M. Latent upregulation of Nlrp3, Nlrc4 and Aim2 differentiates between asymptomatic and symptomatic Trichomonas vaginalis infection. Immunol Invest 2022; 51(5): 1127-48.
[http://dx.doi.org/10.1080/08820139.2021.1909062] [PMID: 33866944]

[40] Torres-Guerrero E, Quintanilla-Cedillo MR, Ruiz-Esmenjaud J, Arenas R. Leishmaniasis: A review. F1000 Res 2017; 6: 750.
[http://dx.doi.org/10.12688/f1000research.11120.1] [PMID: 28649370]

[41] CDC. Parasites - leishmaniasis. Epidemiology & Risk Factors. Centers for Disease Control and Prevention 2022.

[42] Albalawi AE, Alyousif MS, Alanazi DA, *et al.* New insights into pathogenesis and immunity of leishmania parasites with emphasis on vaccines. Int J Pharmaceut Res 2021; 13.
[http://dx.doi.org/10.31838/ijpr/2021.13.02.485]

[43] Harrington V, Gurung P. Reconciling protective and pathogenic roles of the NLRP3 inflammasome in leishmaniasis. Immunol Rev 2020; 297(1): 53-66.
[http://dx.doi.org/10.1111/imr.12886] [PMID: 32564424]

[44] Lima-Junior DS, Costa DL, Carregaro V, *et al.* Inflammasome-derived IL-1β production induces nitric oxide-mediated resistance to Leishmania. Nat Med 2013; 19(7): 909-15.
[http://dx.doi.org/10.1038/nm.3221] [PMID: 23749230]

[45] Shio MT, Christian JG, Jung JY, Chang KP, Olivier M. PKC/ROS-mediated NLRP3 inflammasome activation is attenuated by Leishmania zinc-metalloprotease during infection. PLoS Negl Trop Dis 2015; 9(6): e0003868.
[http://dx.doi.org/10.1371/journal.pntd.0003868] [PMID: 26114647]

[46] Charmoy M, Hurrell BP, Romano A, *et al.* The Nlrp3 inflammasome, IL-1β, and neutrophil recruitment are required for susceptibility to a nonhealing strain of *Leishmania major* in C57BL/6 mice. Eur J Immunol 2016; 46(4): 897-911.
[http://dx.doi.org/10.1002/eji.201546015] [PMID: 26689285]

[47] Gurung P, Karki R, Vogel P, *et al.* An NLRP3 inflammasome-triggered Th2-biased adaptive immune response promotes leishmaniasis. J Clin Invest 2015; 125(3): 1329-38.
[http://dx.doi.org/10.1172/JCI79526] [PMID: 25689249]

[48] Gupta G, Santana AKM, Gomes CM, *et al.* Inflammasome gene expression is associated with immunopathology in human localized cutaneous leishmaniasis. Cell Immunol 2019; 341: 103920.
[http://dx.doi.org/10.1016/j.cellimm.2019.04.008] [PMID: 31078283]

[49] Chaves MM, Marques-da-Silva C, Monteiro APT, Canetti C, Coutinho-Silva R. Leukotriene B4 modulates P2X7 receptor-mediated Leishmania amazonensis elimination in murine macrophages. J Immunol 2014; 192(10): 4765-73.

[http://dx.doi.org/10.4049/jimmunol.1301058] [PMID: 24729618]

[50]   Lefèvre L, Lugo-Villarino G, Meunier E, *et al.* The C-type lectin receptors dectin-1, MR, and SIGNR3 contribute both positively and negatively to the macrophage response to Leishmania infantum. Immunity 2013; 38(5): 1038-49.
[http://dx.doi.org/10.1016/j.immuni.2013.04.010] [PMID: 23684988]

[51]   de Carvalho RVH, Andrade WA, Lima-Junior DS, *et al.* Leishmania lipophosphoglycan triggers caspase-11 and the non-canonical activation of the NLRP3 inflammasome. Cell Rep 2019; 26(2): 429-437.e5.
[http://dx.doi.org/10.1016/j.celrep.2018.12.047] [PMID: 30625325]

[52]   Saresella M, Basilico N, Marventano I, *et al.* Leishmania infantum infection reduces the amyloid β_{42}-stimulated NLRP3 inflammasome activation. Brain Behav Immun 2020; 88: 597-605.
[http://dx.doi.org/10.1016/j.bbi.2020.04.058] [PMID: 32335194]

[53]   Lecoeur H, Prina E, Rosazza T, *et al.* Targeting macrophage histone H3 modification as a leishmania strategy to dampen the NF-κB/NLRP3-mediated inflammatory response. Cell Rep 2020; 30(6): 1870-1882.e4.
[http://dx.doi.org/10.1016/j.celrep.2020.01.030] [PMID: 32049017]

[54]   Dey R, Joshi AB, Oliveira F, *et al.* Gut microbes egested during bites of infected sand flies augment severity of leishmaniasis *via* inflammasome-derived IL-1β. Cell Host Microbe 2018; 23(1): 134-143.e6.
[http://dx.doi.org/10.1016/j.chom.2017.12.002] [PMID: 29290574]

[55]   Zahid A, Li B, Kombe AJK, Jin T, Tao J. Pharmacological inhibitors of the NLRP3 inflammasome. Front Immunol 2019; 10: 2538.
[http://dx.doi.org/10.3389/fimmu.2019.02538] [PMID: 31749805]

[56]   Novais FO, Carvalho AM, Clark ML, *et al.* CD8+ T cell cytotoxicity mediates pathology in the skin by inflammasome activation and IL-1β production. PLoS Pathog 2017; 13(2): e1006196.
[http://dx.doi.org/10.1371/journal.ppat.1006196] [PMID: 28192528]

[57]   Santos D, Campos TM, Saldanha M, *et al.* IL-1β production by intermediate monocytes is associated with immunopathology in cutaneous leishmaniasis. J Invest Dermatol 2018; 138(5): 1107-15.
[http://dx.doi.org/10.1016/j.jid.2017.11.029] [PMID: 29246797]

[58]   Ewald SE, Chavarria-Smith J, Boothroyd JC. NLRP1 is an inflammasome sensor for Toxoplasma gondii. Infect Immun 2014; 82(1): 460-8.
[http://dx.doi.org/10.1128/IAI.01170-13] [PMID: 24218483]

[59]   Gorfu G, Cirelli KM, Melo MB, *et al.* Dual role for inflammasome sensors NLRP1 and NLRP3 in murine resistance to Toxoplasma gondii. MBio 2014; 5(1): e01117-13.
[http://dx.doi.org/10.1128/mBio.01117-13] [PMID: 24549849]

[60]   Yoon C, Ham YS, Gil WJ, Yang CS. The strategies of NLRP3 inflammasome to combat *Toxoplasma gondii.* Front Immunol 2022; 13: 1002387.
[http://dx.doi.org/10.3389/fimmu.2022.1002387] [PMID: 36341349]

[61]   Awad F, Assrawi E, Jumeau C, *et al.* Impact of human monocyte and macrophage polarization on NLR expression and NLRP3 inflammasome activation. PLoS One 2017; 12(4): e0175336.
[http://dx.doi.org/10.1371/journal.pone.0175336] [PMID: 28403163]

[62]   Zhu L, Qi W, Yang G, *et al.* Toxoplasma gondii rhoptry protein 7 (Rop7) interacts with Nlrp3 and promotes inflammasome hyperactivation in thp-1-Derived macrophages. Cells 2022; 11(10): 1630.
[http://dx.doi.org/10.3390/cells11101630] [PMID: 35626667]

[63]   Rzoqy HA, Al-Hadraawy SK. Role of NLRP3 in patients infected with Toxoplasma gondii parasite. IJHS 2022; 6(S2): 824-38.

[64]   Ma Z, Li Z, Jiang R, *et al.* Virulence-related gene wx2 of Toxoplasma gondii regulated host immune response *via* classic pyroptosis pathway. Parasit Vectors 2022; 15(1): 454.

[http://dx.doi.org/10.1186/s13071-022-05502-5] [PMID: 36471417]

[65]   Brown H, Turner G, Rogerson S, *et al.* Cytokine expression in the brain in human cerebral malaria. J Infect Dis 1999; 180(5): 1742-6.
[http://dx.doi.org/10.1086/315078] [PMID: 10515846]

[66]   Kwiatkowski D, Sambou I, Twumasi P, *et al.* TNF concentration in fatal cerebral, non-fatal cerebral, and uncomplicated Plasmodium falciparum malaria. Lancet 1990; 336(8725): 1201-4.
[http://dx.doi.org/10.1016/0140-6736(90)92827-5] [PMID: 1978068]

[67]   Duewell P, Kono H, Rayner KJ, *et al.* NLRP3 inflammasomes are required for atherogenesis and activated by cholesterol crystals. Nature 2010; 464(7293): 1357-61.
[http://dx.doi.org/10.1038/nature08938] [PMID: 20428172]

[68]   Kalantari P, DeOliveira RB, Chan J, *et al.* Dual engagement of the NLRP3 and AIM2 inflammasomes by plasmodium-derived hemozoin and DNA during malaria. Cell Rep 2014; 6(1): 196-210.
[http://dx.doi.org/10.1016/j.celrep.2013.12.014] [PMID: 24388751]

[69]   Velagapudi R, Kosoko AM, Olajide OA. Induction of neuroinflammation and neurotoxicity by synthetic hemozoin. Cell Mol Neurobiol 2019; 39(8): 1187-200.
[http://dx.doi.org/10.1007/s10571-019-00713-4] [PMID: 31332667]

[70]   Reimer T, Shaw MH, Franchi L, *et al.* Experimental cerebral malaria progresses independently of the Nlrp3 inflammasome. Eur J Immunol 2010; 40(3): 764-9.
[http://dx.doi.org/10.1002/eji.200939996] [PMID: 19950187]

[71]   Dutra FF, Alves LS, Rodrigues D, *et al.* Hemolysis-induced lethality involves inflammasome activation by heme. Proc Natl Acad Sci 2014; 111(39): E4110-8.
[http://dx.doi.org/10.1073/pnas.1405023111] [PMID: 25225402]

[72]   Tiemi Shio M, Eisenbarth SC, Savaria M, *et al.* Malarial hemozoin activates the NLRP3 inflammasome through Lyn and Syk kinases. PLoS Pathog 2009; 5(8): e1000559.
[http://dx.doi.org/10.1371/journal.ppat.1000559] [PMID: 19696895]

[73]   Strangward P, Haley MJ, Albornoz MG, *et al.* Targeting the IL33-NLRP3 axis improves therapy for experimental cerebral malaria. Proc Natl Acad Sci 2018; 115(28): 7404-9.
[http://dx.doi.org/10.1073/pnas.1801737115] [PMID: 29954866]

[74]   Reis AS, Barboza R, Murillo O, *et al.* Inflammasome activation and IL-1 signaling during placental malaria induce poor pregnancy outcomes. Sci Adv 2020; 6(10): eaax6346.
[http://dx.doi.org/10.1126/sciadv.aax6346] [PMID: 32181339]

[75]   Lang T, Lee JPW, Elgass K, *et al.* Macrophage migration inhibitory factor is required for NLRP3 inflammasome activation. Nat Commun 2018; 9(1): 2223.
[http://dx.doi.org/10.1038/s41467-018-04581-2] [PMID: 29884801]

[76]   Medeiros NI, Pinto BF, Elói-Santos SM, *et al.* Evidence of different IL-1β activation pathways in innate immune cells from indeterminate and cardiac patients with chronic Chagas disease. Front Immunol 2019; 10: 800.
[http://dx.doi.org/10.3389/fimmu.2019.00800] [PMID: 31057540]

[77]   Pereira NS, Queiroga TBD, Nunes DF, *et al.* Innate immune receptors over expression correlate with chronic chagasic cardiomyopathy and digestive damage in patients. PLoS Negl Trop Dis 2018; 12(7): e0006589.
[http://dx.doi.org/10.1371/journal.pntd.0006589] [PMID: 30044791]

[78]   Rojas Márquez JD, Ana Y, Baigorrí RE, Stempin CC, Cerban FM. Mammalian target of rapamycin inhibition in Trypanosoma cruzi-infected macrophages leads to an intracellular profile that is detrimental for infection. Front Immunol 2018; 9: 313.
[http://dx.doi.org/10.3389/fimmu.2018.00313] [PMID: 29515594]

[79]   Rodriguez T, Pacheco-Fernández T, Vázquez-Mendoza A, *et al.* MGL1 receptor plays a key role in the control of T. cruzi infection by increasing macrophage activation through modulation of ERK1/2,

c-Jun, NF-κB and NLRP3 pathways. Cells 2020; 9(1): 108.
[http://dx.doi.org/10.3390/cells9010108] [PMID: 31906385]

[80]   Paroli AF, Gonzalez PV, Díaz-Luján C, *et al.* NLRP3 inflammasome and caspase-1/11 pathway
       orchestrate different outcomes in the host protection against Trypanosoma cruzi acute infection. Front
       Immunol 2018; 9: 913.
       [http://dx.doi.org/10.3389/fimmu.2018.00913] [PMID: 29774028]

[81]   Queiroga TBD, Pereira NS, Silva DD, *et al.* Virulence of Trypanosoma cruzi Strains is related to the
       differential expression of innate immune receptors in the heart. Front Cell Infect Microbiol 2021; 11:
       696719.
       [http://dx.doi.org/10.3389/fcimb.2021.696719] [PMID: 34336720]

[82]   World health organization. Schistosomiasis. 2022. Available from:https://www.who.int/news-
       room/fact-sheets/detail/schistosomiasis

[83]   Lu YQ, Zhong S, Meng N, Fan YP, Tang WX. NLRP3 inflammasome activation results in liver
       inflammation and fibrosis in mice infected with Schistosoma japonicum in a Syk-dependent manner.
       Sci Rep 2017; 7(1): 8120.
       [http://dx.doi.org/10.1038/s41598-017-08689-1] [PMID: 28808303]

[84]   Meng N, Xia M, Lu YQ, *et al.* Activation of NLRP3 inflammasomes in mouse hepatic stellate cells
       during *Schistosoma J.* infection. Oncotarget 2016; 7(26): 39316-31.
       [http://dx.doi.org/10.18632/oncotarget.10044] [PMID: 27322427]

[85]   Ritter M. Novel C-type lectin-mediated signalling mechanisms that activate the NLRP3 inflammasome
       and IL-1β production: consequences for TH 2 polarized immune responses. Technische Universität
       München 2012.

[86]   Ritter M, Gross O, Kays S, *et al. Schistosoma mansoni* triggers Dectin-2, which activates the Nlrp3
       inflammasome and alters adaptive immune responses. Proc Natl Acad Sci 2010; 107(47): 20459-64.
       [http://dx.doi.org/10.1073/pnas.1010337107] [PMID: 21059925]

[87]   Chen TTW, Cheng PC, Chang KC, *et al.* Activation of the NLRP3 and AIM2 inflammasomes in a
       mouse model of *Schistosoma mansoni* infection. J Helminthol 2020; 94: e72.
       [http://dx.doi.org/10.1017/S0022149X19000622] [PMID: 31412958]

[88]   Zhang WJ, Fang ZM, Liu WQ. NLRP3 inflammasome activation from Kupffer cells is involved in
       liver fibrosis of Schistosoma japonicum-infected mice *via* NF-κB. Parasit Vectors 2019; 12(1): 29.
       [http://dx.doi.org/10.1186/s13071-018-3223-8] [PMID: 30635040]

[89]   Lam HYP, Liang TR, Peng SY. Ameliorative effects of Schisandrin B on Schistosoma mansoni-
       induced hepatic fibrosis *in vivo*. PLoS Negl Trop Dis 2021; 15(6): e0009554.
       [http://dx.doi.org/10.1371/journal.pntd.0009554] [PMID: 34161342]

CHAPTER 7

The NLRP3 Inflammasome as a Target for Anti-inflammatory Drugs

Adekunle Babajide Rowaiye[1,2,*], Oni Solomon Oluwasunmibare[3], Umar Suleiman Abubakar[4], Priscilla Aondona[5], Lorretha Chinonye Emenyeonu[6] and Tarimoboere Agbalalah[5,7]

[1] *Department of Agricultural Biotechnology, National Biotechnology Development Agency, Abuja, Nigeria*

[2] *Department of Pharmaceutical Science, North Carolina Central University, Durham, NC 27707, USA*

[3] *Bioresources Development Centre, Isanlu, National Biotechnology Development Agency, Abuja, Nigeria*

[4] *Bioresources Development Centre, Kano, National Biotechnology Development Agency, Abuja, Nigeria*

[5] *Department of Medical Biotechnology, National Biotechnology Development Agency, Abuja, Nigeria*

[6] *Bioresources Development Centre, Owode, National Biotechnology Development Agency, Abuja, Nigeria*

[7] *Department of Anatomy, Faculty of Basic Medical Sciences, Baze University, Abuja, Nigeria*

Abstract: The Nod-like receptor protein 3 (NLRP3) inflammasome plays a vital role in the nonspecific immune response to inflammatory triggers such as cellular infections, injury, or stressors, and it has also been associated with several inflammation-related diseases. NLRP3 inflammasome activation results in the production of proinflammatory cytokines, contributing to an increased risk of inflammatory conditions, such as cardiovascular, metabolic, infectious, and neurodegenerative diseases. Several signaling pathways and cellular events involved in the NLRP3 inflammasome assembly and activation have been studied, and inhibitory mechanisms have been identified. NLRP3 inflammasome inhibition decreases inflammation and inflammasome-mediated cell death. In prospecting for novel anti-inflammatory therapeutics, signaling molecules upstream or downstream on the NLRP3 inflammasome pathway can serve as viable drug targets. Effective inhibition of these molecules culminates in the downregulation of the expression of proinflammatory cytokines like interleukin-1beta (IL-1β) and IL-18. This chapter elucidates the various

* **Corresponding author Adekunle Babajide Rowaiye:** Department of Agricultural Biotechnology, National Biotechnology Development Agency, Abuja, Nigeria and Department of Pharmaceutical Science, North Carolina Central University, Durham, NC 27707, USA;
E-mail: adekunlerowaiye@gmail.com

Puneetpal Singh (Ed.)
All rights reserved-© 2024 Bentham Science Publishers

classes of NLRP3 inflammasome inhibitors, their resultant anti-inflammatory effects, and various mechanisms of action.

Keywords: Cytokines, Inflammasome, Inflammation, Inhibition, NLRP3.

INTRODUCTION

Inflammasomes are protein complexes that can trigger the activation of powerful inflammatory mediators, which are essential components of the innate immune system. Upon cellular infections, injury, or stressors, inflammasome components aggregate and oligomerize, forming a stable complex. This activation of inflammasome results in the splitting of procaspase-1 to caspase-1 (the active form). This consequently promotes the production and secretion of several proinflammatory cytokines, precipitating a series of inflammatory reactions [1, 2].

Aim2 (absent in melanoma 2), NLRP1, NLRP3, and NLRP4 inflammasomes are the four known inflammasomes, and among these, NLRP3 inflammasome is crucial in determining immune responses and also modulating the integrity of intestinal homeostasis in many prevalent inflammatory disorders [3].

The NLRP3 inflammasome, which is named after the NLRP3 protein in the complex, a member of the NLR family, is currently the most well-characterized inflammasome [4]. NLRP3 is a cytosolic protein of 115 kDa that is expressed in epithelial cells, dendritic cells, neutrophils, monocytes, osteoblasts, and lymphocytes, where they regulate the activation of proteolytic enzyme caspase-1 [5, 6]. It has three domains, which are PYD (N- terminal pyrin domain), NACHT (central nucleotide- binding and oligomerization domain), and LRR (C-terminal leucine-rich repeat) [7]. The NLRP3 inflammasome is made up of the NLRP3 scaffold, procaspase-1, and the adapter protein apoptosis-associated Speck-like protein containing a Caspase recruitment domain (ASC) [8, 9]. The NLRP3 inflammasome can either be primed or activated by two independent pathways [10].

NLRP3 Inflammasome Activation

The priming signal pathway is mediated by Pathogen-Associated Molecular Patterns (PAMPs) from bacteria or viruses or sterile Damage-Associated Molecular Patterns (DAMPs), which bind with and trigger the Toll-like receptors (TLRs) on cell surfaces [10]. In response to activation, TLR triggers the intracellular domains of Toll-interleukin 1 receptor (TIR) [11, 12] by two adapter molecules, namely TIR domain-containing adaptor protein (TIRAP) and MyD88. The interaction of these two adapter molecules activates the TNF receptor-associated factor 6 (TRAF6) [13] and IL-1 receptor-associated kinases (IRAKs)

[14]. TRAF6 then activates the MAPK [15] pathway and IκB kinase [16, 17]. An activated IκB kinase leads to the phosphorylation, ubiquitination, and dissociation of IκBα from the nuclear factor kappa-light-chain-enhancer of activated B cells (NF-κB) [10]. The NF-κB translocates to the nucleus after the dissociation and destruction of the IκB protein, attaches to particular DNA sequences known as response elements, and increases the cytosolic expression of the inactive NLRP3 molecule and cytokine precursors like pro-IL-1 and pro-IL-18. [10, 18].

The activation signal pathway can be triggered by numerous PAMP- or DAMP-mediated mechanisms culminating in the development of the NLRP3 inflammasome complex. The most well-characterized and extensively researched PAMP is lipopolysaccharide (LPS), which is found in the outer layer of gram-negative bacteria's cell membrane [19]. Some of the various DAMP-associated molecular mechanisms that trigger the formation of the NLRP3 inflammasome complex include the production of reactive oxygen species (ROS) due to mitochondrial oxidative stress [20 - 22], pore formation and efflux of ATP potassium ions through ATP-gated P2X7 channel [23, 24] and lysosomal membrane damage which causes the release of cathepsin B [20, 25]. Upon the activation of the LRR domain of NLRP3, oligomerization of its monomers takes place through the NACHT domain with the subsequent triggering of the PYD domain to bind to the ASC. This facilitates the recruitment of the procaspase-1 protein through the Caspase recruitment domain (CARD) of the ASC [26]. Procaspase-1 becomes active caspase-1 after being activated by the NLRP3 inflammasome, which causes the intracellular maturation of pro-IL-1 and pro-I--18 cytokine precursors. When mature IL-1 and IL-18 are transported outside the cell, a series of inflammatory responses and pyroptotic cell death are triggered [17]. The activated caspase-1 cleaves gasdermin D (GSDMD), a pyroptosis substrate, at Asp276 by proteolytic processing to form a cytotoxic GSDMD-N domain and consequently creates GSDMD pore on the cell membrane where the cytokines can be released [27, 28].

The NLRP3 inflammasome is seen as a viable target in the development of innovative anti-inflammatory drugs for the treatment of various disorders related to inflammation, as it plays an essential role in modulating pathological processes [29]. The development of NLRP3-specific inhibitors can be made possible by understanding the intricate mechanisms of NLRP3 activation and can be used to treat a variety of NLRP3-related disorders [30].

The aberrant activation of the NLRP3 inflammasome has been associated with a number of disorders, including Type 2 diabetes (T2D), prion disease, Alzheimer's disease, atherosclerosis, metabolic syndrome, cardiovascular diseases, neurodegenerative diseases, and some infectious diseases, sparking intense clinical interest in investigating potential NLRP3 inflammasome inhibitors [30, 31]. Recent research has identified a number of NLRP3 inflammasome pathway inhibitors, which have been demonstrated in both *in vitro* and *in vivo* animal models of NLRP3-linked diseases. While some of these inhibitors specifically target the NLRP3 protein, others focus on other inflammasome components.

Because it minimizes off-target immunosuppressive effects and thereby decreases tissue destruction, direct targeting of the NLRP3 protein may be a significant alternative [31]. Important amino acid residues in the functional domains of NLRP3 may be phosphorylated or serve as a covalent binding site in the direct inhibition, which directly regulates NLRP3 activity [32]. The academia and pharmaceutical industry have paid close attention to the use of drugs to alter the activity of NLRP3, and the NLRP3 inflammasome has been the focus of several documented inhibitors [33, 34].

INHIBITORS OF THE NLRP3 INFLAMMASOME

Natural Product Inhibitors of NLRP3 Inflammasomes

Some natural products, which include flavonoids, alkaloids, and terpenes, have been reported by several workers to inhibit NLRP3 inflammasome Table **1**. They include:

Table 1. Drugs or potential drug candidates that inhibit the NLRP3 inflammasome.

Name	Mechanism of Action	Stage of Development
Casticin (Flavonoid)	Prevents the translocation of NF-κB subunit p65 [37]	Natural product
Isoliquiritigenin (Flavonoid)	Activates NRF2/ downregulate NF-κB [39]	Natural product
Quercetin (Flavonoid)	Activates SIRT1/NLRP3 pathway [42]	Natural product
Pelargonidin (Flavonoid)	Activates NRF2 [46]	Natural product
Lycorine (alkaloid)	Inhibits NLRP3 inflammasome activation [49]	Natural product
Tetramethylpyrazine (alkaloid)	Inhibits NLRP3 inflammasome activation [54]	Natural product
Berberine (alkaloid)	Upregulates NRF2 & blocks NEK7-NLRP3 interaction [58, 60]	Natural product
Coptisine (alkaloid)	Inhibits the NF-kB pathway & prevents caspase-1 activation [62]	Natural product
Parthenolide (terpene)	Blocks the NF-κB signaling pathway [63]	Natural product
Oridonin (terpene)	Inhibits NLRP3 inflammasome activation [75]	Natural product

(Table 1) cont.....

Name	Mechanism of Action	Stage of Development
Artemisinin (terpene)	Inhibits interaction between NLRP3 and NEK7 [82]	Natural product
Sweroside (terpene)	Activates SIRT1 [86]	Natural product
Triptolide (terpene)	Inhibits the NF-kB pathway [93]	Natural product
MCC950 (SM)	Inhibits NLRP3-ATPase activity [33]	Phase II clinical trials (Failed)
Glitazone (SM)	Inhibits NLRP3-ATPase activity [104]	Approved antidiabetic drug
Dapansutrile (SM)	Inhibits NLRP3-ATPase activity [109]	Phase II clinical trials
INF39 (SM)	Inhibits NLRP3-ATPase activity [114]	Preclinical
Tranilast (SM)	Inhibits NLRP3-ATPase activity [116]	Phase II clinical trials
FC11A-2 (SM)	Inhibits caspase 1 activation [119]	Preclinical
Glyburide (SM)	Inhibits K^+ ATP channels [121]	Approved antidiabetic drug
Imipramine (SM)	Inhibits the formation of TXNIP-NLRP3 complex [128]	Approved tricyclic antidepressant
Verapamil (SM)	Inhibits the formation of TXNIP-NLRP3 complex [131]	Approved calcium channel blocker
16673-34-0 (SM)	Inhibits ASC oligomerization [133]	Preclinical
Disulfiram (SM)	Inhibits GSDMD [135]	Approved alcohol addiction treatment drug
Necrosulfonamide (SM)	Inhibits GSDMD [137]	Preclinical
NT-0167 (SM)	Inhibits NLRP3 directly [142]	Phase I clinical trials
Ibrutinib (SM)	Inhibits NLRP3 directly [104]	Approved antineoplastic drug
FhFDM-1 (peptide)	Blocks lysosomal-associated activation of NLRP3 inflammasome [150]	Preclinical
Gly-Pro-Ala (peptide)	Blocks NLRP3-ASC interaction [152]	Preclinical
ASC$^{PYD/H2-H3}$ (peptide)	Inhibits NLRP3 directly [153]	Preclinical
Phoenixin-14 (peptide)	Inhibits NLRP3 inflammasome activation [155]	Preclinical
Adiponectin peptide	Inhibits NLRP3 inflammasome activation [156]	Preclinical
GW-A2 (peptide)	Inhibits NLRP3 inflammasome activation [157]	Preclinical
APC and PAR-derived peptides	Suppress inflammasome activity [158]	Preclinical
Stapled peptides	Block ASC oligomerization [159]	Preclinical

(Table 1) cont.....

Name	Mechanism of Action	Stage of Development
Pralnacasan (peptidomimetic)	Inhibits caspase-1 [162]	Phase II clinical trials (Failed)
Belnacasan (peptidomimetic)	Inhibits caspase-1 [162]	Phase II clinical trials (Failed)
β-hydroxybutyrate	Inhibits inflammasome activation [17]	Endogenous
Dopamine	Blocks NLRP3 inflammasome activation [173]	Endogenous
VIP (peptide)	Decreases the expressions of NLRP3 [175]	Endogenous
SIRT1	Inhibits the activation of NF-κB [176]	Endogenous
A20	Blocks the NF-kB pathway & inhibits NLRP3 inflammasome priming & activation [179]	Endogenous
Spata2	Deubiquitinates PLK4 & blocks NLRP3-NEK interaction [182]	Endogenous

Flavonoids

Flavonoids are known to exhibit several pharmacological properties which include antimicrobial, antioxidant, anti-inflammatory, antifibrotic, and cardioprotective. The anti-inflammatory properties of flavonoids can be attributed to their ability to suppress the production of pro-inflammatory cytokines, such as IL-1β, IL-6, and IL-18, and control signaling pathways linked with inflammation which include the AP-1, NF-B, TLR, and MAPK pathways [35]. Casticin, isoliquiritigenin, quercetin, dihydroquercetin, and pelargonidin are some flavonoids that have been found to have anti-inflammatory and antifibrotic properties by blocking NLRP3 inflammasome activation [36].

Casticin

Casticin, a compound derived from the Chinese herb *Vitex rotundifolia,* has anti-inflammatory properties and induces the apoptosis of cancer cells. *In vitro* experiments revealed that casticin demonstrated anti-inflammatory activities by inhibiting the production of proinflammatory chemokines, cytokines, and ICAM-1 through the suppression of the PI3K/Akt and MAPK signaling pathways and inhibiting the translocation of NF-κB subunit p65 in IL-1 β-stimulated A549 human pulmonary epithelial cells and by translocating the NF-κB subunit p65 [37].

Casticin also suppresses fibrosis. It prevents the activation of the hypoxia-inducible factors 1 (HIF-1) /NLRP3 inflammasome in knee osteoarthritis (KOA) rats, reducing synovial fibrosis, inflammation, and hypoxia [38]. Casticin is very effective in inhibiting IL-1β, IL-18, TGF-β, COL1A1, and TIMP-1 by suppressing NLRP3 components in primary synovial fibroblasts [36].

Isoliquiritigenin

The flavonoid isoliquiritigenin (ISLQ) has a distinctive chalcone chemical structure [39]. Found in the herb licorice botanically known as *Glycyrrhiza glabra,* ISLQ has been known to alleviate neuroinflammation. When administered intraperitoneally in rats after intracerebral hemorrhage (ICH), ISLQ improved early neurological deficits and brain impairments [39]. The mechanism behind the neuroprotective properties of ISLQ is the triggering of the nuclear factor erythroid-2 related factor 2 (NRF2)-mediated antioxidant system and the downregulation of the NF-κB and NLRP3 inflammasome pathways [39].

In streptozotocin-induced diabetic male rats, ISLQ treatment decreased inflammation and attenuated collagen buildup while maintaining renal function and architecture and restoring renal oxidant-antioxidant balance. Specifically, ISLQ decreased the expression of Sirtuin-1 (SIRT1), NLRP3, NF-κB, and inflammatory mediators such as TNF-α and IL-1β. As a result, ISLQ has an inhibitory effect on diabetic nephropathy (DNE), which is characterized by microvascular disorders and linked to a disrupted redox balance [40].

ISLQ has been shown to have protective properties against carrageenan-induced lung damage and pleurisy in mice. Carrageenan-induced histopathological damage, as well as the levels of inflammatory cell exudation, pro-inflammatory cytokines and protein leakage, were all considerably reduced in mice given intraperitoneal injections of ISLQ. ISLQ's capacity to suppress the NLRP3/NF-κB pathway served as evidence of its anti-inflammatory properties [41]. ISLQ suppresses the expression of fibrosis-related genes in the stromal vascular fraction of obese adipose tissue and macrophages by targeting the NLRP3 inflammasome [36].

Quercetin

One of the most common dietary flavonoids is quercetin [42]. Quercetin has been demonstrated to improve neuroinflammation in aging mice by modulating the SIRT1/NLRP3 pathway [42]. Quercetin administered orally improves the memory and spatial learning deficits seen in aging rats in the Morris water maze test. The decrease in the protein levels of the astrocyte marker (GFAP) and inflammatory markers (IL-1β, IL-18, and cleaved-caspase 1) was indicative of the rise in SIRT1 expression and prevention of neuroinflammation [42]. This has been proven to improve diabetes mellitus and protect against cognitive damage caused by diabetic encephalopathy in mice *via* the SIRT1/NLRP3 pathway. Also, quercetin upregulates the production of SIRT1 and downregulates the production of proteins associated with the NLRP3 inflammasome, which include NLRP3, cleaved Caspase-1, adaptor protein ASC, and the pro-inflammatory mediators IL-1β and IL-18 [43].

In fructose-induced U937 and THP-1 macrophages, quercetin has also been shown to reduce ROS production and subsequent NLRP3 inflammasome activation by regulating the intracellular Thioredoxin-interacting protein (TXNIP), a protein that binds to NLRP3 to increase NLRP3 inflammasome activation [44]. Similar to quercetin, dihydroquercetin inhibits the expression of the proteins fibronectin and collagen IV that are linked to renal fibrosis in high glucose-stimulated rat kidney mesangial and human kidney 2 (HK-2) cells. This inhibition of mitochondrial ROS generation and NLRP3 inflammasome activation may be related to the reduction in renal fibrosis [45].

Pelargonidin

Blueberries, berries, strawberries, and red radishes all contain the natural anthocyanidin pelargonidin (PEL), which has been shown to have a positive impact on health [46]. The dose-dependent, anti-fibrotic effect of pelargonidin may be associated with its suppression of the ROS-NLRP3-IL-1β signaling axis through the NRF2 activation. Pelargonidin inhibits NLRP3 inflammasome activation, decreases COL1A1 and the generation of TIMP1 in TGF--β challenged hepatic stellate cells, and attenuates cellular oxidative stress in CCl4-induced liver fibrosis [46].

Other phenolic compounds that prevent the activation of the NLRP3 inflammasome include curcumin, ellagic acid, ferulic acid, gallic acid, paeonol, phloretin, polydatin, pterostilbene, resveratrol, salidroside, salvianolic acid B, and icariin [36, 47].

Alkaloids

Different classes of alkaloids have been found to have antioxidant, anti-inflammatory, antitumor, and immunoregulatory properties [48]. Additionally, it has been demonstrated that some of these alkaloids block the NLRP3 inflammasome activation in order to exert antifibrotic effects.

Lycorine

Lycorine is an alkaloid isolated from the Amaryllidaceae family of plants [49] with several beneficial biological properties, which include inhibiting inflammation, oxidative stress, apoptosis, and fibrosis [50]. Following the intraperitoneal injection of lycorine, TNF-α, IL-1β, and IL-6 were significantly reduced in mice with isoproterenol-induced cardiac dysfunction. This was achieved by the involvement of the NF-κB signaling pathway. Collagen I and collagen III, two fibrotic factors, were elevated by isoproterenol and lowered by lycorine therapy by suppressing the stimulation of the Smad signaling pathway. According to the findings, lycorine may be utilized to treat cardiac dysfunction and enhance the prognosis for people with heart failure [50, 51].

Lycorine demonstrated its inhibitory activity against bleomycin (BLM)-induced pulmonary inflammation and idiopathic pulmonary fibrosis (IPF) in mice by suppressing the activation of the NLRP3 inflammasome [49]. Experimental findings revealed that lycorine decreased the production of active Caspase-1 and the secretion of lactate dehydrogenase (LDH) in mice suffering from acute lung injury (ALI) induced by BLM. Additionally, *in vitro* tests revealed that lycorine prevented bone marrow-derived macrophages (BMDMs) from pyroptosis and LPS/Nigericin- or LPS/ATP-induced activation of the NLRP3 inflammasome. By targeting the pyrin domain (PYD), specifically on Thr53, Leu9, and Leu50, lycorine mechanically disrupts the binding of NLRP3 to ASC [49].

Tetramethylpyrazine

It was found that the traditional Chinese herb *Rhizoma Ligustici Chuanxiong* contains the amide alkaloid Tetramethylpyrazine (TMP) [52]. It is a natural compound that protects against neuroinflammation [53]. Research suggests that TMP may have similar antidepressant effects on mice under chronic unexpected mild stress (CUMS), and the TLR4-NF-B-NLRP3 signaling pathway of the brain may be inhibited by TMP [53]. It has been proven that TMP has a protective effect against renal ischemia; it ameliorates acute kidney injury and enhances renal function in renal ischemia/reperfusion injury (RIRI) rats. Its mechanism of action may be connected to the inhibition of NLRP3/HIF-1α and apoptosis, which results in the decrease in NLRP3 expression in renal tissues [54].

Additionally, it has been shown that TMP inhibits platelet-derived growth factor (PDGF)-treated HSCs and increases the production of pro-IL-1β, pro-IL-18, and cleaved IL-1β by controlling the PDGFβ receptor (PDGF- R)/NLRP3/caspase-1 pathway [55]. TMP reduces diabetes-related endothelial adhesion and elevated platelet response in T2DM rats by preventing NLRP3 inflammasome activation. In T2DM rats, TMP significantly reduced prothrombotic phenotypes and the expression of vascular adhesion molecules and inflammatory markers. Additionally, TMP suppressed the NLRP3 inflammasome and decreased the adherence of human umbilical vein endothelial cells (HUVEC) to platelets and monocytes *in vitro* [52].

Berberine

Berberine is an isoquinoline alkaloid derived from a traditional Chinese herb, *Coptis chinensis* [56]. It can be used to treat a variety of inflammatory conditions by inhibiting the activation of the NLRP3 inflammasome [57]. Berberine can be a promising drug candidate for the treatment of gouty arthritis. It was discovered that berberine reduced the levels of intracellular ROS, downregulated the expression of NLRP3, IL-1β, caspase 1, Kelch-like ECH–associated protein 1 (Keap1), and TXNIP, and upregulated the NRF2 expression in MSU crystal-stimulated RAW 264.7 macrophages. Berberine also significantly reduced IL-1β, TNF-α, and the activity of articular elastase in MSU crystal-induced rats in a dose-dependent manner [58].

Insulin resistance and inflammation induced by obesity can be treated with berberine. Empirical evidence revealed that berberine strongly inhibited NLRP3 inflammasome activation induced by saturated fatty acid palmitate (PA) and IL-1β production in macrophages, which was one of the most critical mediators in the adipose tissue's sensitivity to insulin [59]. NEK7 is considered a crucial target of berberine in the management of inflammatory disorders associated with NLRP3. Activity-based protein profiling has demonstrated that berberine directly binds to the NEK7 protein *via* the hydrogen bond formed by 2,3-methylenedioxy and residue arginine 121 (R121). The precise location of R121 in the crucial domain involved in the NEK7-NLRP3 binding enables berberine to selectively inhibit this interaction and thus inhibit the production of IL-1β, without affecting the TLR4 and NF-κB signaling pathways [60].

Coptisine

Coptisine is an isoquinoline alkaloid obtained from the Chinese herb, *Coptis chinensis,* which is used for the traditional treatment of colitis [61]. Coptisine adopts a favorable conformation to elicit its inhibitory activity at the active site of caspase-1. By preventing the activation of caspase-1, coptisine significantly reduced the output of mature IL-1β in RAW264.7 macrophages treated with LPS and ATP, MSU or nigericin. Coptisine suppressed inflammasome priming by reducing the expression of NLRP3 by the inactivation of the NF-κB pathway in addition to preventing the assembly of NLRP3 inflammasome by altering the interaction between ASC and pro-caspase-1 [62]. Furthermore, coptisine reduced *in vivo* NLRP3 inflammasome activation, which in turn prevented MSU-mediated mice paw edema and LPS-mediated IL-1β production. Coptisine prevents NLRP3 inflammasome activation by inhibiting caspase-1, and this makes it possible to treat gouty arthritis caused by NLRP3 inflammasome involvement [62].

Also, 8-oxocoptisine (OCOP) is a derivative of coptisine. NLRP3 inflammasome suppression and the protective effect of OCOP against colitis in mice induced by dextran sulphate sodium (DSS) may be closely connected. OCOP therapy reduces inflammatory cytokines, such as IFN-γ, TNF-α, TGF-β, IL-1β, IL-6, and IL-18. This suggests that OCOP would be a more viable option for the treatment of colitis in the future [61].

Terpenes or Terpenoids

Parthenolide

Parthenolide, a sesquiterpene lactone, is the major secondary metabolite obtained from the leaves of the feverfew plant, *Tanacetum parthenium*. Ethnomedicinally, it is used orally for the management of various inflammatory conditions, such as fever, arthritis, migraine, and stomach ache. More recently, the anticancer properties of parthenolide have been explored which include its anti-metastatic, anti-angiogenic, anti-inflammatory, antinociceptive, and chemotherapeutic activities [63].

The activities of parthenolide are likely due to its α-methylene γ-lactone ring and an epoxide moiety that can bind to the nucleophilic sites of biologically important molecules [63]. Parthenolide inhibits NLRP3-induced pyroptosis by blocking the NF-κB signaling pathway, which is its main anti-inflammatory property. This is done by either indirectly interacting with IKK activity through increased expression of IκB kinase or directly interacting with the p65 subunit of NF-κB to downregulate its phosphorylation [63 - 65]. NF-B, a key regulator of innate immunity and inflammatory processes, is affected by Parthenolide, which leads to the inhibition of the transcription of proinflammatory cytokines, such as IL-1β, IL-6, TNF-α, and adhesion molecules (E-selectin, ICAM), and enzymes including nitric oxide synthase (iNOS) and the inducible forms of cyclooxygenase (COX-2) [66 - 68].

Additionally, parthenolide can inhibit caspase-1 activation through the alkylation of cysteine residues on caspase-1, thereby reducing its protease activity and also inhibiting the ATPase activity of NLRP3 through cysteine modifications [63 - 65].

Oridonin

An ent-kaurane diterpenoid, Oridonin, was initially discovered in the herb *Rabdosia rubescens* [69]. Numerous disease models, such as cardiac hypertrophy [70], acute myeloid leukemia [71], pleurisy [72], neuritis [69], osteoarthritis [73], and colitis have been used to study the effectiveness of oridonin [74].

Oridonin disrupts the binding between NEK7 and NLRP3 by covalently attaching to the Cys279 residue in the NLRP3's NACHT domain. This inhibits the assembly and activation of the NLRP3 inflammasome [75, 76]. Oridonin demonstrates its anti-inflammatory activity in a dose-dependent manner in cardiac remodeling, myocardial fibrosis, and hepatic fibrosis caused by carbon tetrachloride [77].

It has been demonstrated that oridonin significantly reduces cardiac enzymes and the severity of myocardial infarction [78]. Oridonin can significantly lower the levels of CK-MB and cTnI induced by I/R, the severity of myocardial infarction, the levels of IL-1β, IL-18, and TNF-α, thereby inhibiting the inflammatory damage and the proteins associated with the NLRP3 inflammatory pathway, such as Caspase-1, NLRP3, and IL-1β [79].

Artemisinin

Artemisinin is a sesquiterpenoid isolated from the Chinese plant *Artemisia annua.* Apart from its antimalarial activity, artemisinin and some of its derivatives have been reported to demonstrate antifibrotic properties [80]. This compound can modulate the NF-κB/NLRP3 pathway and attenuate tubulointerstitial fibrosis in subtotal nephrectomized rats.This is in line with the results observed in Ang II-treated human kidney 2 (HK-2) cells [81].

In uric acid-induced inflammation, artemisinin has been shown to suppress the binding between NLRP3 and NEK7, thus inhibiting the the activation of NLRP3 inflammasome. When LPS and monosodium urate (MSU) crystals were used to activate macrophages, artemisinin reduced the intracellular K+efflux. In mice with arthritis caused by MSU crystals, artemisinin reduced swelling in the feet and ankles [82].

Artemisinin also shows cardioprotective effects. It has been demonstrated that artemisinin can improve cardiac function and lessen adriamycin-induced cardiotoxicity, which may be related to the regulation of NF-κB and TNF-α. This suggests that artemisinin's anti-inflammatory property is linked to decreased myocardial injury [83]. Rats administered with artemisinin intragastrically demonstrated less severe myocardial I/R injury due to the inhibition of the activation of NLRP3 inflammasome, as shown by decreased cleaved caspase-1, NLRP3, ASC, and IL-1β [84].

Sweroside

Sweroside is a monoterpene glucoside isolated from *Manea altissima* [85]. It has been shown to have anti-inflammatory activity, as revealed by the activation of

SIRT1 in LPS-induced ALI in mice and the inhibition of LPS-induced inflammation through SIRT-1 mediated FOXO1 and NF-κB signaling pathways in RAW264.7 cells [86, 87]. *In vivo,* sweroside has been proven to reduce the incidence of arrhythmias induced by aconitine and also, *in vitro*, reduce the cardiotoxicity of aconitine in the H9c2 cardiomyoblast cell line [88]. Sweroside prevents non-alcoholic steatohepatitis by inhibiting the NLRP3 inflammasome activation through reduced production of cleaved Caspase-1, NLRP3, and IL-1β. It also prevents cardiac I/R injury by reducing oxidative stress and pyroptosis, in part by modulating the keap1/Nrf2 pathway [89, 90].

Triptolide

Triptolide is a diterpene isolated from a Chinese medicinal plant *Tripterygium wilfordii.* It has been shown to have anti-inflammatory activity due to the suppression of ROS, NF-κB, and the ERK1/2 pathway [91, 92]. Triptolide was demonstrated to significantly reduce cardiac inflammation, enhance left ventricular function, and suppress NF-κB protein expression in rats with experimental diabetic cardiomyopathy, suggesting that triptolide's myocardial protection is connected to its anti-inflammatory activity [93]. Triptolide can improve myocardial fibrosis through the inhibition of the NLRP3 inflammasome [94]. It can enhance cardiac diastolic and systolic functions, drastically improve TAC-induced myocardial remodeling, prevent the release of NLRP3 inflammasomes and other downstream pro-inflammatory mediators, such as IL-1β and IL-18, and also inhibit the TGF-β1 pathway [95].

Other Terpenoids

Glycyrrhizin, saikosaponin A and anemoside B4 are triterpenoids that have been reported to demonstrate strong antifibrotic activity by suppressing the activation of NLRP3 inflammasome. Glycyrrhizin decreases the accumulation of bile acids, thus inhibiting NLRP3 inflammasome activation to alleviate liver fibrosis [96]. Saikosaponin A exerts its inhibitory effects by suppressing the stimulation of pancreatic stellate cells, thereby inhibiting autophagy and the activation of the NLRP3 inflammasome *via* the AMPK/mTOR pathway [97]. Anemoside B4 lowers the production of NLRP3, ASC, caspase-1, IL-1β, and IL-18 and enhances the production of two major podocytes (nephrin and podocin), suggesting that anemoside B4 protects against renal injury induced by adenine [98]. Other terpenoids that can downregulate the expression of NLRP3 and NF-κB are betulin, celastrol, dioscin, diosgenin, geniposide, and ginsenoside Rg3 [47].

SMALL MOLECULE DRUGS

Inhibitors of NLRP3-ATPase Activity

MCC950

MCC950 is a small-molecule inhibitor of the NLRP3 pathway that is specific and highly potent. At nanomolar concentrations, it is able to prevent NLRP3 activation [33]. MCC950 is the most well-studied of the NLRP3 inflammasome inhibitors, as it has been validated in numerous *in vivo* and species disease models [33]. To stop Bacillus cereus-induced mortality, MCC950 inhibits the NLRP3 inflammasome that is triggered by K^+ efflux induced by haemolysin BL [99]. MCC950 lowers the inflammatory response in the spontaneous murine colitis model when administered orally at a dose of 40 mg/kg [100].

Also, in experimental autoimmune encephalomyelitis, which is the murine model of multiple sclerosis, intraperitoneal injection of MCC950 at a dose of 10 mg/kg reduces T cell-mediated inflammatory response and IL-1β signaling [33]. It has also been proven that MCC950 is effective in treating murine ulcerative colitis. In colonic explants, MCC950 significantly suppressed the production of proinflammatory mediators, such as IFN-γ, TNF-α, IL-1β, IL6, IL17, IL-18, chemokine MIP1α, and nitric oxide. This raises the prospect of a novel treatment for inflammatory bowel illnesses in people [100]. MCC950 specifically inhibits ATP hydrolysis by directly interacting with the WALKER B motif on the NACHT domain of NLRP3. It induces conformational changes in NLRP3, blocking ASC oligomerization, and preventing NLRP3 activation and, consequently, the assembly of inflammasome [32, 33].

It is postulated that MCC950 targets NEK7 to suppress NLRP3 activation [33]. MCC950's intracellular inhibitory activity is limited. It does not inhibit inflammasome priming, potassium efflux, calcium signaling, and mitochondrial production, which induce inflammasome assembly [17, 33, 101]. When tested against LPS-dependent TNF-α production, MCC950 failed to block TNF-α production because it was facilitated by lipopolysaccharide-induced TNF-alpha factor (LITAF) rather than an inflammasome. This demonstrates the specificity of MCC950 [17, 33, 102].

MCC950 is currently under clinical trials. However, phase II clinical trials evaluating MCC950's effectiveness in rheumatoid arthritis (RA) treatment were tragically halted due to liver damage [103]. However, in a single-dose pharmacokinetic trial, MCC7840, another sulfonylurea with a chemical structure identical to MCC950, showed improved ADME properties, including a longer half-life and a greater maximum concentration [104].

Glitazone

Also known as CY-09, Glitazone has demonstrated significant therapeutic benefits for numerous disorders, such as cryopyrin-associated autoinflammatory syndrome (CAPS) in animal models, T2D, hepatic tissue damage induced by thioacetamide, and acute kidney injury induced by ischemia/reperfusion [105, 106]. In *in vivo* mouse models and *ex vivo* cultures of human cells, Glitazone was discovered to inhibit NLRP3 directly [105]. Glitazone suppresses caspase-1 activation and subsequent IL-1β production in BMDMs once they are primed with LPS using ATP, MSU, and nigericin, suggesting that Glitazone's activity is independent of the priming signal [17]. Through the suppression of NLRP3 in thrombosis mice, Glitazone also strongly controls the outside-in signaling of human platelet-specific integrin, αIIbβ3 [107].

Glitazone has a similar mechanism of action to that of MCC950. Also, at the WALKER A motif on the NACHT domain of NLRP3, Glitazone binds specifically at Cys172 residue, blocking NLRP3-ATPase activity and inhibiting ATP hydrolysis. Furthermore, this inhibits oligomerization and suppresses NLRP3 inflammasome assembly and activation [104, 105]. On the contrary, the binding of Glitazone affects neither AIM2 nor NLRC4 inflammasomes [105].

Dapansutrile (OLT1177)

A subclass of -sulfonyl nitrile called OLT1177 was created during the synthesis of methionine and chlorinating agents. When human monocyte-derived macrophages are treated with OLT1177 at 1 M, it specifically suppresses the production of IL-1β and IL-18 mediated by NLRP3 but not by NLRC4 or AIM2 inflammasome. When given orally to healthy volunteers for 8 days, 1000 mg of OLT1177 was well tolerated [108]. In a mouse MS model, OLT1177, administered prophylactically through the oral route, greatly decreases the infiltration of macrophages and CD4+ T cells into the spinal cord as well as the secretion of pro-inflammatory cytokines downstream of NLRP3. Treatment with OLT1177 decreases IL-1β and NLRP3 synovial expressions, which are caused by joint inflammation brought about by MSU crystals [109]. OTL1177 decreases sterile colitis and maintains contractile function in mice with ischemia-reperfusion injury in a dose-dependent manner [110]. In a murine Alzheimer's disease (AD) model, OTL1177 treatment also significantly restores synaptic plasticity and lowers sterile inflammation [111]. According to the findings of a phase IIa clinical open-label study on anti-inflammatory properties, OTL1177, administered through the oral route, reduced joint discomfort in gout flare patients. Additionally, no side effects of OTL1177 were seen during the clinical investigation [112].

The first NLRP3 inhibitor to complete the phase I clinical trial in 2012 is OLT1177, registered by Olatec (Clinical Trials Identifier: NCT01636141). The ATPase activity of NLRP3 is inhibited by OLT1177, which also stops NLRP3 and ASC from interacting [109]. Olatec has just begun the investigation into COVID-19 infection after completing phase II of the clinical trials of OLT1177 on acute gouty arthritis, osteoarthritis, and cardiovascular conditions [104]. The results from these trials have not yet been made public.

INF39

The ATPase activity of NLRP3 is irreversibly inhibited by the non-toxic acrylate derivative INF39 [113]. INF39 only inhibits the NLRP3 inflammasome activation and not AIM2 or NLRC4 inflammasomes [113]. Specifically, INF39 inhibits NEK7-NLRP3 binding and subsequently suppresses the formation of the NLRP3 inflammasome complex [113]. It has been demonstrated that INF39 has no effect on the membrane potential of the mitochondria, K^+ efflux, or ROS generation and no direct inhibitory effect on GSDMD [113]. Findings reveal that direct NLRP3 inflammasome inhibition with INF39 reduces systemic and bowel inflammatory changes more effectively than the inhibition of caspase-1 or IL-1 receptor and can be a viable technique for treating bowel inflammation [114].

In BMDMs primed with LPS, treatment with INF39 inhibits caspase-1 activation and IL-1β release at micromolar dosage. According to BRET analysis, INF39 modifies activated NLRP3 confirmation in a K+-independent manner. Rats with DNBS (2,4-dinitrobenzenesulfonic acid)-induced colitis respond favorably to the oral treatment by INF39 [115].

Tranilast

Tranilast, also identified as N-(3',4'-dimethoxycinnamoyl) anthranilic acid, is a traditional anti-allergic medication that works well in many fibrosis models. Tranilast inhibits the oligomerization of NLRP3 by attaching to the NACHT domain. The mechanism of action of tranilast therapy involves NLRP3 ubiquitination and inactivation but not of NLRC4, AIM2, or other NLRs [116]. In the apolipoprotein E- and low-density lipoprotein receptor-deficient murine atherosclerosis model, tranilast prevents NLRP3 inflammasome assembly [117].

In a group of 24 patients with quiescent CD, oral therapy with tranilast at 200 mg/time/three times per day delayed the onset of symptomatic intestinal stricture in a four-year prospective pilot study [104]. A phase II clinical trial (ClinicalTrials.gov Identifier: NCT03923140) on the treatment of Cryopyrin-Associated Periodic Syndrome (CAPS) with tranilast was performed [118].

Other inhibitors of NLRP3-ATPase activity include Bay 11-7082 and 3,4-Methylenedioxy-β-nitrostyrene (MNS) [17]

Inhibitors of Caspase 1

FC11A-2: A novel benzo [d] imidazole derivate, FC11A-2 (1-ethyl-5-meth-l-2-phenyl-1H-benzo[d]imidazole), was investigated *in vivo* for its potential to inhibit the NLRP3 inflammasome against DSS-induced colitis in mice as well as in THP-1 cells. FC11A-2 inhibits the NLRP3 inflammasome by specifically suppressing caspase-1 activation [119].

By preventing pro-caspase-1 self-cleavage, FC11A-2 decreases the levels of IL-1β and IL-18 production [119].

Inhibitors of K⁺ ATP Channels

Glyburide belongs to the sulfonylurea class of drugs, and it is used to lower blood sugar in T2D patients [120]. Through its cyclohexylurea group, glyburide binds to the sulfonylurea receptor 1 (SUR1) on the membranes of potassium ATP-dependent (KATP) channel beta cells. This stimulates the closure of the KATP channels, increases intracellular potassium and calcium ion concentrations, and consequently stimulates insulin secretion [121].

Glyburide is an approved antidiabetic drug with well-documented anti-inflammatory properties. It effectively reduces pulmonary inflammation and injury by inhibiting the NLRP3 inflammasome activation and, as a result blocks the expression of IL-18 and IL-1β in lung tissues [122]. In BMDMs, glyburide prevents NLRP3 inflammasome activation induced by PAMPs, DAMPs, and crystals, which further prevents caspase-1 activation and 1L-1β production [10]. On the contrary, glyburide is not able to inhibit the activation of caspase-1 in *Salmonella typhimurium*-infected BMDMs. This is because they function upstream of the P2X7 receptor, which means they do not need NLRP3 for caspase-1 activation [10].

Glyburide has also been known to prevent the stimulation of the Cryopyrin/NALP3/NLRP3 inflammasome, which is activated by microbial ligands, DAMPs, and crystals. Alzheimer's disease, gouty arthritis, and silicosis have all been linked to abnormal cryopyrin activity [123].

Inhibitors Formation of TXNIP-NLRP3 Complex

These drugs disrupt the binding between NLRP3 and TXNIP, consequently inactivating the NLRP3 inflammasome [124]. Imipramine and verapamil are additional inhibitors that control TXNIP/NLRP3 inflammasome activity, suggesting they may be used as drug candidates to treat inflammatory diseases.

Imipramine

Imipramine is a tricyclic antidepressant that increases serotonin and norepinephrine levels in the brain [125]. This drug has been shown to exert anti-inflammatory activities in microglial and astrocyte cultures. Imipramine is an acid sphingomyelinase (ASM) activity inhibitor, *i.e.*, it possesses the ability to suppress the release of inflammatory cytokines from macrophages [126]. Inflammation and challenges with systemic immunity have been linked to increased ASM activity [127]. Studies have shown that imipramine exerts activity on the TXNIP/NLRP3 inflammasome pathway. The assessment of the effect of imipramine on the NLRP3 inflammasome complex in *in vitro* THP-1 cells induced by ATP in major depressive disorder patients showed that treatment led to NLRP3 inflammasome inhibition [128]. Another study found that imipramine treatment inhibited the upregulation of TXNIP, NLRP3, and Caspase 1 mRNA in LPS/ATP-induced J774A1 cells and THP-1 macrophages [129]. These research findings imply that imipramine plays a role in mitigating the TXNIP/NLRP3 inflammasome complex.

Verapamil

Verapamil, also known as TXNIP siRNA, is a non-dihydropyridine calcium channel blocker [130] and a TXNIP expression inhibitor [131]. In J774A1 cells and THP-1 macrophages, verapamil was observed to successfully inhibit the upregulation of TXNIP and NLRP3 mRNAs [129]. In a randomized controlled trial that evaluated the effect of verapamil in T2DM patients, it was observed that verapamil led to better control of T2DM by downregulating TXNIP gene expression [132]. Furthermore, in animal models, verapamil administration has been shown to reduce pro-inflammatory cytokine concentration and improve hepatic meta-inflammation by attenuating TXNIP/NLRP3 pathways in mice with non-alcoholic fatty liver disease induced by a high-fat diet [131].

Inhibitors of ASC Oligomerization

16673-34-0

16673-34-0 is a byproduct of glyburide synthesis, and it has been demonstrated to suppress the activation of NLRP3 inflammasome [133]. The inhibitory effect of 16673-34-0 on the NLRP3 inflammasome in mice models of ischemia/reperfusion injury and acute peritonitis has been investigated *in vitro* and *in vivo,* and it has been shown to reduce the activity of caspase-1 and IL-1β and IL-18 secretion

[133]. After ischemia/reperfusion injury, molecule 16673-34-0 caused a 90% suppression of inflammasome activity in the heart of mice, as determined by caspase-1 activity. This resulted in a decrease in infarct size as determined by troponin levels and pathology [133].

Inhibitors of GSDMD

These drugs block the GSDMD pore formation and prevent IL-1β release [104, 134]. GSDMD-targeted drugs are still under development.

Disulfiram

Disulfiram was discovered in a recent screening for GSDMD inhibitors utilizing a fluorogenic liposome leakage assay. It covalently modifies the GSDMD Cys191 residue to inhibit GSDMD [135]. In LPS-primed human monocytic THP-1 cells, the thiol-reactive drug disulfiram, also known as Antabuse, was discovered to block nigericin-induced NLRP3-mediated pyroptosis and inflammatory cytokine production [134]. Used to treat alcoholism, Disulfiram is a drug that blocks acetaldehyde dehydrogenase [118]. At higher concentrations, Disulfiram also prevents TLR-induced priming, thus reducing the production of ASC specks and the protease activity of caspases 1 and 11. With "μM potency," disulfiram was demonstrated to suppress pyroptosis in human and murine myeloid cells and to stop the release of IL-1β from these cells [135]. At a dosage of 50 mg/kg, it greatly delayed mortality when administered intraperitoneally to mice that had been exposed to LPS [118].

Others

Necrosulfonamide (NSA) was discovered to be a potent inhibitor of pyroptosis. The findings of a study suggested that NSA enhanced the multiplication and differentiation of osteoblasts through the inhibition of the NLRP3/caspase-1/GSDMD pyroptosis pathway [136]. Additionally, it reduced TNF-α, IL-1β, and IL-6 secretion and negated the effects of Lipopolysaccharide/adenosine triphosphate (LPS/ATP) on the activity of alkaline phosphatase (ALP) and the mRNA expression of genes involved in osteoblast differentiation [136]. Specifically, NSA inhibited pyroptosis by targeting the Cys191 residue of GSDMD [137]. Cys191 in the human GSDMD (equivalent to Cys192 in the mouse) is assumed to be essential for the development of GSDMD pores and oligomerization of the protein [138].

A cell-permeable inhibitor called Z-VAD-FMK was initially produced to irreversibly bind and inhibit inflammatory caspases [139]. The tripeptide VAD serves as a binding agent, whereas FMK is the warhead that can stably inhibit the catalytic activity by forming a covalent link with the catalytic cysteines [140]. Bay 11-7082 and LDC7559 are also the inhibitors of GSDMD.

Direct Inhibitors of NLRP3

IFM2427, developed by IFM Therapeutics, is a peripheral inhibitor of NLRP3 that interacts with NLRP3 directly. In phase I clinical trial, IFM2427 was examined for the treatment of fibrosis, neuroinflammation, and inflammatory disorders [104]. Two oral inhibitors of NLRP3 developed by Inflazome are Inzomelid (Clinical Trials Identifier: NCT04086602) and Somalix, which are intended for the treatment of cryopyrin-associated autoinflammatory syndrome (CAPS) and ca rdiovascular diseases, respectively. Inzolemid has completed the phase I clinical trial. Somalix and IFM-2427 have completed phase II clinical trials [141]. Clinical studies on NodThera's NT-0167, which targets chronic inflammatory disorders characterized by the hyperactivation of the NLRP3 inflammasome, such as inflammatory bowel diseases (IBD) and neurological diseases, have advanced. NT-0167 is currently in phase I clinical trial [142].

Ibrutinib

Ibrutinib is an approved antineoplastic drug, and it is a direct inhibitor of NLRP3. It suppresses the dephosphorylation of Ser5 in the NLRP3's pyrin domain, which is mediated by PP2A [104]. Upon B cell receptor activation, Bruton's tyrosine kinase (Btk) becomes activated by other protein tyrosine kinases (PTKs), which triggers downstream transcription factors essential for the proliferation and differentiation of B cells [143]. Btk travels to the plasma membrane by forming a membrane-bound complex with phosphatidylinositol-3,4,5 (PIP3) [144]. It then undergoes step-by-step activation through transphosphorylation, followed by autophosphorylation [145].

Peptides, Peptidomimetic Drugs, and Proteins that Inhibit the NLRP3 Inflammasome Pathway

Several human diseases have been associated with impaired protein-protein interactions in cell signaling. Given the role played by NLRP3 inflammasome in inflammatory responses in the human body, efforts to find potential inhibitors of the inflammasome are ongoing [146]. Furthermore, reports suggest that NLRP3 inflammasome activation can be inhibited directly by binding to NLRP3 or indirectly by hindering the components of the inflammasome and related signaling pathways, which include potassium efflux, ROS, and mtDNA production, amongst others [147].

Peptides

The prospective use of peptides as therapeutic agents for inflammatory-related diseases has continually evolved due to their high selectivity and potency, as well as low toxicity [148]. Several studies of clinical importance have been conducted on peptides to establish possible inhibitory effects on inflammatory diseases [148]. However, information on peptide inhibition of NLRP3 inflammasome is limited. Some peptides that can potentially inhibit the NLRP3 inflammasome include:

Fasciola hepatica-Derived Molecule-1 (FhHDM-1)

FhHDM-1 is an immunomodulatory peptide derived from the Helminth Defense Molecule (HDM) sequence of *Fasciola hepatica*. It has demonstrated strong anti-inflammatory properties in clinically relevant models of disorders like diabetes, multiple sclerosis, asthma, and acute lung injury, increasing the possibility of the development of novel anti-inflammatory therapeutics [149]. In a pre-clinical study, Alvarado *et al.* in 2017 [150] reported that FhFDM-1 inhibited lysosomal-associated stimulation of NLRP3 inflammasome in BMDMs primed with lipopolysaccharide (LPS). This was achieved by inhibiting the lysosomal lumen's acidification and thus decreasing the activity of cathepsin B and the NLRP3 inflammasome. FhHDM-1 decreased the production of IL-1β in macrophages stimulated with NLRP3 activator NanoSiO$_2$ and alum. FhFDM-1 is thus indicated for possible use in the treatment of liver flukes [150].

Gly-Pro-Ala (GPA)

GPA is generally regarded as a peptide with the capacity to regulate oxidative stress and cell death in inflammatory diseases [151]. GPA exhibits an indirect inhibition of NLRP3 inflammasome. In ATP-treated macrophages, results of studies revealed that the NLRP3-ASC interaction was blocked, and this suppressed the assembly of the NLRP3 inflammasome [152]. In further investigations using mice with colitis induced by dextran sulfate sodium (DSS), GPA suppressed ROS production by increasing the phosphorylation of AMPK with a resultant inhibiting effect on NLRP3 inflammasome activation [152].

ASC$^{PYD/H2-H3}$

The peptide ASC$^{PYD/H2-H3}$ has been found to bind specifically to the Pyrin domain of NLRP3 and suppress NLRP3 inflammasome activation. Sušjan *et al.*, 2020 [153] reported that with ASC$^{PYD/H2-H3}$ peptide, the release of cytokines, activation of caspase-1, and formation of ASC speck were inhibited in BMDMs primed with LPS and activated with nanoparticles of silica (nanoSiO$_2$). In addition, a significant reduction of neutrophil count and suppressed NLRP3-driven inflammation were observed in mice with silica-induced peritonitis [153]. These findings highlight the potential of ASC$^{PYD/H2-H3}$ peptide to serve as a basis for the production of novel drugs for NLRP3 inflammasome-induced peritonitis [153].

Phoenixin-14

Phoenixin-14, a pleiotropic neuropeptide and an isoform of phoenixin, was first isolated in 2013 from the hypothalamus of a rat and is involved in bodily functions, such as reproduction and pain [154, 155]. In mouse astrocytes, the neuropeptide was shown to reduce LPS-induced cell death by increasing the activity of superoxide dismutase (SOD). Additionally, phoenixin-14 suppressed the high mobility group box 1 (HMGB1)-mediated expression of NLRP3 inflammasome as evidenced by the decreased levels of IL-1β and caspase-1 [155].

Adiponectin Peptide (APNp)

APNp is a synthetic peptide based on the functional area in the globular domain of adiponectin and was synthesized to augment the limitation of blood-brain barrier permeability exhibited by adiponectin [156]. *In vitro* investigations using primary astrocytes treated with oxygen-glucose deprivation and reintroduction (OGD-R) revealed that APNp elevated the phosphorylation of GSK-3β (Ser9) and AMPK (Thr172) inhibited NLRP3 inflammasome activation. Moreover, results from *in vivo* experiments using mice with transient middle cerebral artery occlusion (tMCAO) suggested a marked reduction in apoptosis, as well as decreased levels of GSH-Px and SOD [156]. These findings propose APNp for the treatment of cerebral ischemia [156].

GW-A2

GW-A2 is a cationic antimicrobial peptide (AMP) of synthetic origin that exhibits both antimicrobial and anti-inflammatory properties [157]. In LPS-activated macrophages, GW-A2 inhibited NLRP3 inflammasome activation, as seen by the suppressed production of IL-1β and inhibited the activation of caspase-1 [157]. The results of an *in vivo* study revealed that GW-A2 significantly reduced the levels of TNF-α, IL-1β, and IL-6 in the serum as well as the expression of COX-2, iNOS, and NLRP3 in the liver and lungs, demonstrating the anti-inflammatory properties of GW-A2 [157].

Other Peptides

The activity of the natural anti-coagulant Activated Protein C (APC) and Protease-activated receptor (PAR)-derived peptides on NLRP3 has been recently characterized. Findings from pre-clinical research using differentiated THP-1 cells and primary monocytes both from humans demonstrate that APC, P1(47-66), and P3(42-65) significantly reduced the activity of caspase-1 and consequently inhibited NLRP3 inflammasome [158]. Furthermore, the potential of the PAR-derived peptides to produce a synergistic anti-inflammatory effect can be maximized for therapeutic benefits [158].

Stapled peptides are peptides with strategically positioned hydrocarbon chains to enhance pharmacological attributes, such as affinity for target and resistance to protease. Targeting the apoptosis-associated speck-like protein (ASC), Pal *et al.,* 2019 [159] designed α-helical stapled peptides that bind to the pyrin domain (PYD) and interfere with NLRP3-induced ASC oligomerization. Resultantly, this reduces caspase-1 activation as well as the production of interleukin IL-1β from human monocytes/macrophages.

Peptidomimetics

Peptidomimetics are structural and functional analogs of naturally occurring peptides that have the same biological effects as those peptides when they engage with a biological target [160, 161].

Pralnacasan (VX-740) and its structural analog Belnacasan (VX-765) are peptidomimetic inhibitors of caspase-1. Being prodrugs, they are converted to their corresponding aldo-acids by plasma esterases [162]. They act by covalently modifying the catalytic cysteine residue found in the active site of caspase-1, blocking the caspase-1 and preventing it from cleaving pro-IL-1β/18 [163].

To address the challenges of low bioavailability and toxicity with peptidic caspase inhibitors, fully synthetic peptide-mimetic prodrugs like VX-740 and VX-765 were developed. These prodrugs are metabolically transformed into VRT-18858 and VRT-043198 in the cytosol *via* esterase activity, both of which function as reversible inhibitors of caspase-1 and the associated inflammatory caspases 4 and 5 [118, 164].

In two animal models of osteoarthritis, VX-740 was found to alleviate joint damage, and it also inhibited colitis induced by DSS [164, 165]. However, the phase 2 clinical trial of VX-740 in patients with rheumatoid arthritis was terminated as a result of the discovery of hepatotoxicity in long-term follow-up animal studies [118, 162]. On the contrary, VX-765 greatly decreased the secretion of inflammatory mediators in models of skin inflammation and rheumatoid arthritis. In two mouse models of epilepsy, VX-765 was shown to diminish both acute seizures and chronic epileptic activity [118, 166]. Additionally, it was demonstrated that it reduced amyloid beta deposition and neuroinflammation in mice with Alzheimer's disease, enhancing cognition [118, 167]. Although VX765 has a good safety record, its key goals were not met in phase 2 clinical trials in patients with drug-resistant partial epilepsy (ClinicalTrials.gov Identifier: NCT01501383) [118].

Exogenous Proteins

Several other proteins modulate certain targets downstream of the NLRP3 pathway. They include IL-1R antagonist (Anakinra) [10], monoclonal antibodies that target IL-1ß (Canakinumab) [168], anti-IL-18 receptor monoclonal antibodies [168], and IL-18 binding protein (Rilonacept) [10]. All these inhibit immune signaling and exert anti-inflammatory effects [10].

Endogenous NLRP3 Inhibitors

β-hydroxybutyrate

During the process of metabolizing fatty acids, the liver produces the ketone body β-hydroxybutyrate (BHB). In mouse BMDMs, BHB has been demonstrated to inhibit NLRP3 inflammasome activation in a dose-dependent manner [17]. In another study using human monocytes, BHB also demonstrated inhibitory activity against NLRP3 inflammasome by suppressing K^+ efflux, ASC oligomerization, and speck formation. This led to a reduction in the expression of IL-1β and IL-18, suggesting that BHB could be used to treat NLRP3-mediated chronic inflammatory disorders [17].

The endogenous NLRP3 inflammasome inhibitory activity of BHB also has antidepressant and anti-anxiety effects [169, 170]. The pathophysiology of depression has been proven to have a strong relationship with neuroinflammation. In a rodent model of depression, BHB administered directly to the brain induced an antidepressant effect, possibly *via* anti-inflammatory mechanisms, and enhanced hypothalamus-pituitary-adrenal axis responses [169]. Rat models of post-traumatic stress disorder (PTSD) usually show increased serum levels of TNF-α and IL-1β due to exposure to single-prolonged stress (SPS). Repeated BHB treatment reduced the anxiety-related behaviors in rat models exposed to SPS and suppressed TNF-α. BHB may, therefore, provide a cutting-edge therapeutic option for the treatment of PTSD [170].

Dopamine

1-methyl-4-phenyl-1,2,3,6-tetrahydropyridine (MPTP), an environmental neurotoxic pollutant, has been linked to both the pathology of human and animal models of Parkinson's disease (PD) [171]. PD is a classic neurodegenerative disease marked by the death of dopamine neurons found in the substantia nigra region [172]. Dopamine's function as an immunomodulator has been investigated in an MPTP-PD model, and it has been shown that dopamine regulated immunological response by acting as an endogenous inhibitor of the NLRP3 inflammasome pathway. Furthermore, dopamine has been shown to suppress MPTP-induced neuroinflammation by blocking NLRP3 inflammasome activation *via* dopamine D1 receptor (DRD1) signaling [173]. In DRD1 signaling, a secondary messenger, cyclic adenosine monophosphate (cAMP), interacts with NLRP3 and facilitates its ubiquitination and degradation through the E3 ubiquitin ligase MARCH7. Empirical data suggests that dopamine through DRD1 signaling inhibits NLRP3 inflammasome-dependent inflammation and peritoneal inflammation induced by monosodium urate crystal (MSU). Also, it inhibits systemic inflammation induced by LPS and neurotoxin-induced neuroinflammation [173].

Vasoactive Intestinal Peptide (VIP)

VIP, a peptide made by immune cells, has a broad range of immunological effects that modulate the homeostasis of the immune system. VIP has been recognized as a strong anti-inflammatory agent, and it has been demonstrated to inhibit the production of inflammatory chemokines and cytokines from dendritic cells, macrophages, and microglia [174].

In mice having acute lung injury induced by LPS, Zhou *et al.*, 2020 [175] reported that Lentivirus-carrying VIP (Lenti-VIP) downregulated caspase-1 p10 expression in lung tissues as well as IL-1β levels. Additionally, *in vitro* investigations using primary peritoneal macrophages primed with LPS revealed that VIP notably decreased the expressions of pro-IL-1β and NLRP3 and suppressed the generation of ROS. This serves as a platform for further studies on the potential therapeutic use of VIP for NLRP3 inflammasome-associated diseases.

Sirtuin 1 (SIRT1)

The activation of SIRT1 is connected to the downregulation of IL-1β. Research findings reveal that treatment with resveratrol, a SIRT1 activator, inhibited IL-1β expression induced by radiation in a concentration-dependent manner. In contrast, nicotinamide's inhibition of SIRT1 significantly increased IL-1β expression induced by radiation [176]. The fact that SIRT1 limits NF-κB's transactivation potential by deacetylating it, which then inhibits the transcription of NLRP3, suggests that this impact is caused by SIRT1-mediated inhibition of the activation of NLRP3 inflammasome [176]. Together, the findings show that SIRT1 inhibits inflammation by controlling the production of NLRP3 in mesenchymal stem cells, partially *via* the NF-κB pathway [176].

Polydatin also activates SIRT1. The treatment of hyperuricemic rats with polydatin reduced the concentrations of uric acid and creatinine in blood and urine, which suppressed the production of pro-inflammatory mediators in serum and kidney. Western blot investigations showed that polydatin inhibited NF-κB p65 translocation, breakdown of IκBα, and inflammasome component protein levels (caspase-1, ASC, and NLRP3), which in turn lowered IL-1β release. Notably, polydatin therapy boosted SIRT1 expression and activated the AMPK protein. When used in combination, polydatin may be used for the possible treatment of gout by suppressing the activation of the renal NF-κB/NLRP3 inflammasome *via* the AMPK/SIRT1 pathway [177]. In another study, treatment with a SIRT1 activator decreased the levels of IL-1β in the serum and the expression levels of C-reactive protein (CRP) and monocyte chemotactic protein-1 (MCP-1) in collared arteries of rabbits. This shows that NLRP3 inflammasome activation promotes endothelial inflammation and that SIRT1 controls the inflammatory response in part by controlling NLRP3 inflammasome activity in vascular endothelial cells [178].

A20

A20 also plays an important role in inhibiting NLRP3 inflammasome [179]. The mononuclear phagocytes of the central nervous system (CNS), known as microglia, play a crucial role in both the maintenance of CNS homeostasis and CNS disease. It has been proven that the NF-κB regulatory protein, A20, is essential for controlling microglia activation in both normal and pathological CNS physiology [179]. Mice with microglia lacking A20 show an increase in microglial cell count and changes in how microglia regulate neuronal synaptic function. Mice with microglia-confined A20 loss undergo significant microglia activation, neuroinflammation, and mortality after receiving a sublethal dose of lipopolysaccharide [179].

Due to increased IL-1β secretion and CNS inflammation caused by hyperactivated NLRP3 inflammasome, microglia A20 deficiency also worsens multiple sclerosis (MS)-like diseases. Also, with the validation of the expression of IL-1β and the NLRP3 inflammasome signature in MS patients' brains and cerebrospinal fluid, it is suggested that A20 plays an important role in the regulation of microglia activation and neuroinflammation [179].

Spermatogenesis-Associated Protein 2 (Spata2)

Spata 2 is a centrosomal protein that has been linked with the activity of the deubiquitination enzyme CYLD [180]. Ubiquitin also contributes to intracellular signaling and the apoptosis of other proteins [181]. In the analysis of their investigations, Yang *et al.,* 2020 [182] reported that using a mouse model, Spata2 reduced cytokine levels, such as IL-1β in BMDMs with LPS-induced septic shock. Moreover, mice with alum-induced peritonitis and Spata2 knocked out had increased neutrophils in the peritoneal fluid. Mechanistic studies reveal that Spata2 acts by recruiting CYLD deubiquitinase to the centrosome to deubiquitinate polo-like kinase 4 (PLK4), a process that facilitates the binding to and phosphorylation of NEK7 at SER204 by PLK4 and blocks NLRP3-NEK interaction [182]. In a recent study, thiolutin was suggested to inhibit deubiquitination and activate the NLRP3 inflammasome by suppressing the BRCC3-containing isopeptidase complex [183]. Thus, targeting the deubiquitination of NLRP3 could be a foundation for the creation of innovative pharmaceuticals to treat disorders related to the NLRP3 inflammasome [183].

CONCLUSION

The NLRP3 inflammasome has been linked to a number of inflammation-related disorders and has been the subject of numerous recent research efforts. Consequently, various treatment approaches have been proposed to prevent the NLRP3 inflammasome from being assembled and activated. The bioactive molecules that can be engaged as NLRP3 inflammasome inhibitors include natural products, small molecules, peptides, peptidomimetics, and proteins, which are at different stages of clinical development to ensure efficacy and safety. Some endogenous inhibitors have also been identified as viable drug targets. All these provide a foundation for the rational design of novel therapeutics for inflammation-related diseases.

REFERENCES

[1]   Yaribeygi H, Katsiki N, Butler AE, Sahebkar A. Effects of antidiabetic drugs on NLRP3 inflammasome activity, with a focus on diabetic kidneys. Drug Discov Today 2019; 24(1): 256-62.
       [http://dx.doi.org/10.1016/j.drudis.2018.08.005] [PMID: 30086405]

[2]   Rai RC. Host inflammatory responses to intracellular invaders: Review study. Life Sci 2020; 240: 117084.
       [http://dx.doi.org/10.1016/j.lfs.2019.117084] [PMID: 31759040]

[3]   Próchnicki T, Latz E. Inflammasomes on the crossroads of innate immune recognition and metabolic control. Cell Metab 2017; 26(1): 71-93.
       [http://dx.doi.org/10.1016/j.cmet.2017.06.018] [PMID: 28683296]

[4]   Inoue M, Shinohara ML. NLRP3 inflammasome and MS/EAE. Autoimmune Dis 2013; 2013: 1-8.
       [http://dx.doi.org/10.1155/2013/859145] [PMID: 23365725]

[5]   Zhong Y, Kinio A, Saleh M. Functions of NOD-like receptors in human diseases. Front Immunol 2013; 4: 333.
       [http://dx.doi.org/10.3389/fimmu.2013.00333] [PMID: 24137163]

[6]   Wang Z, Zhang S, Xiao Y, *et al.* NLRP3 inflammasome and inflammatory diseases. Oxid Med Cell Longev 2020; 2020: 4063562.
       [PMID: 32148650]

[7]   Halle A, Hornung V, Petzold GC, *et al.* The NALP3 inflammasome is involved in the innate immune

response to amyloid-β. Nat Immunol 2008; 9(8): 857-65.
[http://dx.doi.org/10.1038/ni.1636] [PMID: 18604209]

[8]   Ito M, Shichita T, Okada M, *et al.* Bruton's tyrosine kinase is essential for NLRP3 inflammasome activation and contributes to ischaemic brain injury. Nat Commun 2015; 6(1): 7360.
[http://dx.doi.org/10.1038/ncomms8360] [PMID: 26059659]

[9]   Inoue M, Shinohara ML. The role of interferon-β in the treatment of multiple sclerosis and experimental autoimmune encephalomyelitis - in the perspective of inflammasomes. Immunology 2013; 139(1): 11-8.
[http://dx.doi.org/10.1111/imm.12081] [PMID: 23360426]

[10]   Zahid A, Li B, Kombe AJK, Jin T, Tao J. Pharmacological inhibitors of the NLRP3 inflammasome. Front Immunol 2019; 10: 2538.
[http://dx.doi.org/10.3389/fimmu.2019.02538] [PMID: 31749805]

[11]   O'Neill LAJ, Golenbock D, Bowie AG. The history of Toll-like receptors - redefining innate immunity. Nat Rev Immunol 2013; 13(6): 453-60.
[http://dx.doi.org/10.1038/nri3446] [PMID: 23681101]

[12]   Vaure CÃ, Liu Y. A comparative review of toll-like receptor 4 expression and functionality in different animal species. Front Immunol 2014; 5: 316.
[http://dx.doi.org/10.3389/fimmu.2014.00316] [PMID: 25071777]

[13]   De Nardo D, Balka KR, Cardona Gloria Y, Rao VR, Latz E, Masters SL. Interleukin-1 receptor–associated kinase 4 (IRAK4) plays a dual role in myddosome formation and Toll-like receptor signaling. J Biol Chem 2018; 293(39): 15195-207.
[http://dx.doi.org/10.1074/jbc.RA118.003314] [PMID: 30076215]

[14]   Küppers R. IRAK4 inhibition to shut down TLR signaling in autoimmunity and MyD88-dependent lymphomas. J Exp Med 2015; 212(13): 2184.
[http://dx.doi.org/10.1084/jem.21213insight1]

[15]   Pennini ME, Perkins DJ, Salazar AM, Lipsky M, Vogel SN. Complete dependence on IRAK4 kinase activity in TLR2, but not TLR4, signaling pathways underlies decreased cytokine production and increased susceptibility to Streptococcus pneumoniae infection in IRAK4 kinase-inactive mice. J Immunol 2013; 190(1): 307-16.
[http://dx.doi.org/10.4049/jimmunol.1201644] [PMID: 23209321]

[16]   Sugiyama K, Muroi M, Kinoshita M, *et al.* NF-κB activation *via* MyD88-dependent Toll-like receptor signaling is inhibited by trichothecene mycotoxin deoxynivalenol. J Toxicol Sci 2016; 41(2): 273-9.
[http://dx.doi.org/10.2131/jts.41.273] [PMID: 26961612]

[17]   Kinra M, Nampoothiri M, Arora D, Mudgal J. Reviewing the importance of TLR-NLRP3-pyroptosis pathway and mechanism of experimental NLRP3 inflammasome inhibitors. Scand J Immunol 2022; 95(2): e13124.
[http://dx.doi.org/10.1111/sji.13124] [PMID: 34861056]

[18]   Concetti J, Wilson CL. NFKB1 and cancer: Friend or foe? Cells 2018; 7(9): 133.
[http://dx.doi.org/10.3390/cells7090133] [PMID: 30205516]

[19]   Bertani B, Ruiz N. Function and biogenesis of lipopolysaccharides. Ecosal Plus 2018; 8(1): 2018.
[http://dx.doi.org/10.1128/ecosalplus.ESP-0001-2018] [PMID: 30066669]

[20]   Heid ME, Keyel PA, Kamga C, Shiva S, Watkins SC, Salter RD. Mitochondrial reactive oxygen species induces NLRP3-dependent lysosomal damage and inflammasome activation. J Immunol 2013; 191(10): 5230-8.
[http://dx.doi.org/10.4049/jimmunol.1301490] [PMID: 24089192]

[21]   Gurung P, Lukens JR, Kanneganti TD. Mitochondria: Diversity in the regulation of the NLRP3 inflammasome. Trends Mol Med 2015; 21(3): 193-201.
[http://dx.doi.org/10.1016/j.molmed.2014.11.008] [PMID: 25500014]

[22]   Rowaiye AB, Onuh OA, Oli AN, Okpalefe OA, Oni S, Nwankwo EJ. The pandemic COVID-19: A tale of viremia, cellular oxidation and immune dysfunction. Pan Afr Med J 2020; 36: 188.
[http://dx.doi.org/10.11604/pamj.2020.36.188.23476] [PMID: 32952832]

[23]   Perregaux D, Gabel CA. Interleukin-1 beta maturation and release in response to ATP and nigericin. Evidence that potassium depletion mediated by these agents is a necessary and common feature of their activity. J Biol Chem 1994; 269(21): 15195-203.
[http://dx.doi.org/10.1016/S0021-9258(17)36591-2] [PMID: 8195155]

[24]   Pétrilli V, Papin S, Dostert C, Mayor A, Martinon F, Tschopp J. Activation of the NALP3 inflammasome is triggered by low intracellular potassium concentration. Cell Death Differ 2007; 14(9): 1583-9.
[http://dx.doi.org/10.1038/sj.cdd.4402195] [PMID: 17599094]

[25]   Okada M, Matsuzawa A, Yoshimura A, Ichijo H. The lysosome rupture-activated TAK1-JNK pathway regulates NLRP3 inflammasome activation. J Biol Chem 2014; 289(47): 32926-36.
[http://dx.doi.org/10.1074/jbc.M114.579961] [PMID: 25288801]

[26]   Duncan JA, Bergstralh DT, Wang Y, *et al.* Cryopyrin/NALP3 binds ATP/dATP, is an ATPase, and requires ATP binding to mediate inflammatory signaling. Proc Natl Acad Sci 2007; 104(19): 8041-6.
[http://dx.doi.org/10.1073/pnas.0611496104] [PMID: 17483456]

[27]   Shi J, Zhao Y, Wang K, *et al.* Cleavage of GSDMD by inflammatory caspases determines pyroptotic cell death. Nature 2015; 526(7575): 660-5.
[http://dx.doi.org/10.1038/nature15514] [PMID: 26375003]

[28]   Kayagaki N, Stowe IB, Lee BL, *et al.* Caspase-11 cleaves gasdermin D for non-canonical inflammasome signalling. Nature 2015; 526(7575): 666-71.
[http://dx.doi.org/10.1038/nature15541] [PMID: 26375259]

[29]   Mao L, Kitani A, Similuk M, *et al.* Loss-of-function CARD8 mutation causes NLRP3 inflammasome activation and Crohn's disease. J Clin Invest 2018; 128(5): 1793-806.
[http://dx.doi.org/10.1172/JCI98642] [PMID: 29408806]

[30]   Yang Y, Wang H, Kouadir M, Song H, Shi F. Recent advances in the mechanisms of NLRP3 inflammasome activation and its inhibitors. Cell Death Dis 2019; 10(2): 128.
[http://dx.doi.org/10.1038/s41419-019-1413-8] [PMID: 30755589]

[31]   Haque ME, Akther M, Jakaria M, Kim IS, Azam S, Choi DK. Targeting the microglial NLRP3 inflammasome and its role in Parkinson's disease. Mov Disord 2020; 35(1): 20-33.
[http://dx.doi.org/10.1002/mds.27874] [PMID: 31680318]

[32]   Tapia-Abellán A, Angosto-Bazarra D, Martínez-Banaclocha H, *et al.* MCC950 closes the active conformation of NLRP3 to an inactive state. Nat Chem Biol 2019; 15(6): 560-4.
[http://dx.doi.org/10.1038/s41589-019-0278-6] [PMID: 31086329]

[33]   Coll RC, Hill JR, Day CJ, *et al.* MCC950 directly targets the NLRP3 ATP-hydrolysis motif for inflammasome inhibition. Nat Chem Biol 2019; 15(6): 556-9.
[http://dx.doi.org/10.1038/s41589-019-0277-7] [PMID: 31086327]

[34]   Mak'Anyengo R, Duewell P, Reichl C, *et al.* Nlrp3-dependent IL-1β inhibits CD103+ dendritic cell differentiation in the gut. JCI Insight 2018; 3(5): e96322.
[http://dx.doi.org/10.1172/jci.insight.96322] [PMID: 29515025]

[35]   Yi YS. Regulatory roles of flavonoids on inflammasome activation during inflammatory responses. Mol Nutr Food Res 2018; 62(13): 1800147.
[http://dx.doi.org/10.1002/mnfr.201800147] [PMID: 29774640]

[36]   Ding N, Wei B, Fu X, Wang C, Wu Y. Natural products that target the NLRP3 inflammasome to treat fibrosis. Front Pharmacol 2020; 11: 591393.
[http://dx.doi.org/10.3389/fphar.2020.591393] [PMID: 33390969]

[37]   Liou CJ, Huang WC. Casticin inhibits interleukin-1β-induced ICAM-1 and MUC5AC expression by blocking NF-κB, PI3K-Akt, and MAPK signaling in human lung epithelial cells. Oncotarget 2017; 8(60): 101175-88.
[http://dx.doi.org/10.18632/oncotarget.20933] [PMID: 29254155]

[38]   Li X, Mei W, Huang Z, *et al.* Casticin suppresses monoiodoacetic acid-induced knee osteoarthritis through inhibiting HIF-1α/NLRP3 inflammasome signaling. Int Immunopharmacol 2020; 86: 106745.
[http://dx.doi.org/10.1016/j.intimp.2020.106745] [PMID: 32622201]

[39]   Zeng J, Chen Y, Ding R, *et al.* Isoliquiritigenin alleviates early brain injury after experimental intracerebral hemorrhage *via* suppressing ROS- and/or NF-κB-mediated NLRP3 inflammasome activation by promoting Nrf2 antioxidant pathway. J Neuroinflammation 2017; 14(1): 119.
[http://dx.doi.org/10.1186/s12974-017-0895-5] [PMID: 28610608]

[40]   Alzahrani S, Zaitone SA, Said E, *et al.* Protective effect of isoliquiritigenin on experimental diabetic nephropathy in rats: Impact on Sirt-1/NFκB balance and NLRP3 expression. Int Immunopharmacol 2020; 87: 106813.
[http://dx.doi.org/10.1016/j.intimp.2020.106813] [PMID: 32707499]

[41]   Gao Y, Lv X, Yang H, Peng L, Ci X. Isoliquiritigenin exerts antioxidative and anti-inflammatory effects *via* activating the KEAP-1/Nrf2 pathway and inhibiting the NF-κB and NLRP3 pathways in carrageenan-induced pleurisy. Food Funct 2020; 11(3): 2522-34.
[http://dx.doi.org/10.1039/C9FO01984G] [PMID: 32141447]

[42]   Li H, Chen FJ, Yang WL, Qiao HZ, Zhang SJ. Quercetin improves cognitive disorder in aging mice by inhibiting NLRP3 inflammasome activation. Food Funct 2021; 12(2): 717-25.
[http://dx.doi.org/10.1039/D0FO01900C] [PMID: 33338087]

[43]   Hu T, Lu XY, Shi JJ, *et al.* Quercetin protects against diabetic encephalopathy *via* SIRT1/NLRP3 pathway in db/db mice. J Cell Mol Med 2020; 24(6): 3449-59.
[http://dx.doi.org/10.1111/jcmm.15026] [PMID: 32000299]

[44]   Choe JY, Kim SK. Quercetin and ascorbic acid suppress fructose-induced NLRP3 inflammasome activation by blocking intracellular shuttling of TXNIP in human macrophage cell lines. Inflammation 2017; 40(3): 980-94.
[http://dx.doi.org/10.1007/s10753-017-0542-4] [PMID: 28326454]

[45]   Ding S, Wang H, Wang M, Bai L, Yu P, Wu W. Resveratrol alleviates chronic "real-world" ambient particulate matter-induced lung inflammation and fibrosis by inhibiting NLRP3 inflammasome activation in mice. Ecotoxicol Environ Saf 2019; 182: 109425.
[http://dx.doi.org/10.1016/j.ecoenv.2019.109425] [PMID: 31295660]

[46]   Shi YS, Li XX, Li HT, Zhang Y. Pelargonidin ameliorates CCl_4-induced liver fibrosis by suppressing the ROS-NLRP3-IL-1β axis *via* activating the Nrf2 pathway. Food Funct 2020; 11(6): 5156-65.
[http://dx.doi.org/10.1039/D0FO00660B] [PMID: 32432601]

[47]   Hua F, Shi L, Zhou P. Phenols and terpenoids: natural products as inhibitors of NLRP3 inflammasome in cardiovascular diseases. Inflammopharmacology 2022; 30(1): 137-47.
[http://dx.doi.org/10.1007/s10787-021-00918-4] [PMID: 35039992]

[48]   Liu C, Yang S, Wang K, *et al.* Alkaloids from Traditional Chinese Medicine against hepatocellular carcinoma. Biomed Pharmacother 2019; 120: 109543.
[http://dx.doi.org/10.1016/j.biopha.2019.109543] [PMID: 31655311]

[49]   Liang Q, Cai W, Zhao Y, *et al.* Lycorine ameliorates bleomycin-induced pulmonary fibrosis *via* inhibiting NLRP3 inflammasome activation and pyroptosis. Pharmacol Res 2020; 158: 104884.
[http://dx.doi.org/10.1016/j.phrs.2020.104884] [PMID: 32428667]

[50]   Wu J, Fu Y, Wu Y, Wu Z, Wang Z, Li P. Lycorine ameliorates isoproterenol-induced cardiac dysfunction mainly *via* inhibiting inflammation, fibrosis, oxidative stress and apoptosis. Bioengineered 2021; 12(1): 5583-94.

[http://dx.doi.org/10.1080/21655979.2021.1967019] [PMID: 34515620]

[51] Schimmel K, Jung M, Foinquinos A, *et al.* Natural compound library screening identifies new molecules for the treatment of cardiac fibrosis and diastolic dysfunction. Circulation 2020; 141(9): 751-67.
[http://dx.doi.org/10.1161/CIRCULATIONAHA.119.042559] [PMID: 31948273]

[52] Zhang H, Chen H, Wu X, *et al.* Tetramethylpyrazine alleviates diabetes-induced high platelet response and endothelial adhesion *via* inhibiting NLRP3 inflammasome activation. Phytomedicine 2022; 96: 153860.
[http://dx.doi.org/10.1016/j.phymed.2021.153860] [PMID: 34836743]

[53] Fu S, Wang J, Hao C, Dang H, Jiang S. Tetramethylpyrazine ameliorates depression by inhibiting TLR4-NLRP3 inflammasome signal pathway in mice. Psychopharmacology 2019; 236(7): 2173-85.
[http://dx.doi.org/10.1007/s00213-019-05210-6] [PMID: 30847567]

[54] Sun W, Li A, Wang Z, *et al.* Tetramethylpyrazine alleviates acute kidney injury by inhibiting NLRP3/HIF-1α and apoptosis. Mol Med Rep 2020; 22(4): 2655-64.
[http://dx.doi.org/10.3892/mmr.2020.11378] [PMID: 32945382]

[55] Wang Q, Wei S, Zhou S, *et al.* Hyperglycemia aggravates acute liver injury by promoting liver-resident macrophage NLRP 3 inflammasome activation *via* the inhibition of AMPK / MTOR -mediated autophagy induction. Immunol Cell Biol 2020; 98(1): 54-66.
[http://dx.doi.org/10.1111/imcb.12297] [PMID: 31625631]

[56] Song D, Hao J, Fan D. Biological properties and clinical applications of berberine. Front Med 2020; 14(5): 564-82.
[http://dx.doi.org/10.1007/s11684-019-0724-6] [PMID: 32335802]

[57] Sarbadhikary P, George BP, Abrahamse H. Inhibitory role of berberine, an isoquinoline alkaloid, on NLRP3 inflammasome activation for the treatment of inflammatory diseases. Molecules 2021; 26(20): 6238.
[http://dx.doi.org/10.3390/molecules26206238] [PMID: 34684819]

[58] Dinesh P, Rasool M. Berberine, an isoquinoline alkaloid suppresses TXNIP mediated NLRP3 inflammasome activation in MSU crystal stimulated RAW 264.7 macrophages through the upregulation of Nrf2 transcription factor and alleviates MSU crystal induced inflammation in rats. Int Immunopharmacol 2017; 44: 26-37.
[http://dx.doi.org/10.1016/j.intimp.2016.12.031] [PMID: 28068647]

[59] Zhou H, Feng L, Xu F, *et al.* Berberine inhibits palmitate-induced NLRP3 inflammasome activation by triggering autophagy in macrophages: A new mechanism linking berberine to insulin resistance improvement. Biomed Pharmacother 2017; 89: 864-74.
[http://dx.doi.org/10.1016/j.biopha.2017.03.003] [PMID: 28282788]

[60] Zeng Q, Deng H, Li Y, *et al.* Berberine directly targets the NEK7 protein to block the NEK7–NLRP3 interaction and exert anti-inflammatory activity. J Med Chem 2021; 64(1): 768-81.
[http://dx.doi.org/10.1021/acs.jmedchem.0c01743] [PMID: 33440945]

[61] Ai G, Huang Z, Cheng J. Gut microbiota-mediated transformation of coptisine into a novel metabolite 8-oxocoptisine: Insight into its superior anti-colitis effect. Front Pharmacol 2021; 12: 409.
[http://dx.doi.org/10.3389/fphar.2021.639020]

[62] Wu J, Luo Y, Jiang Q, *et al.* Coptisine from Coptis chinensis blocks NLRP3 inflammasome activation by inhibiting caspase-1. Pharmacol Res 2019; 147: 104348.
[http://dx.doi.org/10.1016/j.phrs.2019.104348] [PMID: 31336157]

[63] Koprowska K, Czyż M. Molecular mechanisms of parthenolide's action: Old drug with a new face. Postepy Hig Med Dosw 2010; 64: 100-14.
[PMID: 20354259]

[64] Juliana C, Fernandes-Alnemri T, Wu J, *et al.* Anti-inflammatory compounds parthenolide and Bay 11-

7082 are direct inhibitors of the inflammasome. J Biol Chem 2010; 285(13): 9792-802.
[http://dx.doi.org/10.1074/jbc.M109.082305] [PMID: 20093358]

[65]   Saadane A, Masters S, DiDonato J, Li J, Berger M. Parthenolide inhibits IkappaB kinase, NF-kappaB activation, and inflammatory response in cystic fibrosis cells and mice. Am J Respir Cell Mol Biol 2007; 36(6): 728-36.
[http://dx.doi.org/10.1165/rcmb.2006-0323OC] [PMID: 17272824]

[66]   Dawood M, Ooko E, Efferth T. Collateral sensitivity of parthenolide *via* NF-κB and HIF-α inhibition and epigenetic changes in drug-resistant cancer cell lines. Front Pharmacol 2019; 10: 542.
[http://dx.doi.org/10.3389/fphar.2019.00542] [PMID: 31164821]

[67]   Liu T, Zhang L, Joo D, Sun SC. NF-κB signaling in inflammation. Signal Transduct Target Ther 2017; 2: 1-9.
[http://dx.doi.org/10.1038/sigtrans.2017.23]

[68]   Zinatizadeh MR, Schock B, Chalbatani GM, Zarandi PK, Jalali SA, Miri SR. The nuclear factor kappa B (NF-kB) signaling in cancer development and immune diseases. Genes Dis 2021; 8(3): 287-97.
[http://dx.doi.org/10.1016/j.gendis.2020.06.005] [PMID: 33997176]

[69]   Xu L, Li L, Zhang CY, Schluesener H, Zhang ZY. Natural diterpenoid oridonin ameliorates experimental autoimmune neuritis by promoting anti-inflammatory macrophages through blocking notch pathway. Front Neurosci 2019; 13: 272.
[http://dx.doi.org/10.3389/fnins.2019.00272] [PMID: 31001070]

[70]   Xu M, Wan C, Huang S, *et al.* Oridonin protects against cardiac hypertrophy by promoting P21-related autophagy. Cell Death Dis 2019; 10(6): 403.
[http://dx.doi.org/10.1038/s41419-019-1617-y] [PMID: 31127082]

[71]   Shi M, Deng Y, Yu H, *et al.* Protective effects of oridonin on acute liver injury *via* impeding posttranslational modifications of interleukin-1 receptor-associated kinase 4 (IRAK4) in the toll-like receptor 4 (TLR4) signaling pathway. Mediators Inflamm 2019; 2019: 1-11.
[http://dx.doi.org/10.1155/2019/7634761] [PMID: 31611735]

[72]   Yang H, Huang J, Gao Y, Wen Z, Peng L, Ci X. Oridonin attenuates carrageenan-induced pleurisy *via* activation of the KEAP-1/Nrf2 pathway and inhibition of the TXNIP/NLRP3 and NF-κB pathway in mice. Inflammopharmacology 2020; 28(2): 513-23.
[http://dx.doi.org/10.1007/s10787-019-00644-y] [PMID: 31552548]

[73]   Jia T, Cai M, Ma X, Li M, Qiao J, Chen T. Oridonin inhibits IL-1β-induced inflammation in human osteoarthritis chondrocytes by activating PPAR-γ. Int Immunopharmacol 2019; 69: 382-8.
[http://dx.doi.org/10.1016/j.intimp.2019.01.049] [PMID: 30776647]

[74]   Wang M, Xu B, Liu L, Wang D. Oridonin attenuates dextran sulfate sodium-induced ulcerative colitis in mice *via* the Sirt1/NF-κB/p53 pathway. Mol Med Rep 2022; 26: 1-7.
[http://dx.doi.org/10.3892/mmr.2022.12888] [PMID: 36321784]

[75]   He H, Jiang H, Chen Y, *et al.* Oridonin is a covalent NLRP3 inhibitor with strong anti-inflammasome activity. Nat Commun 2018; 9(1): 2550.
[http://dx.doi.org/10.1038/s41467-018-04947-6] [PMID: 29959312]

[76]   Sharif H, Wang L, Wang WL, *et al.* Structural mechanism for NEK7-licensed activation of NLRP3 inflammasome. Nature 2019; 570(7761): 338-43.
[http://dx.doi.org/10.1038/s41586-019-1295-z] [PMID: 31189953]

[77]   Liu H, Gu C, Liu M, Liu G, Wang Y. NEK7 mediated assembly and activation of NLRP3 inflammasome downstream of potassium efflux in ventilator-induced lung injury. Biochem Pharmacol 2020; 177: 113998.
[http://dx.doi.org/10.1016/j.bcp.2020.113998] [PMID: 32353421]

[78]   Zhang J, Zhou Y, Sun Y, *et al.* Beneficial effects of Oridonin on myocardial ischemia/reperfusion injury: Insight gained by metabolomic approaches. Eur J Pharmacol 2019; 861: 172587.

[http://dx.doi.org/10.1016/j.ejphar.2019.172587] [PMID: 31377155]

[79]   Lu C, Chen C, Chen A, *et al.* Oridonin attenuates myocardial ischemia/reperfusion injury *via* downregulating oxidative stress and NLRP3 inflammasome pathway in mice. Evid Based Complement Alternat Med 2020; 2020: 1-9.
[http://dx.doi.org/10.1155/2020/7395187] [PMID: 32565873]

[80]   Wang Y, Wang Y, You F, Xue J. Novel use for old drugs: The emerging role of artemisinin and its derivatives in fibrosis. Pharmacol Res 2020; 157: 104829.
[http://dx.doi.org/10.1016/j.phrs.2020.104829] [PMID: 32360483]

[81]   Wen Y, Pan MM, Lv LL, *et al.* Artemisinin attenuates tubulointerstitial inflammation and fibrosis *via* the NF-κB/NLRP3 pathway in rats with 5/6 subtotal nephrectomy. J Cell Biochem 2019; 120(3): 4291-300.
[http://dx.doi.org/10.1002/jcb.27714] [PMID: 30260039]

[82]   Kim SK, Choe JY, Park KY. Anti-inflammatory effect of artemisinin on uric acid-induced NLRP3 inflammasome activation through blocking interaction between NLRP3 and NEK7. Biochem Biophys Res Commun 2019; 517(2): 338-45.
[http://dx.doi.org/10.1016/j.bbrc.2019.07.087] [PMID: 31358323]

[83]   Aktaş İ, Özmen Ö, Tutun H, Yalçın A, Türk A. Artemisinin attenuates doxorubicin induced cardiotoxicity and hepatotoxicity in rats. Biotech Histochem 2020; 95(2): 121-8.
[http://dx.doi.org/10.1080/10520295.2019.1647457] [PMID: 32064961]

[84]   Wang F, Gao Q, Yang J, *et al.* Artemisinin suppresses myocardial ischemia-reperfusion injury *via* NLRP3 inflammasome mechanism. Mol Cell Biochem 2020; 474(1-2): 171-80.
[http://dx.doi.org/10.1007/s11010-020-03842-3] [PMID: 32729005]

[85]   Gousiadou C, Kokubun T, Gotfredsen CH, Jensen SR. Further iridoid glucosides in the genus Manulea *(Scrophulariaceae)*. Phytochemistry 2015; 109: 43-8.
[http://dx.doi.org/10.1016/j.phytochem.2014.10.004] [PMID: 25457503]

[86]   Wang R, Dong Z, Lan X, Liao Z, Chen M. Sweroside alleviated LPS-induced inflammation *via* SIRT1 mediating NF-κB and FOXO1 signaling pathways in RAW264. 7 cells. Molecules 2019; 24(5): 872.
[http://dx.doi.org/10.3390/molecules24050872] [PMID: 30823686]

[87]   Wang J, Cai X, Ma R, Lei D, Pan X, Wang F. Anti-inflammatory effects of sweroside on LPS-induced ALI in mice *via* activating SIRT1. Inflammation 2021; 44(5): 1961-8.
[http://dx.doi.org/10.1007/s10753-021-01473-4] [PMID: 33913051]

[88]   Ma LQ, Yu Y, Chen H, *et al.* Sweroside alleviated aconitine-induced cardiac toxicity in H9c2 cardiomyoblast cell line. Front Pharmacol 2018; 9: 1138.
[http://dx.doi.org/10.3389/fphar.2018.01138] [PMID: 30410440]

[89]   Yang G, Jang JH, Kim SW, *et al.* Sweroside prevents non-alcoholic steatohepatitis by suppressing activation of the NLRP3 inflammasome. Int J Mol Sci 2020; 21(8): 2790.
[http://dx.doi.org/10.3390/ijms21082790] [PMID: 32316419]

[90]   Li J, Zhao C, Zhu Q, *et al.* Sweroside protects against myocardial ischemia–reperfusion injury by inhibiting oxidative stress and pyroptosis partially *via* modulation of the Keap1/Nrf2 axis. Front Cardiovasc Med 2021; 8: 650368.
[http://dx.doi.org/10.3389/fcvm.2021.650368] [PMID: 33816579]

[91]   Yang B, Yan P, Yang GZ, Cao HL, Wang F, Li B. Triptolide reduces ischemia/reperfusion injury in rats and H9C2 cells *via* inhibition of NF□κB, ROS and the ERK1/2 pathway. Int J Mol Med 2018; 41(6): 3127-36.
[http://dx.doi.org/10.3892/ijmm.2018.3537] [PMID: 29512681]

[92]   Tong L, Zhao Q, Datan E, *et al.* Triptolide: Reflections on two decades of research and prospects for the future. Nat Prod Rep 2021; 38(4): 843-60.
[http://dx.doi.org/10.1039/D0NP00054J] [PMID: 33146205]

[93]   Wen HL, Liang ZS, Zhang R, Yang K. Anti-inflammatory effects of triptolide improve left ventricular function in a rat model of diabetic cardiomyopathy. Cardiovasc Diabetol 2013; 12(1): 50.
[http://dx.doi.org/10.1186/1475-2840-12-50] [PMID: 23530831]

[94]   Pan XC, Liu Y, Cen YY, *et al.* Dual role of triptolide in interrupting the NLRP3 inflammasome pathway to attenuate cardiac fibrosis. Int J Mol Sci 2019; 20(2): 360.
[http://dx.doi.org/10.3390/ijms20020360] [PMID: 30654511]

[95]   Li R, Lu K, Wang Y, *et al.* Triptolide attenuates pressure overload-induced myocardial remodeling in mice *via* the inhibition of NLRP3 inflammasome expression. Biochem Biophys Res Commun 2017; 485(1): 69-75.
[http://dx.doi.org/10.1016/j.bbrc.2017.02.021] [PMID: 28202417]

[96]   Yan T, Wang H, Cao L, *et al.* Glycyrrhizin alleviates nonalcoholic steatohepatitis *via* modulating bile acids and meta-inflammation. Drug Metab Dispos 2018; 46(9): 1310-9.
[http://dx.doi.org/10.1124/dmd.118.082008] [PMID: 29959134]

[97]   Cui L, Li C, Zhuo Y, *et al.* Saikosaponin A inhibits the activation of pancreatic stellate cells by suppressing autophagy and the NLRP3 inflammasome *via* the AMPK/mTOR pathway. Biomed Pharmacother 2020; 128: 110216.
[http://dx.doi.org/10.1016/j.biopha.2020.110216] [PMID: 32497863]

[98]   Gong Q, He LL, Wang ML, *et al.* Anemoside B4 protects rat kidney from adenine-induced injury by attenuating inflammation and fibrosis and enhancing podocin and nephrin expression. Evid Based Complement Alternat Med 2019; 2019: 1-11.
[http://dx.doi.org/10.1155/2019/8031039] [PMID: 31275420]

[99]   Mathur A, Feng S, Hayward JA, *et al.* A multicomponent toxin from Bacillus cereus incites inflammation and shapes host outcome *via* the NLRP3 inflammasome. Nat Microbiol 2018; 4(2): 362-74.
[http://dx.doi.org/10.1038/s41564-018-0318-0] [PMID: 30531979]

[100] Perera AP, Fernando R, Shinde T, *et al.* MCC950, a specific small molecule inhibitor of NLRP3 inflammasome attenuates colonic inflammation in spontaneous colitis mice. Sci Rep 2018; 8(1): 8618.
[http://dx.doi.org/10.1038/s41598-018-26775-w] [PMID: 29872077]

[101] Gaidt MM, Ebert TS, Chauhan D, *et al.* Human monocytes engage an alternative inflammasome pathway. Immunity 2016; 44(4): 833-46.
[http://dx.doi.org/10.1016/j.immuni.2016.01.012] [PMID: 27037191]

[102] Coll RC, Robertson AAB, Chae JJ, *et al.* A small-molecule inhibitor of the NLRP3 inflammasome for the treatment of inflammatory diseases. Nat Med 2015; 21(3): 248-55.
[http://dx.doi.org/10.1038/nm.3806] [PMID: 25686105]

[103] Mullard A. NLRP3 inhibitors stoke anti-inflammatory ambitions. Nat Rev Drug Discov 2019; 18(6): 405-7.
[http://dx.doi.org/10.1038/d41573-019-00086-9] [PMID: 31160775]

[104] Chen QL, Yin HR, He QY, Wang Y. Targeting the NLRP3 inflammasome as new therapeutic avenue for inflammatory bowel disease. Biomed Pharmacother 2021; 138: 111442.
[http://dx.doi.org/10.1016/j.biopha.2021.111442] [PMID: 33667791]

[105] Jiang H, He H, Chen Y, *et al.* Identification of a selective and direct NLRP3 inhibitor to treat inflammatory disorders. J Exp Med 2017; 214(11): 3219-38.
[http://dx.doi.org/10.1084/jem.20171419] [PMID: 29021150]

[106] Pan LL, Liang W, Ren Z, *et al.* Cathelicidin-related antimicrobial peptide protects against ischaemia reperfusion-induced acute kidney injury in mice. Br J Pharmacol 2020; 177(12): 2726-42.
[http://dx.doi.org/10.1111/bph.14998] [PMID: 31976546]

[107] Qiao J, Wu X, Luo Q, *et al.* NLRP3 regulates platelet integrin αIIbβ3 outside-in signaling, hemostasis and arterial thrombosis. Haematologica 2018; 103(9): 1568-76.

[http://dx.doi.org/10.3324/haematol.2018.191700] [PMID: 29794149]

[108]   Marchetti C, Swartzwelter B, Gamboni F, *et al.* OLT1177, a β-sulfonyl nitrile compound, safe in humans, inhibits the NLRP3 inflammasome and reverses the metabolic cost of inflammation. Proc Natl Acad Sci 2018; 115(7): E1530-9.
[http://dx.doi.org/10.1073/pnas.1716095115] [PMID: 29378952]

[109]   Marchetti C, Swartzwelter B, Koenders MI, *et al.* NLRP3 inflammasome inhibitor OLT1177 suppresses joint inflammation in murine models of acute arthritis. Arthritis Res Ther 2018; 20(1): 169.
[http://dx.doi.org/10.1186/s13075-018-1664-2] [PMID: 30075804]

[110]   Toldo S, Mauro AG, Cutter Z, *et al.* The NLRP3 inflammasome inhibitor, OLT1177 (dapansutrile), reduces infarct size and preserves contractile function after ischemia reperfusion injury in the mouse. J Cardiovasc Pharmacol 2019; 73(4): 215-22.
[http://dx.doi.org/10.1097/FJC.0000000000000658] [PMID: 30747785]

[111]   Lonnemann N, Hosseini S, Marchetti C, *et al.* The NLRP3 inflammasome inhibitor OLT1177 rescues cognitive impairment in a mouse model of Alzheimer's disease. Proc Natl Acad Sci 2020; 117(50): 32145-54.
[http://dx.doi.org/10.1073/pnas.2009680117] [PMID: 33257576]

[112]   Klück V, Jansen TLTA, Janssen M, *et al.* Dapansutrile, an oral selective NLRP3 inflammasome inhibitor, for treatment of gout flares: an open-label, dose-adaptive, proof-of-concept, phase 2a trial. Lancet Rheumatol 2020; 2(5): e270-80.
[http://dx.doi.org/10.1016/S2665-9913(20)30065-5] [PMID: 33005902]

[113]   Shi H, Gao Y, Dong Z, *et al.* GSDMD-mediated cardiomyocyte pyroptosis promotes myocardial I/R injury. Circ Res 2021; 129(3): 383-96.
[http://dx.doi.org/10.1161/CIRCRESAHA.120.318629] [PMID: 34015941]

[114]   Pellegrini C, Fornai M, Colucci R, *et al.* A comparative study on the efficacy of NLRP3 inflammasome signaling inhibitors in a pre-clinical model of bowel inflammation. Front Pharmacol 2018; 9: 1405.
[http://dx.doi.org/10.3389/fphar.2018.01405] [PMID: 30559669]

[115]   Cocco M, Pellegrini C, Martínez-Banaclocha H, *et al.* Development of an acrylate derivative targeting the NLRP3 inflammasome for the treatment of inflammatory bowel disease. J Med Chem 2017; 60(9): 3656-71.
[http://dx.doi.org/10.1021/acs.jmedchem.6b01624] [PMID: 28410442]

[116]   Huang Y, Jiang H, Chen Y, *et al.* Tranilast directly targets NLRP 3 to treat inflammasome-driven diseases. EMBO Mol Med 2018; 10(4): e8689.
[http://dx.doi.org/10.15252/emmm.201708689] [PMID: 29531021]

[117]   Chen S, Wang Y, Pan Y, *et al.* Novel role for tranilast in regulating NLRP3 ubiquitination, vascular inflammation, and atherosclerosis. J Am Heart Assoc 2020; 9(12): e015513.
[http://dx.doi.org/10.1161/JAHA.119.015513] [PMID: 32476536]

[118]   Chauhan D, Vande Walle L, Lamkanfi M. Therapeutic modulation of inflammasome pathways. Immunol Rev 2020; 297(1): 123-38.
[http://dx.doi.org/10.1111/imr.12908] [PMID: 32770571]

[119]   Liu W, Guo W, Wu J, *et al.* A novel benzo[d]imidazole derivate prevents the development of dextran sulfate sodium-induced murine experimental colitis *via* inhibition of NLRP3 inflammasome. Biochem Pharmacol 2013; 85(10): 1504-12.
[http://dx.doi.org/10.1016/j.bcp.2013.03.008] [PMID: 23506741]

[120]   Riddle MC. Editorial: sulfonylureas differ in effects on ischemic preconditioning--is it time to retire glyburide? J Clin Endocrinol Metab 2003; 88(2): 528-30.
[http://dx.doi.org/10.1210/jc.2002-021971] [PMID: 12574174]

[121]   Gribble FM, Reimann F. Sulphonylurea action revisited: The post-cloning era. Diabetologia 2003;

46(7): 875-91.
[http://dx.doi.org/10.1007/s00125-003-1143-3] [PMID: 12819907]

[122]   Yang J, Yang J, Huang X, *et al.* Glibenclamide alleviates LPS-induced acute lung injury through nlrp3 inflammasome signaling pathway. Mediators Inflamm 2022; 2022: 1-12.
[http://dx.doi.org/10.1155/2022/8457010] [PMID: 35185385]

[123]   Lamkanfi M, Mueller JL, Vitari AC, *et al.* Glyburide inhibits the Cryopyrin/Nalp3 inflammasome. J Cell Biol 2009; 187(1): 61-70.
[http://dx.doi.org/10.1083/jcb.200903124] [PMID: 19805629]

[124]   Zhao Y, Guo Q, Zhu Q, *et al.* Flavonoid VI-16 protects against DSS-induced colitis by inhibiting Txnip-dependent NLRP3 inflammasome activation in macrophages *via* reducing oxidative stress. Mucosal Immunol 2019; 12(5): 1150-63.
[http://dx.doi.org/10.1038/s41385-019-0177-x] [PMID: 31152156]

[125]   Khakpai F, Ramezanikhah M, Valizadegan F, Zarrindast MR. Synergistic effect between imipramine and citicoline upon induction of analgesic and antidepressant effects in mice. Neurosci Lett 2021; 760: 136095.
[http://dx.doi.org/10.1016/j.neulet.2021.136095] [PMID: 34216716]

[126]   Carpinteiro A, Edwards MJ, Hoffmann M, *et al.* Pharmacological inhibition of acid sphingomyelinase prevents uptake of SARS-CoV-2 by epithelial cells. Cell Rep Med 2020; 1(8): 100142.
[http://dx.doi.org/10.1016/j.xcrm.2020.100142] [PMID: 33163980]

[127]   Yoshida S, Noguchi A, Kikuchi W, Fukaya H, Igarashi K, Takahashi T. Elevation of serum acid sphingomyelinase activity in children with acute respiratory syncytial virus bronchiolitis. Tohoku J Exp Med 2017; 243(4): 275-81.
[http://dx.doi.org/10.1620/tjem.243.275] [PMID: 29238000]

[128]   Alcocer-Gómez E, Casas-Barquero N, Williams MR, *et al.* Antidepressants induce autophagy dependent-NLRP3-inflammasome inhibition in Major depressive disorder. Pharmacol Res 2017; 121: 114-21.
[http://dx.doi.org/10.1016/j.phrs.2017.04.028] [PMID: 28465217]

[129]   Jiang J, Shi Y, Cao J, Lu Y, Sun G, Yang J. Role of ASM/Cer/TXNIP signaling module in the NLRP3 inflammasome activation. Lipids Health Dis 2021; 20(1): 19.
[http://dx.doi.org/10.1186/s12944-021-01446-4] [PMID: 33612104]

[130]   Steuber TD, Lee J, Holloway A, Andrus MR. Nondihydropyridine calcium channel blockers for the treatment of proteinuria: A review of the literature. Ann Pharmacother 2019; 53(10): 1050-9.
[http://dx.doi.org/10.1177/1060028019843644] [PMID: 30966785]

[131]   Zhou F, Zhang Y, Chen J, Hu Y, Xu Y. Verapamil ameliorates hepatic metaflammation by inhibiting thioredoxin-interacting protein/NLRP3 pathways. Front Endocrinol 2018; 9: 640.
[http://dx.doi.org/10.3389/fendo.2018.00640] [PMID: 30429827]

[132]   Malayeri A, Zakerkish M, Ramesh F, Galehdari H, Hemmati AA, Angali KA. The effect of verapamil on TXNIP gene expression, GLP1R mRNA, FBS, HbA1c, and lipid profile in T2DM patients receiving metformin and sitagliptin. Diabetes Ther 2021; 12(10): 2701-13.
[http://dx.doi.org/10.1007/s13300-021-01145-4] [PMID: 34480721]

[133]   Lipinski MJ, Frias JC. Molecule 16673-34-0. J Cardiovasc Pharmacol 2014; 63(4): 314-5.
[http://dx.doi.org/10.1097/FJC.0000000000000070] [PMID: 24662491]

[134]   Hu JJ, Liu X, Xia S, *et al.* FDA-approved disulfiram inhibits pyroptosis by blocking gasdermin D pore formation. Nat Immunol 2020; 21(7): 736-45.
[http://dx.doi.org/10.1038/s41590-020-0669-6] [PMID: 32367036]

[135]   Hu JJ, Liu X, Zhao J, *et al.* Identification of pyroptosis inhibitors that target a reactive cysteine in gasdermin D. BioRxiv 2018; 2018: 365908.
[http://dx.doi.org/10.1101/365908]

[136] Zhang J, Wei K. Necrosulfonamide reverses pyroptosis-induced inhibition of proliferation and differentiation of osteoblasts through the NLRP3/caspase-1/GSDMD pathway. Exp Cell Res 2021; 405(2): 112648.
[http://dx.doi.org/10.1016/j.yexcr.2021.112648] [PMID: 34119493]

[137] Rathkey JK, Zhao J, Liu Z, *et al.* Chemical disruption of the pyroptotic pore-forming protein gasdermin D inhibits inflammatory cell death and sepsis. Sci Immunol 2018; 3(26): eaat2738.
[http://dx.doi.org/10.1126/sciimmunol.aat2738] [PMID: 30143556]

[138] Pandey A, Dabhade P, Kumarasamy A. Inflammatory effects of subacute exposure of Roundup in rat liver and adipose tissue. Dose Response 2019; 17: 2.
[http://dx.doi.org/10.1177/1559325819843380] [PMID: 31205454]

[139] Slee EA, Zhu H, Chow SC, MacFARLANE M, Nicholson DW, Cohen GM. Benzyloxycarbonyl-Va-
-Ala-Asp (OMe) fluoromethylketone (Z-VAD.FMK) inhibits apoptosis by blocking the processing of CPP32. Biochem J 1996; 315(1): 21-4.
[http://dx.doi.org/10.1042/bj3150021] [PMID: 8670109]

[140] Ekert PG, Silke J, Vaux DL. Caspase inhibitors. Cell Death Differ 1999; 6(11): 1081-6.
[http://dx.doi.org/10.1038/sj.cdd.4400594] [PMID: 10578177]

[141] Li H, Guan Y, Liang B, *et al.* Therapeutic potential of MCC950, a specific inhibitor of NLRP3 inflammasome. Eur J Pharmacol 2022; 928: 175091.
[http://dx.doi.org/10.1016/j.ejphar.2022.175091] [PMID: 35714692]

[142] Mullard A. Roche snaps up another NLRP3 contender. Nat Rev Drug Discov 2020; 19(11): 744-5.
[PMID: 33020643]

[143] Burger JA, Chiorazzi N. B cell receptor signaling in chronic lymphocytic leukemia. Trends Immunol 2013; 34(12): 592-601.
[http://dx.doi.org/10.1016/j.it.2013.07.002] [PMID: 23928062]

[144] Parmar S, Patel K, Pinilla-Ibarz J. Ibrutinib (imbruvica): A novel targeted therapy for chronic lymphocytic leukemia. P&T 2014; 39(7): 483-519.
[PMID: 25083126]

[145] Akinleye A, Chen Y, Mukhi N, Song Y, Liu D. Ibrutinib and novel BTK inhibitors in clinical development. J Hematol Oncol 2013; 6(1): 59.
[http://dx.doi.org/10.1186/1756-8722-6-59] [PMID: 23958373]

[146] Tang T, Gong T, Jiang W, Zhou R. GPCRs in NLRP3 inflammasome activation, regulation, and therapeutics. Trends Pharmacol Sci 2018; 39(9): 798-811.
[http://dx.doi.org/10.1016/j.tips.2018.07.002] [PMID: 30054020]

[147] Swanson KV, Deng M, Ting JPY. The NLRP3 inflammasome: molecular activation and regulation to therapeutics. Nat Rev Immunol 2019; 19(8): 477-89.
[http://dx.doi.org/10.1038/s41577-019-0165-0] [PMID: 31036962]

[148] La Manna S, Di Natale C, Florio D, Marasco D. Peptides as therapeutic agents for inflammatory-related diseases. Int J Mol Sci 2018; 19(9): 2714.
[http://dx.doi.org/10.3390/ijms19092714] [PMID: 30208640]

[149] Ryan S, Shiels J, Taggart CC, Dalton JP, Weldon S. Fasciola hepatica-derived molecules as regulators of the host immune response. Front Immunol 2020; 11: 2182.
[http://dx.doi.org/10.3389/fimmu.2020.02182] [PMID: 32983184]

[150] Alvarado R, To J, Lund ME, *et al.* The immune modulatory peptide FhHDM-1 secreted by the helminth Fasciola hepatica prevents NLRP3 inflammasome activation by inhibiting endolysosomal acidification in macrophages. FASEB J 2017; 31(1): 85-95.
[http://dx.doi.org/10.1096/fj.201500093r] [PMID: 27682204]

[151] Liu Y, Zhang Y, Feng Q, *et al.* GPA peptide attenuates sepsis-induced acute lung injury in mice *via*

inhibiting oxidative stress and pyroptosis of alveolar macrophage. Oxid Med Cell Longev 2021; 2021: 1-12.
[http://dx.doi.org/10.1155/2021/5589472] [PMID: 34992715]

[152] Deng Z, Ni J, Wu X, Wei H, Peng J. GPA peptide inhibits NLRP3 inflammasome activation to ameliorate colitis through AMPK pathway. Aging 2020; 12(18): 18522-44.
[http://dx.doi.org/10.18632/aging.103825] [PMID: 32950971]

[153] Sušjan P, Lainšček D, Strmšek Ž, Hodnik V, Anderluh G, Hafner-Bratkovič I. Selective inhibition of NLRP3 inflammasome by designed peptide originating from ASC. FASEB J 2020; 34(8): 11068-86.
[http://dx.doi.org/10.1096/fj.201902938RR] [PMID: 32648626]

[154] Yuan T, Sun Z, Zhao W, Wang T, Zhang J, Niu D. Phoenixin: a newly discovered peptide with multi-functions. Protein Pept Lett 2017; 24(6): 472-5.
[PMID: 28176660]

[155] Wang J, Zheng B, Yang S, Tang X, Wang J, Wei D. The protective effects of phoenixin-14 against lipopolysaccharide-induced inflammation and inflammasome activation in astrocytes. Inflamm Res 2020; 69(8): 779-87.
[http://dx.doi.org/10.1007/s00011-020-01355-9] [PMID: 32435966]

[156] Liu H, Wu X, Luo J, *et al.* Adiponectin peptide alleviates oxidative stress and NLRP3 inflammasome activation after cerebral ischemia-reperfusion injury by regulating AMPK/GSK-3β. Exp Neurol 2020; 329: 113302.
[http://dx.doi.org/10.1016/j.expneurol.2020.113302] [PMID: 32275928]

[157] Li LH, Ju TC, Hsieh CY, *et al.* A synthetic cationic antimicrobial peptide inhibits inflammatory response and the NLRP3 inflammasome by neutralizing LPS and ATP. PLoS One 2017; 12(7): e0182057.
[http://dx.doi.org/10.1371/journal.pone.0182057] [PMID: 28750089]

[158] Healy LD, Fernández JA, Mosnier LO, Griffin JH. Activated protein C and PAR1-derived and PAR3-derived peptides are anti-inflammatory by suppressing macrophage NLRP3 inflammasomes. J Thromb Haemost 2021; 19(1): 269-80.
[http://dx.doi.org/10.1111/jth.15133] [PMID: 33049092]

[159] Pal A, Neo K, Rajamani L, *et al.* Inhibition of NLRP3 inflammasome activation by cell-permeable stapled peptides. Sci Rep 2019; 9(1): 4913.
[http://dx.doi.org/10.1038/s41598-019-41211-3] [PMID: 30894604]

[160] Del Gatto A, Cobb SL, Zhang J, Zaccaro L. Editorial: Peptidomimetics: Synthetic tools for drug discovery and development. Front Chem 2021; 9: 802120.
[http://dx.doi.org/10.3389/fchem.2021.802120] [PMID: 34869243]

[161] Li Petri G, Di Martino S, De Rosa M. Peptidomimetics: An overview of recent medicinal chemistry efforts toward the discovery of novel small molecule inhibitors. J Med Chem 2022; 65(11): 7438-75.
[http://dx.doi.org/10.1021/acs.jmedchem.2c00123] [PMID: 35604326]

[162] MacKenzie SH, Schipper JL, Clark AC. The potential for caspases in drug discovery. Curr Opin Drug Discov Devel 2010; 13(5): 568-76.
[PMID: 20812148]

[163] Boxer MB, Shen M, Auld DS, Wells JA, Thomas CJ. A small molecule inhibitor of Caspase 1. Probe Reports from the NIH Molecular Libraries Program 2011.

[164] Rudolphi K, Gerwin N, Verzijl N, van der Kraan P, van den Berg W. Pralnacasan, an inhibitor of interleukin-1β converting enzyme, reduces joint damage in two murine models of osteoarthritis. Osteoarthritis Cartilage 2003; 11(10): 738-46.
[http://dx.doi.org/10.1016/S1063-4584(03)00153-5] [PMID: 13129693]

[165] Bauer C, Loher F, Dauer M, *et al.* The ICE inhibitor pralnacasan prevents DSS-induced colitis in C57BL/6 mice and suppresses IP-10 mRNA but not TNF-α mRNA expression. Dig Dis Sci 2007;

52(7): 1642-52.
[http://dx.doi.org/10.1007/s10620-007-9802-8] [PMID: 17393315]

[166] Maroso M, Balosso S, Ravizza T, *et al.* Interleukin-1β biosynthesis inhibition reduces acute seizures and drug resistant chronic epileptic activity in mice. Neurotherapeutics 2011; 8(2): 304-15.
[http://dx.doi.org/10.1007/s13311-011-0039-z] [PMID: 21431948]

[167] Flores J, Noël A, Foveau B, Lynham J, Lecrux C, LeBlanc AC. Caspase-1 inhibition alleviates cognitive impairment and neuropathology in an Alzheimer's disease mouse model. Nat Commun 2018; 9(1): 3916.
[http://dx.doi.org/10.1038/s41467-018-06449-x] [PMID: 30254377]

[168] Satish M, Agrawal DK. Atherothrombosis and the NLRP3 inflammasome – endogenous mechanisms of inhibition. Transl Res 2020; 215: 75-85.
[http://dx.doi.org/10.1016/j.trsl.2019.08.003] [PMID: 31469975]

[169] Kajitani N, Iwata M, Miura A, *et al.* Prefrontal cortex infusion of beta-hydroxybutyrate, an endogenous NLRP3 inflammasome inhibitor, produces antidepressant-like effects in a rodent model of depression. Neuropsychopharmacol Rep 2020; 40(2): 157-65.
[http://dx.doi.org/10.1002/npr2.12099] [PMID: 32125791]

[170] Yamanashi T, Iwata M, Shibushita M, *et al.* Beta-hydroxybutyrate, an endogenous NLRP3 inflammasome inhibitor, attenuates anxiety-related behavior in a rodent post-traumatic stress disorder model. Sci Rep 2020; 10(1): 21629.
[http://dx.doi.org/10.1038/s41598-020-78410-2] [PMID: 33303808]

[171] Khan MM, Kempuraj D, Thangavel R, Zaheer A. Protection of MPTP-induced neuroinflammation and neurodegeneration by Pycnogenol. Neurochem Int 2013; 62(4): 379-88.
[http://dx.doi.org/10.1016/j.neuint.2013.01.029] [PMID: 23391521]

[172] Wang S, Yuan YH, Chen NH, Wang HB. The mechanisms of NLRP3 inflammasome/pyroptosis activation and their role in Parkinson's disease. Int Immunopharmacol 2019; 67: 458-64.
[http://dx.doi.org/10.1016/j.intimp.2018.12.019] [PMID: 30594776]

[173] Yan Y, Jiang W, Liu L, *et al.* Dopamine controls systemic inflammation through inhibition of NLRP3 inflammasome. Cell 2015; 160(1-2): 62-73.
[http://dx.doi.org/10.1016/j.cell.2014.11.047] [PMID: 25594175]

[174] Gonzalez-Rey E, Delgado M. Role of vasoactive intestinal peptide in inflammation and autoimmunity. Curr Opin Investig Drugs 2005; 6: 1116-23.
[PMID: 16312132]

[175] Zhou Y, Zhang CY, Duan JX, *et al.* Vasoactive intestinal peptide suppresses the NLRP3 inflammasome activation in lipopolysaccharide-induced acute lung injury mice and macrophages. Biomed Pharmacother 2020; 121: 109596.
[http://dx.doi.org/10.1016/j.biopha.2019.109596] [PMID: 31731193]

[176] Fu Y, Wang Y, Du L, *et al.* Resveratrol inhibits ionising irradiation-induced inflammation in MSCs by activating SIRT1 and limiting NLRP-3 inflammasome activation. Int J Mol Sci 2013; 14(7): 14105-18.
[http://dx.doi.org/10.3390/ijms140714105] [PMID: 23880858]

[177] Chen L, Lan Z. Polydatin attenuates potassium oxonate-induced hyperuricemia and kidney inflammation by inhibiting NF-κB/NLRP3 inflammasome activation *via* the AMPK/SIRT1 pathway. Food Funct 2017; 8(5): 1785-92.
[http://dx.doi.org/10.1039/C6FO01561A] [PMID: 28428988]

[178] Li Y, Wang P, Yang X, *et al.* SIRT1 inhibits inflammatory response partly through regulation of NLRP3 inflammasome in vascular endothelial cells. Mol Immunol 2016; 77: 148-56.
[http://dx.doi.org/10.1016/j.molimm.2016.07.018] [PMID: 27505710]

[179] Voet S, Mc Guire C, Hagemeyer N, *et al.* A20 critically controls microglia activation and inhibits inflammasome-dependent neuroinflammation. Nat Commun 2018; 9(1): 2036.

[http://dx.doi.org/10.1038/s41467-018-04376-5] [PMID: 29789522]

[180]   Schlicher L, Wissler M, Preiss F, *et al.* SPATA 2 promotes CYLD activity and regulates TNF -induced NF -κB signaling and cell death. EMBO Rep 2016; 17(10): 1485-97.
[http://dx.doi.org/10.15252/embr.201642592] [PMID: 27458237]

[181]   Guo HJ, Tadi P. Biochemistry, Ubiquitination. StatPearls. StatPearls Publishing 2021.

[182]   Yang XD, Li W, Zhang S, *et al.* PLK 4 deubiquitination by Spata2-CYLD suppresses NEK7-mediated NLRP3 inflammasome activation at the centrosome. EMBO J 2020; 39(2): e102201.
[http://dx.doi.org/10.15252/embj.2019102201] [PMID: 31762063]

[183]   Ren GM, Li J, Zhang XC, *et al.* Pharmacological targeting of NLRP3 deubiquitination for treatment of NLRP3-associated inflammatory diseases. Sci Immunol 2021; 6(58): eabe2933.
[http://dx.doi.org/10.1126/sciimmunol.abe2933] [PMID: 33931568]

CHAPTER 8

The Potential Value of Sputum Level Interleukin-38 and NLRP3 Inflammasome in Severe Childhood Asthma

Agnès Hamzaoui[1], Sabrine Louhaichi[1] and Kamel Hamzaoui[1,*]

[1] *Tunis El Manar University, Medicine Faculty of Tunis, Department of Paediatric and Respiratory Diseases, Abderrahman Mami Hospital, Pavillon B, Ariana, Research Laboratory 19SP02 "Chronic Pulmonary Pathologies: From Genome to Management", Tunisia*

Abstract: Asthma in children is associated with serious exacerbations that are modulated by inflammation. The expression of inflammatory cytokines varies according to the severity of the disease. The transition from the state of exacerbation of the disease to the state of cure always passes through a relationship between inflammatory and anti-inflammatory mediators. This study looks at the expression of IL-38 and NLRP3 inflammasome in severe childhood asthma. NLRP3 inflammasome is upregulated in severe asthma, contrasting with low levels of IL-38. The inflammatory pattern of severe asthma in children is characterized by the expression of IL-17, IL-32, IL-1β, and NLRP3 inflammasome.

Keywords: ELISA, Gene expression, Induced sputum, Immunity, Severe asthma.

INTRODUCTION

Any immune response in the body begins with the pro-inflammatory phase. The regulatory process that follows restores immune homeostasis. Acute inflammation depends mainly on tissue immunity involving macrophages and dendritic cells. Inflammation is limited in time as resolution occurs with the removal of the initial stimulus. Pathogen-associated molecular patterns (PAMPs) interact with pattern recognition receptors (PRR) and danger-associated molecular patterns (DAMPs) receptors to trigger the inflammatory process. Toll-like receptors (TLRs), nucleotide-binding oligomerisation domain (NOD)-like receptors (NLR) and mannose-binding lectin (MBL) [1, 2] constitute the PRRs family. Activation signals include viral, bacterial (*e.g.*, LPS) [3] and cellular products (*e.g.*, nucleic

[*] **Corresponding author Kamel Hamzaoui:** Tunis El Manar University, Medicine Faculty of Tunis, Department of Paediatric and Respiratory Diseases, Abderrahman Mami Hospital, Pavillon B, Ariana, Research Laboratory 19SP02 "Chronic Pulmonary Pathologies: From Genome to Management", Tunisia; E-mail: kamel.hamzaoui@gmail.com

Puneetpal Singh (Ed.)
All rights reserved-© 2024 Bentham Science Publishers

acids) [4]. The inflammasome represents another innate system of immune activation [5, 6]. The release of DAMPs may also be due to several other metabolic triggers, chemical or physical [7]. However, chronic diseases are associated with persistent inflammation that implies continuously recruiting leuco- cytes to the target organ. Significant physiological and structural changes result in tissue remodelling and disease exacerbation. The main cytokines involved in this chronic inflammatory pathway of chronic inflammation are interleukin (IL)-1α, IL-1β, IL-6 and tumour necrosis factor-α (TNF-α). All these pro-inflammatory mediators are confronted with inhibitory mediators such as IL-37, IL-38, and IL-35.

We investigated the mechanisms of asthma. Activated inflammatory responses are major causes and common features of numerous disorders. Nucleotide-binding oligomerization domain (NOD) and leucine-rich repeat (LRR)-containing receptors or NOD-like receptors (NLRs) are inflammasomes that are critical in the initiation of innate immune responses to host-derived danger signals [8]. The activation of many prototypic NLRs, including NLR with a pyrin domain (NLRP) containing NLRP1, NLRP3, and NLRP4, results in the maturation and release of different pro-inflammatory cytokines (IL-1 β, and IL-18) [9]. The process has been suggested to be of great importance in the occurrence of programmed cell death, which is called pyroptosis [10]. As a part of the innate immune system, the NLRP inflammasome regulates the host's defence against harmful threats. Its activation is implicated in inflammatory sites (bronchoalveolar lavage induces sputum).

The NLRP inflammasome is a multi-protein complex that mainly consists of the nucleotide-binding oligomerization domain, leucine-rich repeat, and pyrin domain. All the NLRP (1, 3, 4) AIM2 inflammasomes contain caspase-1. The NLRP3 inflammasome has been deeply studied. Recent results describe the contribution of caspase-4/5 and caspase-11 in the activation of NLRP3 inflammasome in humans [11, 12]. In bronchi, NLRP3 inflammasome is activated [13] in circulating neutrophils, inducing IL-1b and IL-18 production [14]. NLRP3 inflammasome activation has been studied in several pulmonary diseases, including obstructive conditions (COPD and asthma), interstitial lung diseases and neoplasms [15, 16]. The activation of NLRP3 could be inappropriate, leading to persistent inflammation [17]. Despite these observations, the precise role of NLRP3 inflammasome in asthma is not clearly described. The objective of our work is to investigate the NLRP3 inflammasome in asthmatic patients.

Activation of the NLRP3 Inflammasome

NLRP3 inflammasome activation requires two steps: the first signal and a second signal. The first signal is also called the priming signal, which is usually PAMP. Some studies have shown that IL-1 β and TNF-α can also be used as priming signals. They initiate the gene transcription of NLRP3, CASP1, IL-1β and IL-18 through the NF- κB pathway and produce more pro-IL-1 β and pro-IL-18. DAMP and PAMP represent the second signal, which is the activation mechanism, mainly including K^+ efflux and Ca^+ influx, which alter the cellular composition of K^+ and Ca^{2+}. K^+ efflux is triggered by binding the cell membrane of extracellular ATP to the ATP-ligand-gated channel P2X7. The lowering of intracellular K^+ results in Pannexin-1 opening, allowing microbial molecules to penetrate the cytoplasm. These molecules recognized by the LRR are able to activate NLRP3. In addition, perforin causes an outflow of K^+ from the cell, forming pores in the plasma membrane, further promoting the passage of microorganisms into the cell [18]. Other molecules act in a similar way on K^+ efflux, such as membrane attack complex (MAC), silica, alum, and calcium pyrophosphate crystals [19, 20]. The cellular afflux of extracellular Ca^2 also activates NLRP3 [20]. Secondary to lysosome damage, cathepsin E is released into the cytoplasm and activates NLRP3 through LRR [3]. In the same way, DNA released by mitochondrial damage triggers NLRP3 activation [21, 22]. The NADPH oxidase, xanthine oxidase, cytochrome P450, cyclooxygenase and lipoxygenase can also generate ROS to induce NLRP3 activation [23].

Regulation of NLRP3 Inflammasome

The NLRP3 inflammasome includes transcriptional and post-transcriptional regulation and post-translational modification. Transcriptional regulation in cells is under the control of NF-κB, ensuring the functionality of the receptor protein NLRP3 before its activation. NF-κB regulation is linked to the presence of Toll-like receptor (TLR) or tumour necrosis factor (TNF). TNF receptors (TNFRs) suppress the inflammasome activation by blocking TNF. Moreover, type I interferons favour the release of interleukin 10 (IL-10), controlling the production of pro-IL-1β, thus blocking the activation of the inflammasome. miRNAs are responsible for post-transcriptional regulation. When miR-233 binds to the NLRP3 3' untranslated region, NLRP3 receptor proteins are downregulated, thereby blocking inflammasome activation [24, 25]. The inhibition of post-translational modification corresponds to the expression of the iNOS gene induced by type I interferon, leading to the release of ROS by the production of NO. Studies report that the LRR domain of NLRP3 can be ubiquitinated by the membrane-associated protein RING CH VII (WALK-7). Phosphorylation of its Ser291 residue may also negatively regulate NLRP3 activation [26].

NLRP3 in Asthma

Asthma is a respiratory disease with an inflammatory connotation targeting the airways, causing the proliferation of a variety of inflammatory and resident cells (bronchial epithelium, smooth muscle cells, *etc.*). Pathologically, asthma is characterized by mucosa infiltration with polynuclear eosinophils and CD4+T lymphocytes [27]. This persistent inflammation is associated with airway hyperresponsiveness (AHR), defined as a reversible decrease in airflow. Clinically, bronchial disease induces exacerbations, the symptoms of which are wheezes, dyspnoea, chest tightness and cough. Asthma is usually worse at night or very early in the morning. Very early in the course of the disease, the structure of the airway is modified, leading to remodelling with subepithelial fibrosis and muscular hyperplasia. This structural change exaggerates airflow limitation and probably reduces response to inhaled steroids. Numerous studies have suggested the possibility of NLRP3 involvement in asthma inflammation. Cheng *et al.* reported an increase in NLRP3 and its products, caspase-1 and IL-1β, along with IL-18, in bronchoalveolar lavage fluid from mouse models of asthmatic airway inflammation sensitized to ovalbumin (OVA) [28]. In asthmatic patients, IL-1β protein was increased in induced sputum as well as the expression of NLRP3 and NOD-like domain 1 [29].

Activation of NLRP3 Inflammasome in Asthma

A murine model triggered a severe steroid-resistant allergic airway disease associated with chlamydia/haemophilus and ovalbumin (OVA) sensitization [16]. Infection caused by pathogenic microorganisms exaggerated NLRP3, caspase-1 and IL-1β production, inducing inflammation by steroid-resistant neutrophils. Rodríguez-Alcázar and collaborators reported that Charcot-Leyden released by eosinophils binds to the NLRP3 receptor, promoting NLRP3 activation in ASC and IL-1β production and strengthening chronic inflammation [30]. Tsai *et al.* found that Der f1, a dust mite allergen, promotes pyroptosis and IL-1β production by human bronchial epithelial cells (HBECs) *in vitro via* the NLRP3-caspase-1 pathway [31]. Mice treated with OVA and titanium dioxide nanoparticles (NP) expressed high levels of NLRP3 and its downstream products. Similarly, NP silica-treated mice also exhibited more airway inflammation in asthma models through NLRP3 activation [32-33].

NLRP3 inflammasome is activated in the lung through contact with PAMPs and DAMPs, facilitating the production of inflammatory mediators (IL-1β, IL-18) and inducing the chronicity of the inflammation. Tissue damage and fibrosis are also observed. Various NLRP3 inflammasome inhibitors have been described, including direct or indirect inflammasome inhibitors, which block the NLRP3 inflammasome by binding to key targets upstream or downstream of its activation pathway.

In this report, we investigated the role of NLRP3 inflammasome in induced sputum in severe asthma. The role of the NLRP3 inflammasome process was contrasted by the expression of a novel anti-inflammatory mediator, IL-38.

Interleukin-38

IL-38 is a recently discovered cytokine, and is a member of the IL-1 cytokine family that shares some characteristics of IL-1Ra, *i.e.*, binding the same IL-1 receptor type I. The IL1F10 gene is located in the IL-1 family cluster on chromosome 2 in human subjects and mice, between the genes encoding IL-36Ra and IL-1Ra. IL-38 is highly homologous to IL-36Ra and IL-1Ra, suggesting that it might act as an IL-1 family antagonist. IL-38 expression was reported in the skin, tonsil, thymus, spleen, foetal liver, and salivary glands [33]. IL-38 is defined as a cytokine that has a protective role in various pathologies. The effects of IL-38 are similar to IL-36Ra in that it binds to the IL-36 receptor, suppressing specific Th17 manifestations [34].

Asthma

Asthma affects more than 300 million people worldwide. Characterized by variable symptoms of shortness of breath, cough, and chest tightness, asthma is associated with chronic airway inflammation, reversible expiratory airflow limitation, and airway hyperresponsiveness [35, 36]. Severe asthma is defined as a disease inadequately controlled despite a high dose of inhaled steroids associated with a long-acting bronchodilator [37]. It is considered that 10% of adult patients and 2.5% of asthmatic children are severe, suffering from recurrent exacerbations, frequent healthcare visits, hospitalization, and risk of death [38]. They require repetitive glucocorticoid bursts or maintenance of oral glucocorticoids [35]. In these patients, add-on treatment, which may include biological therapies, is needed to reduce the disease burden.

Severe asthma is heterogeneous with several phenotypes depending on onset age (childhood or adulthood), allergy and co-morbidities, such as obesity, gender, lung function limitation, *etc*. These clinical phenotypes are associated with biological diversity with different patterns of airway inflammation. Endotypes are characterized by the increase (or the absence) of eosinophils or neutrophils in sputum and bronchial biopsy. Being easier to use, blood eosinophilia and exhaled NO are considered the biomarkers for eosinophilic asthma, considered as type 2 high-inflammation (type 2–high) asthma. Type 2–low asthma, neutrophilic asthma and paucigranulocytic asthma represent type 2-low phenotypes. More than

50% of severe asthma cases are identified as type 2–high asthma [39-40], the main target of biologics therapy. However, the efficacy of these treatments varies between the patients, and T2 low phenotypes are essentially resistant.

The reactivation of Th2 and Th17 cells is responsible for the appearance of specific symptoms in asthmatic patients. The cytokines secreted by various inflammatory cells interact with the resident cells, inducing the production of mediators considered alarmins (TSLP, IL-33), which leads to the exacerbation of various symptoms. This inflammatory situation can be soothed by conventional treatments. However, in severe forms of asthma, the situation is more complex, and patients respond poorly to bronchodilators due to the presence of mucous plugs in the small airways [41].

Allergic asthma exacerbations in children are provoked by exposure to aeroallergens, mainly represented by dust mites, pollen or pet dander. Allergen presentation stimulates CD4+ T cells and the T2 cascade involving IL-4, IL-5, IL-9, IL-13 and IgE production. This pathway favours eosinophils recruitment and activation, leading to bronchospasm and mucus production. Why a disease that begins early in life persists into adulthood is unclear. Early exposure to allergens during lung and immune system development and maturation causes major modifications in the establishment of the disease [42, 43].

Late-onset asthma is more difficult to explain and is more severe. It is common in women and obese patients [43, 44]. Bronchial inflammation resists inhaled steroids. In fact, a large subset of late-onset asthmatics presents with non-eosinophilic airway inflammation [45]. This may be explained by the impaired epithelial barrier function of the airways associated with the presence of mucus plugs, which promotes the establishment of respiratory pathogens, in turn contributing to the exacerbation of the disease.

Additional information is needed to understand the interactions between the resident microbes and bronchial epithelium. The microbiome is increasingly involved in immune homeostasis, participating through the interactions between the gut and lungs in the onset and the chronicity of asthma. The microbiota plays a major role through its interaction with innate and adaptive immunity. It constitutes a privileged field of research. Microbial colonization takes place during the first three years and is essential to the health of the organism. Many factors are associated with microbiota imbalance, such as caesarean delivery, formula feeding, and antibiotics. Investigations into the gut and respiratory microbiome in asthmatic children have reported a correlation between microbial dysbiosis and asthma in early life. Respiratory system bacteria can rectify the onset and progression of asthma by producing metabolites. However, much remains to be done in the field of research and understanding of the mechanisms. Asthmatic lung displays an increased load of bacteria, and an imbalance favouring proteobacteria, in particular Haemophilus spp. and Moraxella catarrhalis. Lung resident cells identify serial PAMPs on inhaled germs and aeroallergens. In the same way, they are able to detect molecular patterns associated with the damage exhibited by suffering cells. Indeed, epithelial cells express numerous receptors, such as TLRs. Activated lung epithelium produces growth factors, cytokines, chemokines and lipidic factors. This process has also been demonstrated in murine asthma models, with a production of GM-CSF, M-CSF, TGFb, IL-18, and alarmins (TSLP, IL-25 and IL-33) by the epithelium after allergen exposure [46 - 49].

A complete interaction between cytokines and epithelial cells is necessary for the development of T2 inflammation in murine asthma models [50]. In the nasopharynx, the predominant stabilized bacterial communities associate Dolosigranulum species and Moraxella. They are modified by several factors, such as daycare attendance, viruses, and antibiotics treatment [50]. The decrease in bacterial load and diversity can influence the inflammatory phenotypes of asthma [51, 52]. T2 activation induces infiltration of the airways by eosinophils [53, 54]. *Staphylococcus aureus* transforms the immune expression of the respiratory tract mucosa by releasing IL-33, activating innate lymphoid cells (ILC) to produce Th2 mediators, and inducing degranulation of mast cells and maturation B lymphocytes into IgE plasma cells. This process leads to the recruitment of eosinophils, releasing extracellular traps that contribute to aggravating the disease [55, 56].

Microbial diversity is lower in neutrophilic severe asthmatics than in eosinophilic patients, along with a high prevalence of organisms potentially pathogenic, like Haemophilus, and a decrease in airways commensals, like *Streptococcus* [54, 57]. The expression of Th17-associated genes and cytokines production are increased in case of proteobacteria colonization. Th17 mediators induce non-eosinophilic asthma, which responds poorly to corticosteroids [58], while actinobacteria may proliferate in the bronchi of severe eosinophilic asthmatics [14]. *Lactobacillus* and *Clostridium*, which are bifidobacteria, promote Treg subset induction. Clostridium stimulates ILC3 production of IL22 which contributes to strengthening the epithelial adherence and reducing its permeability. Bifidobacteria can stimulate dendritic cell metabolism. Capsular polysaccharide A from Bacteroides fragilis in mice interacts with plasmacytoid dendritic cells and induces IL10 release by helper T cells. In addition, a polysaccharide from Bifidobacterium longum can inhibit Th17 gut and pulmonary pathways [59]. However, colonization alone is not sufficient to modify immunity, as adaptive responses can be modulated through interactions with the gut by bacterial metabolites and released molecules.

The majority of T helper (Th1, Th2, Th17) components and alarmins (IL-33, IL-25, TSLP) have been studied and incriminated in severe asthma. Anti-inflammatory drugs reduced bronchoalveolar lavage (BALF) and induced sputum inflammatory cell count. They also modified IL-4 and IFN-γ production as well as the percentages of Th1, Th2, Th17, and Treg cells in the blood and bronchi and regulated the JAK-STAT signaling pathway through phosphorylation of the STATs. Treatments alleviate airway inflammation by modulating microenvironment homeostasis [60, 61].

However, there is nobiomarker that is able to predict and assess the response to treatment early. Such a marker would be of great help. We investigated NLRP3 inflammasome and IL-38 expression in different phases of asthma in childhood. A total of 72 children with asthma consulting in our department and 30 aged sex-matched healthy subjects were included in this study.

To highlight the role of the NLRP3 inflammasome, we also studies in parallel the expression of IL-38, an anti-inflammatory cytokine associated with a panel of agnostic and anti-agonistic mediators.

STUDY PARTICIPANTS

We studied non-smoking children with severe asthma (n = 22; age; 9.2 ± 2.7; range 7–15) from the Respiratory Medicine Department of Pneumology A. Mami, Ariana (Tunisia). Experiments were conducted in the research laboratory (19SP02: Chronic Pulmonary Pathologies: From Genome to Management). Healthy controls (n = 30; age: 9.6 ± 3.2; range 7–15) were enrolled from the community by advertisement.

Asthma was defined as physician-diagnosed asthma with a history of demonstrated airway hyperreactivity to hypertonic saline (a provocative dose causing a 15% fall in forced expiratory volume in 1 s (FEV1),15 L) and/or a response to bronchodilator of. Participants gave written informed consent. FEV1% was significantly increased in severe asthma (48.5 + 2.7) compared to non-asthmatic controls (114.84 ± 3.9) ($p < 0.0001$). IgE (IU/ml) was elevated in severe asthmatics (616.9 ± 602.3 *vs* 35.5 ± 17.5 in HC) ($p < 0.0001$). Sputum lymphocytes in severe asthma were increased (14.8% ± 6.9%) *vs* HC (3.5% + 3.77%) (p = 0.0007). Similarly, an increase in macrophages (65.9% + 7.8%), neutrophils (47.95% + 12.48%) and eosinophils (1.16% ± 0.92%) was observed as compared to healthy children [(25.7% ± 3.72%), (22.6% ±7.32%) and (0.0% ± 0.02%)]($p < 0.0001$), respectively].

The Ethics Committee of the A. Mami Hospital and the Medicine University of Tunis approved this study.

STUDY DESIGN

The induced sputum was explored for the level of inflammatory cells, the expression of proteins and their genes by ELISA and RT-PCR.

Peripheral blood mononuclear cells (PBMC): Cultured PBMC of 10 severe asthmatics and 10 HC were investigated by RT-PCR analysis for the expression of IL-1β, IL-18, IL-17, IL-32, IL-10 and IFN-γ. Lymphocytes were isolated by Ficoll Hypaque gradient centrifugation (Histopaque; Sigma Aldrich, The Netherlands). PBMCs were cultured for 2 days in RPMI 1640 media with 20 units/ml IL-2 (R&D Systems) and 10% foetal bovine serum. Total RNA was isolated from unfractionated PBMC using an RNeasy Mini kit (Sigma-Aldrich).

RNA extraction and real-time polymerase chain reaction (RT-PCR): Total cellular RNA from sputum cells was isolated by using RNeasy Micro kit extraction columns (Qiagen, Chatsworth, CA, USA). RNA was reverse-transcribed using oligo(dT) 12–18 primer in the presence of RNA guard (both from GE Healthcare, Velizy Villacoublay, France) and Superscript II reverse transcriptase (Invitrogen, Life Technologies Products HTDS. 2035 Carthage Aeroport, Tunis; Tunisia). Quantification of mRNA levels was performed by real-time PCR using the LightCycler PCR (Roche Diagnostics, Indianapolis, Ind.) and Quantit Tect SYBR Green PCR master mix (Qiagen, Chatsworth, CA, USA). Relative quantification of the PCR products was achieved using a standard curve, which was obtained by simultaneously amplifying samples with serial dilutions of the amplicon. The results were analyzed with LightCycler software version 3.5.3 (Roche Diagnostics). Both melting curve analysis and agarose gel electrophoresis were used to assess the specificity of the amplification products as well as primer–dimer formation. Quantification of mRNA encoding endogenous 40S ribosomal protein S9, as a housekeeping gene, was performed and was used to correct variations in cDNA content among samples. The ribosomal protein S9 has recently been ranked in the top 100 best housekeeping genes. Primers were designed to span an intron.The sequences are depicted in Table **1**. Preparations for RT-PCR amplification reactions were carried out with the SYBR Green PCR kit (Bio-rad, USA) and were performed using the 7500 fast Real-Time PCR system (Applied Biosystems, USA). PCR products were verified by melting curve analysis. Relative mRNA levels of target genes were calculated by the $2^{-\delta\delta CT}$ method, as described previously [62].

Enzyme-linked immunosorbent assay (ELISA): Sputum levels of IL-38 and NLRP3 were determined by ELISA following the manufacturer's instructions. Macrophage isolation from sputum: Sputum macrophages were isolated according to the method indicated by Simpson *et al.* [15] *via* negative selection using magnetic cell separation with CD15 microbeads (Miltenyi Biotec, Sydney, Australia), LS cell separation columns and the VarioMACS system according to the manufacturer's instructions (Miltenyi Biotec).

Table 1. Primers sequences of target genes.

IL-1β	5'TGAGGAGCAGCACCCAGAGC-3' 5'-CCGTAGGA CTGGAAAGAGGA-3'	IL-10	5'-GCCTAACATGCTTCGAGATC-3' 5'-TGATGTCTGGGTCTTGGTTC-3'
IL-18	5'-AACACTGGCTGTTCCCACAA-3' 5'TCCAGGTCTCCATTTTCTTCAGG-3'	IFNγ	5'-TTTGGGTTCTCTTGGCTGTT-3' 5'TCCATTATCCGCTACATCTGAA-3'
IL-32	5'-TGAGGAGCAGCACCCAGAGC-3' 5'-CCGTAGGA CTGGAAAGAGGA-3'	IL-35	5'-GCACATTCCCAGAGTTCCT-3' 5'-TTGAGTGTCCGCTGCTTC-3'
IL-17	5'-ACCAATCCCAAAAGGTCCTC-3' 5'-TGGATGGGGACAGAGTTCAT-3'	IL-38	5'-TTATCCTTGTGGGCTCAGTT-3' 5'-AATCCGTTCCCTTGGCTTTT-3'
NLRP3	5'- TTCGGAGATTGTGGTTGGG-3' 5'- GTCACCGAGGGCGTTGTC-3'	β-Actin	5'CCTGACTGACTACCTCATGAG-3' 5'-GACGTAGCACAGCTTCTCTTA-3'
IL-33	5'-GCCTGTCAACAGCAGTCTACTG-3 5'TGTGCTTAGAGAAGCAAGACTC-3'	-	-

Analysis: Data were analysed using Stata software version 11 (StataCorp, College Station, TX, USA).

Results were reported as mean ± SD or median (interquartile range), unless indicated otherwise. Analysis was performed using the two-sample Wilcoxon's rank sum test, and the Kruskal-Wallis test was used for more than two groups. Multiple linear regression was conducted using a stepwise regression with significance level for removal from the model of $p = 0.100$ and significance level for addition to the model of $p = 0.050$. Variables were included in the model when $p < 0.250$ in univariate regression. All the results were reported as significant when $p < 0.05$.

RESULTS

Expression of IL-38 in Sputum of Severe Asthmatic Children

IL-38 in sputum of severe asthmatic patients (30.04 ± 5.64 pg/ml) was lower than that of healthy children (58.93 ± 7.39 pg/ml; $p > 0.005$) (Fig. **1A**). Significant sputum correlation was found between IL-38 protein and IL-38 mRNA in severe asthma ($r = 0.677$; $p = 0.0005$) (Fig. **1**).

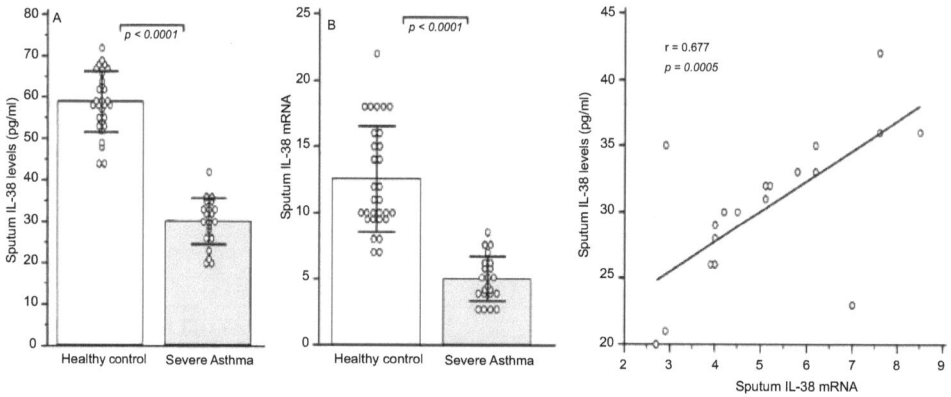

Fig. (1). IL-38 levels in induced sputum of severe childhood asthmatics. (**A**) IL-38 was quantified by ELISA in sputum. (**B**) The relative mRNA level of IL-38 was determined by qRT-PCR in 22 severe asthmatic patients. (**C**) Correlation between sputum IL-38 and mRNA levels of IL-38. Results are expressed as mean ± SD. The statistical analysis was performed using the Mann–Whitney U test. p values are indicated. The correlations were evaluated with the Spearman's nonparametric test.

Expression of Sputum NLRP3 Inflammasome

Sputum levels expressing the NLRP3 inflammasome were higher in severe asthmatics (14.85± 3.20 pg/ml) compared to healthy controls (4.35±3.20 pg/ml; $p < 0.0001$). In the same way, gene expression was increased in severe asthma sputum cells than in non-asthmatic controls ($p = 0.0005$). An inverse correlation was observed between IL-38 and NLRP3 inflammasome in severe asthma (r = -0.686; $p = 0.0004$) (Fig. **2**).

Correlations Between NLRP3 Inflammasome and FEV1%, PNN%, and Macrophages

Fig. (**3**) illustrates the correlations between NLRP3 inflammasomes and FEV1%, PNN% and macrophages. Levels of NLRP3 inflammasome were inversely correlated with FEV1%. The highest positive correlations were found between NLRP3 and PNN%.

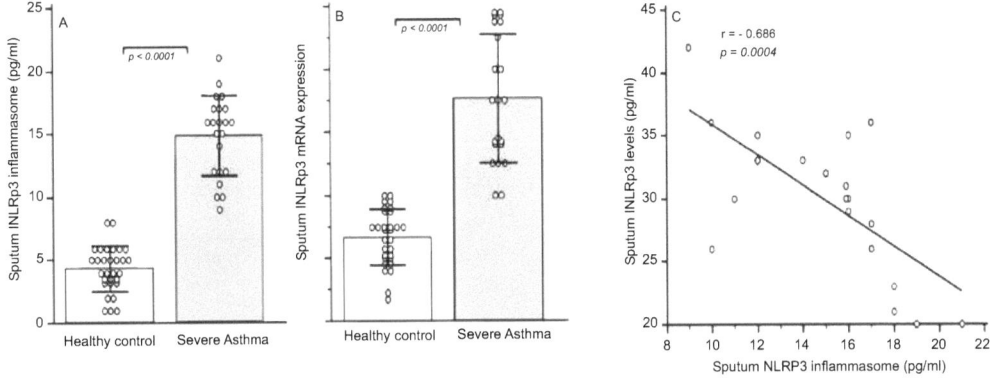

Fig. (2). (**A**) Nucleotide-binding domain, leucine-rich repeat-containing family protein (NLRP)3 and (**B**) Protein level and NLRP3 mRNA expression in severe asthma children.

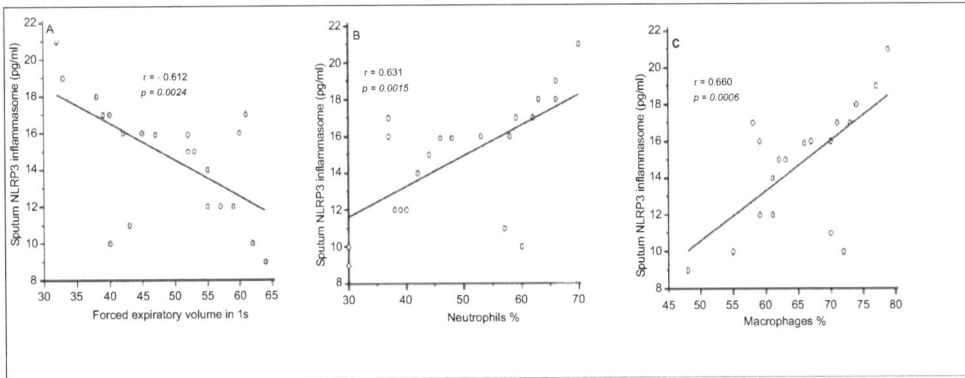

Fig. (3). Correlations between NLRP3 inflammasome and FEV1%, PNN and macrophages.

NLRP3 Inflammasome and IL-1β Gene Expression in Isolated Sputum Macrophages

Isolated sputum macrophages from 7 severe asthmatics and 5 non-asthmatic controls (purity of > 90%) were investigated for IL-1β and NLRP3 inflammasome. Gene expressions of NLRP3 inflammasome and IL-1β were significantly increased in isolated sputum macrophages from severe asthmatic children (Fig. **4**).

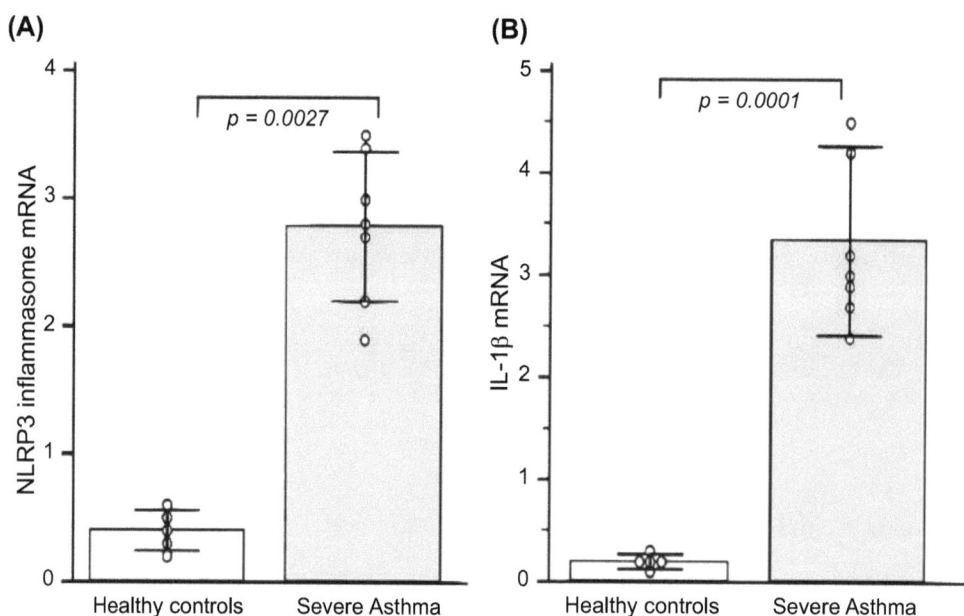

Fig. (4). Gene expressions of (**A**) NLRP3 inflammasome and (**B**) interleukin (IL)-1β were increased in isolated sputum macrophages of severe asthma compared with healthy controls.

Expression of IL-1β, IL-18, IL-17, IL-32, IL-33, IL-35, IL-10 and IFN-γ

Given that IL-38, an anti-inflammatory mediator, is weakly expressed in severe asthmatics and inversely correlated with NLRP3, we proposed to study the expression profile of a panel of inflammatory and suppressor cytokines. Gene expression for the components of IL-1β, IL-18, IL-17, IL-32, IL33, IL-35, IL-10 and IFN-γ were investigated in PBMCs of 10 severe asthmics and 10 healthy controls. IL-1β, IL-18, IL-17, IL-32 and IL-33 were higher in severe asthmics as compared to non-asthmatic controls (Fig. **5A, B, C, D, G**), while antagonistic cytokines (IL-10, IFNγ and IL-35) were significantly observed in healthy controls (Fig. **5E, F, H**) as compared to severe asthmatic patients.

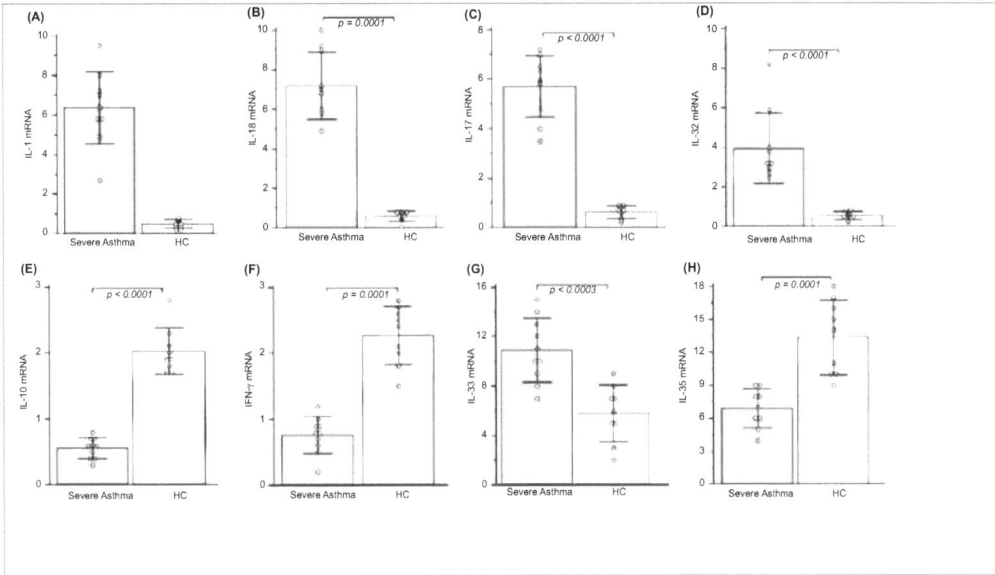

Fig. (5). Representation of PBMCs mRNA expression of IL-1β, IL-18, IL-17, IL-32, IL-33, IL-10, IL-35 and IFN-γ related gene expression: Statistical significance between the two groups was assessed using the Wilcoxon–Mann–Whitney test.

DISCUSSION

We reported that children with severe asthma express low levels of IL38 protein and mRNA in sputum as compared to healthy subjects. The decrease in IL-38 is contrasted by an increased expression of the NLRP3 inflammasome. Our study is the first to describe IL-38 and NLRP3 inflammasome in induced sputum of children with severe asthma. The levels of NLRP3 inflammasome were inversely correlated to FEV1% in asthmatics, while the percentages of neutrophils and macrophages were positively associated with the expression of the NLRP3 inflammasome, suggesting that the high number of these cells would be in some way a source of exacerbation of asthma. To trace a possible inflammatory profile of asthmatic children, we studied the expression of five pro-inflammatory cytokines (IL-1β, IL-17, IL-18, IL-33, IL-32) and three anti-inflammatory cytokines (IL-10, IFN-γ and IL-35) at the level of mononuclear cells of the peripheral circulation.

IL-38 cytokine, a member of the IL-1 family, is released after activation by several immune cells, such as lymphocytes and macrophages, and regulates inflammation negatively. The multiplicity of cells (nuclear cells, macrophages, lymphocytes) to simultaneously produce anti- and pro-inflammatory cytokines shows an immunological imbalance favouring asthma exacerbation. Certain cytokines are known to secrete both agonistic and antagonistic mediators. The sputum microenvironment includes numerous defensive cells, among which T lymphocytes, polynuclear cells and macrophages associated with resident cells exert an essential role in the modulation of inflammation in severe asthma. Levels of anti-inflammatory mediators, such as TGF-β or IL-10, together with proinflammatory cytokines production, such as IL-6, establish the pathway of the immune response towards he regulation with Treg or inflammation with Th17. IL-17-producing Treg that are in the transitional state (RORγt⁺Foxp3⁺) represents the centre of the polarized Treg/Th17 cell axis. IL-6 separating RORγt from FOXP3 favours Th17 differentiation. JAK-STAT pathway influences T cell polarization through several cytokine receptors [63, 64]. Foxp3 is essential to Tregs differentiation and persistence. Therefore, miRNAs that regulate Foxp3 expression could be important in Tregs modulation [65]. Some cytokines may affect Treg or IL-17-producing cells through phosphorylation of STAT3 or STAT5. IL-1β, IL-6, and IL-10 activate STAT3 suppressing Foxp3 expression contrasting with IL-2, IL-15, IL-27, and IL-35 that stabilize Foxp3 expression through STAT5 stimulation [66-67]. These cytokines may also enhance the expression of miRNAs that regulate STAT3 activators and modulators [68].

There is growing interest in investigating IL-38 in asthmatic children. Chu *et al.* observed an increased expression of circulating IL-38, suggesting its involvement in asthma [69]. They reported that serum concentrations of IL-5, IL-6, IL-38, IL-17, IFNγ, periostin, IL-1β and IL-13 were significantly higher in asthma patients compared to control subjects, independent of corticosteroid therapy. The authors did not classify their patients according to asthma severity. We speculate that the contrast between our results and those of Chu *et al.* is due to the different compartmental inflammation processes, where cytokines are expressed differently in sputum and peripheral circulation. This suggests a different regulation of IL-38 production in bronchial mucosa and blood cells. Our hypothesis was that IL-38 levels in induced sputum reflected the immune balance between the inflammatory and suppressive inflammatory cytokines. IL-38 which binds to IL-36R, can inhibit inflammation as described in several immunological diseases. Sputum IL-38 protein and mRNA levels were lower in severe asthmatics than in healthy controls. Expression of innate and adaptive cytokines that promote inflammation was increased in sputum from severe asthmatics. IL-1, NLRP3, IL-17 and IL-32 levels were inversely correlated with IL-38. IL-17 and IL-1 are known as actors of alternative pathways in the asthma inflammatory process. More recently, NLRP3 inflammasome and IL-32 were involved in severe asthma in line with the presence of activated macrophages and PNNs in the sputum [14].

Interest in the NLRP inflammasomes has increased over recent years, but little is understood about the role of inflammasome activation in the airways of patients with asthma. Its expression in severe asthma has not been described yet. The reduced number of clinical studies limits our knowledge about the role of inflammasome in asthma. It has been reported in a mouse model that the NLPR3 inflammasome was necessary to develop the neutrophilic bronchi inflammation provoked by pollution particles with a diameter of less than 10 mm [70], demonstrating that nonmicrobial stimuli can trigger the accumulation of neutrophils in the airway. Other studies showed that NLRP3 inflammasome activation and upregulation of its cascade products in the lungs of a mouse model of asthma were correlated to increased AHR, neutrophil infiltration, and mucus hypersecretion of the airways. Moreover, retinoid-RORgt mRNA expression was increased, and Foxp3 mRNA expression was decreased. On the contrary, treatment with NLRP3 inhibitors significantly decreased AHR, bronchial inflammation, and inverted Th17/Treg cell ratio [71]. The authors suggested that the NLRP3 pathway is important to neutrophilic asthma inflammation, which could be inhibited, representing a potential new way of treatment [71]. Our results for NLRP3 match with Simpson's report on a positive correlation between sputum neutrophils and NLRP3 in neutrophilic asthma [1]. The simultaneous increase of IL-1β and NLRP3, together with several inflammatory mediators, was described in severe asthma [72 - 74]. It was not surprising to find high values of NLRP3 inflammasome protein and mRNA. Moreover, a negative correlation was observed between IL-38 and the values of NLPR3 inflammasome in the induced sputum.

Yang *et al.* observed that miR-146a-5p reduces allergic bronchial inflammation as it inhibits NLRP3 inflammasome activation in macrophages. Allergic mice that were treated with miR-146a-5p, an inhibitor of NLRP3 inflammasome activation, showed an anti-inflammatory M2 polarization of pulmonary macrophages by targeting the TIRAP/NF-κB pathway, thus reducing inflammatory responses [75]. More recently, Simpson *et al.* [14] reported an increase in NLRP3 gene expression of sputum cells in neutrophilic asthmatics, along with the detection of NLRP3 and caspase-1 protein in neutrophils and macrophages. NLRP3 inflammasome expression was elevated in asthma, particularly in neutrophilic patients, potentially due to innate signals. Sputum IL-1 protein levels were correlated with neutrophil recruitment and activation.

We have studied the protein and mRNA expression of IL-1β and NLRP3 in the sputum and showed that significant correlations exist with airway macrophages and neutrophils from patients with severe asthma. This suggests that severe asthma may be partly driven by the release of NLRP3 and IL-1β from both macrophages and neutrophils. Mankan *et al.* [76] demonstrated the presence of a functional NLRP3 inflammasome in neutrophils, while others reported that genetic variations in NLRP3 delayed neutrophils, negatively influencing inflammation resolution [77]. Further work is necessary to precisely understand the role of the neutrophil inflammasome during asthma inflammation.

A panel of agonist and antagonist parameters was studied in the peripheral circulation of severe asthmatic children to have an immune profile compared to non-asthmatic children, focusing particularly on the expression of NLRP3 inflammasome. The results showed an exaggerated expression of inflammatory cytokine genes contrasted by a low expression of IL-10, IFN-g and IL-35. IL-1β is essential to the pathogenesis of several diseases. It plays an important role in severe asthma. IL-1β expression is always associated with elevated values of IL-32, IL-17 and the NLRP3 inflammasome. IL-1β-targeted therapies have been successfully used in several inflammatory conditions [78]; however, the role of the IL-1 members has been poorly investigated in severe asthma [79]. Neutrophils represent the main cellular drivers of IL-1β [80] and were always positively correlated to NLRP3 inflammasome. The increase of IL-17 in the sputum of severe asthmaticcould be linked to the increase of NLRP3 inflammasome. Liu *et al.* studied the effect of IL17A on the biological behaviour of lung cancer cells. They reported that IL-17A enhanced NLRP3 expression, caspase-1 activity and IL-1β production, promoting cell migration and epithelial-mesenchymal transition process favouring invasion. All of these pathological processes were alleviated by NLRP3 blockade [81].

CONCLUSION

In this chapter, we reported recent findings related to the composition, activation, and regulation of the NLRP3 inflammasome. In addition, we also summarized our latest research results on NLRP3 involvement in severe asthma. Inhalation of molecular patterns of PAMPs and DAMPs induces lung activation of the NLRP3 inflammasome, promoting the release of a cascade of inflammatory mediators, such as IL-1β, IL-18, IL-32 and IL-33. These factors maintain chronic inflammation. Currently, several NLRP3 inflammasome inhibitors have been described, that target different sites of its activation pathway. With an improved understanding of the mechanism of NLRP3 inflammasome activation, new treatment strategies could be developed.

Our study showed the gene expression of inflammatory and anti-inflammatory mediators in the induced sputum in the context of exacerbation of the disease. We reported an important contribution of polynuclear and macrophage cells to NLRP3 inflammasome secretion and a probable predominance of agonistic cytokines. Taken together, these findings may drive further studies on the balance between immunosuppressive and inflammatory processes in severe asthmatic children.

In conclusion, our observations highlight the potential relevance of the cytokines and the inflammasome studied, as well as the possibility of their use in clinical applications. However, the puzzling but expected results obtained for IL-38 and NLRP3 inflammasome increase the need for future experimental and clinical research to clarify their role in severe asthma in children. We are aware of several limitations in our study, including relatively small sample size and restriction to a single-centre population, which are likely to limit the statistical power. Moreover, due to the small number of asthmatic patients and the lack of patients in the remission phase of asthma at baseline, their selection as a separate group for statistical analysis and comparisons was unavailable. Therefore, replication of multi-centre studies with a greater number of enrolled individuals will be beneficial.

REFERENCES

[1]   El-Zayat SR, Sibaii H, Mannaa FA. Toll-like receptors activation, signaling, and targeting: An overview. Bull Natl Res Cent 2019; 43(1): 187.
[http://dx.doi.org/10.1186/s42269-019-0227-2]

[2]   Kawasaki T, Kawai T. Toll-like receptor signaling pathways. Front Immunol 2014; 5: 461.
[http://dx.doi.org/10.3389/fimmu.2014.00461] [PMID: 25309543]

[3]   Hennessy C, McKernan DP. Anti-viral pattern recognition receptors as therapeutic targets. Cells 2021; 10(9): 2258.
[http://dx.doi.org/10.3390/cells10092258] [PMID: 34571909]

[4]   Kimura Y, Tsukui D, Kono H. Uric acid in inflammation and the pathogenesis of atherosclerosis. Int J Mol Sci 2021; 22(22): 12394.
[http://dx.doi.org/10.3390/ijms222212394] [PMID: 34830282]

[5]   Kanneganti TD. The inflammasome: Firing up innate immunity. Immunol Rev 2015; 265(1): 1-5.
[http://dx.doi.org/10.1111/imr.12297] [PMID: 25879279]

[6]   Zheng D, Liwinski T, Elinav E. Inflammasome activation and regulation: Toward a better understanding of complex mechanisms. Cell Discov 2020; 6(1): 36.
[http://dx.doi.org/10.1038/s41421-020-0167-x] [PMID: 32550001]

[7]   Roh JS, Sohn DH. Damage-associated molecular patterns in inflammatory diseases. Immune Netw 2018; 18(4): e27.
[http://dx.doi.org/10.4110/in.2018.18.e27] [PMID: 30181915]

[8]   Yuan M, Jiang Z, Bi G, *et al.* Pattern-recognition receptors are required for NLR-mediated plant immunity. Nature 2021; 592(7852): 105-9.
[http://dx.doi.org/10.1038/s41586-021-03316-6] [PMID: 33692546]

[9]   Toldo S, Abbate A. The NLRP3 inflammasome in acute myocardial infarction. Nat Rev Cardiol 2018; 15(4): 203-14.
[http://dx.doi.org/10.1038/nrcardio.2017.161] [PMID: 29143812]

[10]   Sok SPM, Ori D, Wada A, *et al.* 1′-Acetoxychavicol acetate inhibits NLRP3-dependent inflammasome activation *via* mitochondrial ROS suppression. Int Immunol 2021; 33(7): 373-86.
[http://dx.doi.org/10.1093/intimm/dxab016] [PMID: 33830232]

[11]   Zhang WJ, Chen SJ, Zhou SC, Wu SZ, Wang H. Inflammasomes and fibrosis. Front Immunol 2021; 12: 643149.
[http://dx.doi.org/10.3389/fimmu.2021.643149] [PMID: 34177893]

[12]   Mandell JT, de Rivero Vaccari JP, Sabater AL, Galor A. The inflammasome pathway: A key player in ocular surface and anterior segment diseases. Surv Ophthalmol 2023; 68(2): 280-9.
[http://dx.doi.org/10.1016/j.survophthal.2022.06.003] [PMID: 35798189]

[13]   Alcazar CGM, Paes VM, Shao Y, *et al.* The association between early-life gut microbiota and childhood respiratory diseases: A systematic review. Lancet Microbe 2022; 3(11): e867-80.
[http://dx.doi.org/10.1016/S2666-5247(22)00184-7] [PMID: 35988549]

[14]   Simpson JL, Daly J, Baines KJ, *et al.* Airway dysbiosis: *Haemophilus influenzae* and *Tropheryma* in poorly controlled asthma. Eur Respir J 2016; 47(3): 792-800.
[http://dx.doi.org/10.1183/13993003.00405-2015] [PMID: 26647445]

[15]   Lachowicz-Scroggins ME, Dunican EM, Charbit AR, *et al.* Extracellular DNA, neutrophil extracellular traps, and inflammasome activation in severe asthma. Am J Respir Crit Care Med 2019; 199(9): 1076-85.
[http://dx.doi.org/10.1164/rccm.201810-1869OC] [PMID: 30888839]

[16]   Kim RY, Pinkerton JW, Essilfie AT, *et al.* Role for NLRP3 inflammasome-mediated, IL-1β-dependent responses in severe, steroid-resistant asthma. Am J Respir Crit Care Med 2017; 196(3): 283-97.
[http://dx.doi.org/10.1164/rccm.201609-1830OC] [PMID: 28252317]

[17]   De Nardo D, De Nardo CM, Latz E. New insights into mechanisms controlling the NLRP3 inflammasome and its role in lung disease. Am J Pathol 2014; 184(1): 42-54.
[http://dx.doi.org/10.1016/j.ajpath.2013.09.007] [PMID: 24183846]

[18]   Parzych K, Zetterqvist AV, Wright WR, Kirkby NS, Mitchell JA, Paul-Clark MJ. Differential role of pannexin-1/ATP/ P2X$_7$ axis in IL-1β release by human monocytes. FASEB J 2017; 31(6): 2439-45.
[http://dx.doi.org/10.1096/fj.201600256] [PMID: 28246166]

[19]   Triantafilou K, Hughes TR, Triantafilou M, Morgan BP. The complement membrane attack complex triggers intracellular Ca2+ fluxes leading to NLRP3 inflammasome activation. J Cell Sci 2013; 126(Pt 13): jcs.124388.
[http://dx.doi.org/10.1242/jcs.124388] [PMID: 23613465]

[20]   Murakami T, Ockinger J, Yu J, *et al.* Critical role for calcium mobilization in activation of the NLRP3 inflammasome. Proc Natl Acad Sci 2012; 109(28): 11282-7.
[http://dx.doi.org/10.1073/pnas.1117765109] [PMID: 22733741]

[21]   Zorov DB, Juhaszova M, Sollott SJ. Mitochondrial reactive oxygen species (ROS) and ROS-induced ROS release. Physiol Rev 2014; 94(3): 909-50.
[http://dx.doi.org/10.1152/physrev.00026.2013] [PMID: 24987008]

[22]   Zhou R, Yazdi AS, Menu P, Tschopp J. A role for mitochondria in NLRP3 inflammasome activation. Nature 2011; 469(7329): 221-5.
[http://dx.doi.org/10.1038/nature09663] [PMID: 21124315]

[23]   Sarniak A, Lipińska J, Tytman K, Lipińska S. Endogenous mechanisms of reactive oxygen species (ROS) generation. Postepy Hig Med Dosw 2016; 70(0): 1150-65.
[http://dx.doi.org/10.5604/17322693.1224259] [PMID: 27892899]

[24]   Xu W, Wang Y, Ma Y, Yang J. MiR-223 plays a protecting role in neutrophilic asthmatic mice through the inhibition of NLRP3 inflammasome. Respir Res 2020; 21(1): 116.
[http://dx.doi.org/10.1186/s12931-020-01374-4] [PMID: 32423405]

[25]   Guo S, Chen R, Zhang L, *et al.* microRNA-22-3p plays a protective role in a murine asthma model through the inhibition of the NLRP3–caspase-1–IL-1β axis. Exp Physiol 2021; 106(8): 1829-38.
[http://dx.doi.org/10.1113/EP089575] [PMID: 33932961]

[26] Yan Y, Jiang W, Liu L, *et al.* Dopamine controls systemic inflammation through inhibition of NLRP3 inflammasome. Cell 2015; 160(1-2): 62-73.
[http://dx.doi.org/10.1016/j.cell.2014.11.047] [PMID: 25594175]

[27] Boulet LP, Reddel HK, Bateman E, Pedersen S, FitzGerald JM, O'Byrne PM. The Global Initiative for Asthma (GINA): 25 years later. Eur Respir J 2019; 54(2): 1900598.
[http://dx.doi.org/10.1183/13993003.00598-2019] [PMID: 31273040]

[28] Cheng C, Wu H, Wang M, *et al.* Estrogen ameliorates allergic airway inflammation by regulating activation of NLRP3 in mice. Biosci Rep 2019; 39(1): BSR20181117.
[http://dx.doi.org/10.1042/BSR20181117] [PMID: 30373775]

[29] Wood LG, Li Q, Scott HA, *et al.* Saturated fatty acids, obesity, and the nucleotide oligomerization domain–like receptor protein 3 (NLRP3) inflammasome in asthmatic patients. J Allergy Clin Immunol 2019; 143(1): 305-15.
[http://dx.doi.org/10.1016/j.jaci.2018.04.037] [PMID: 29857009]

[30] Rodríguez-Alcázar JF, Ataide MA, Engels G, *et al.* Charcot–Leyden crystals activate the NLRP3 inflammasome and cause IL-1β inflammation in human macrophages. J Immunol 2019; 202(2): 550-8.
[http://dx.doi.org/10.4049/jimmunol.1800107] [PMID: 30559319]

[31] Tsai YM, Chiang KH, Hung JY, *et al.* Der f1 induces pyroptosis in human bronchial epithelia *via* the NLRP3 inflammasome. Int J Mol Med 2018; 41(2): 757-64.
[PMID: 29207030]

[32] Kim BG, Lee PH, Lee SH, Park MK, Jang AS. Effect of TiO$_2$ nanoparticles on inflammasome-mediated airway inflammation and responsiveness. Allergy Asthma Immunol Res 2017; 9(3): 257-64.
[http://dx.doi.org/10.4168/aair.2017.9.3.257] [PMID: 28293932]

[33] Palomo J, Dietrich D, Martin P, Palmer G, Gabay C. The interleukin (IL)-1 cytokine family - Balance between agonists and antagonists in inflammatory diseases. Cytokine 2015; 76(1): 25-37.
[http://dx.doi.org/10.1016/j.cyto.2015.06.017] [PMID: 26185894]

[34] Garlanda C, Dinarello CA, Mantovani A. The interleukin-1 family: Back to the future. Immunity 2013; 39(6): 1003-18.
[http://dx.doi.org/10.1016/j.immuni.2013.11.010] [PMID: 24332029]

[35] Global Initiative for Asthma. 2021 GINA report, global strategy for asthma management and prevention. 2021. Available from:https://ginasthma.org/gina-reports

[36] Hsieh A, Assadinia N, Hackett TL. Airway remodeling heterogeneity in asthma and its relationship to disease outcomes. Front Physiol 2023; 14: 1113100.
[http://dx.doi.org/10.3389/fphys.2023.1113100] [PMID: 36744026]

[37] Asthma that is difficult to treat is considered to be severe when control remains poor despite measures that adequately address each of these three variables.. Available from:https://ginasthma.org/wp-content/uploads/2019/04/GINA-Severe-asthma-Pocket-Guide-v2.0-wms-1.pdf

[38] Settipane RA, Kreindler JL, Chung Y, Tkacz J. Evaluating direct costs and productivity losses of patients with asthma receiving GINA 4/5 therapy in the United States. Ann Allergy Asthma Immunol 2019; 123(6): 564-572.e3.
[http://dx.doi.org/10.1016/j.anai.2019.08.462] [PMID: 31494235]

[39] Woodruff PG, Modrek B, Choy DF, *et al.* T-helper type 2-driven inflammation defines major subphenotypes of asthma. Am J Respir Crit Care Med 2009; 180(5): 388-95.
[http://dx.doi.org/10.1164/rccm.200903-0392OC] [PMID: 19483109]

[40] Frøssing L, Silberbrandt A, Von Bülow A, Backer V, Porsbjerg C. The prevalence of subtypes of type 2 inflammation in an unselected population of patients with severe asthma. J Allergy Clin Immunol Pract 2021; 9(3): 1267-75.
[http://dx.doi.org/10.1016/j.jaip.2020.09.051] [PMID: 33039645]

[41]   Dunican EM, Elicker BM, Gierada DS, *et al.* Mucus plugs in patients with asthma linked to eosinophilia and airflow obstruction. J Clin Invest 2018; 128(3): 997-1009.
[http://dx.doi.org/10.1172/JCI95693] [PMID: 29400693]

[42]   de Kleer IM, Kool M, de Bruijn MJW, *et al.* Perinatal activation of the interleukin-33 pathway promotes type 2 immunity in the developing lung. Immunity 2016; 45(6): 1285-98.
[http://dx.doi.org/10.1016/j.immuni.2016.10.031] [PMID: 27939673]

[43]   Saglani S, Gregory LG, Manghera AK, *et al.* Inception of early-life allergen-induced airway hyperresponsiveness is reliant on IL-13(+)CD4(+) T cells. Sci Immunol 2018; 3: 4128.

[44]   Pakkasela J, Ilmarinen P, Honkamäki J, *et al.* Age-specific incidence of allergic and non-allergic asthma. BMC Pulm Med 2020; 20(1): 9.
[http://dx.doi.org/10.1186/s12890-019-1040-2] [PMID: 31924190]

[45]   Lameire S, Hammad H. Lung epithelial cells: Upstream targets in type 2-high asthma. Eur J Immunol 2023; 53(11): 2250106.
[http://dx.doi.org/10.1002/eji.202250106] [PMID: 36781404]

[46]   Ximenez C, Torres J. Development of Microbiota in Infants and its Role in Maturation of Gut Mucosa and Immune System. Arch Med Res 2017; 48(8): 666-80.
[http://dx.doi.org/10.1016/j.arcmed.2017.11.007] [PMID: 29198451]

[47]   Alcazar CGM, Paes VM, Shao Y, *et al.* The association between early-life gut microbiota and childhood respiratory diseases: A systematic review. Lancet Microbe 2022; 3(11): e867-80.
[http://dx.doi.org/10.1016/S2666-5247(22)00184-7] [PMID: 35988549]

[48]   Renz H, Brandtzaeg P, Hornef M. The impact of perinatal immune development on mucosal homeostasis and chronic inflammation. Nat Rev Immunol 2012; 12(1): 9-23.
[http://dx.doi.org/10.1038/nri3112] [PMID: 22158411]

[49]   Arrieta MC, Stiemsma LT, Amenyogbe N, Brown EM, Finlay B. The intestinal microbiome in early life: Health and disease. Front Immunol 2014; 5: 427.
[http://dx.doi.org/10.3389/fimmu.2014.00427] [PMID: 25250028]

[50]   Ver Heul A, Planer J, Kau AL. The human microbiota and asthma. Clin Rev Allergy Immunol 2019; 57(3): 350-63.
[http://dx.doi.org/10.1007/s12016-018-8719-7] [PMID: 30426401]

[51]   Chung KF. Airway microbial dysbiosis in asthmatic patients: A target for prevention and treatment? J Allergy Clin Immunol 2017; 139(4): 1071-81.
[http://dx.doi.org/10.1016/j.jaci.2017.02.004] [PMID: 28390574]

[52]   Sverrild A, Kiilerich P, Brejnrod A, *et al.* Eosinophilic airway inflammation in asthmatic patients is associated with an altered airway microbiome. J Allergy Clin Immunol 2017; 140(2): 407-417.e11.
[http://dx.doi.org/10.1016/j.jaci.2016.10.046] [PMID: 28042058]

[53]   Barcik W, Boutin RCT, Sokolowska M, Finlay BB. The role of lung and gut microbiota in the pathology of asthma. Immunity 2020; 52(2): 241-55.
[http://dx.doi.org/10.1016/j.immuni.2020.01.007] [PMID: 32075727]

[54]   Taylor SL, Leong LEX, Choo JM, *et al.* Inflammatory phenotypes in patients with severe asthma are associated with distinct airway microbiology. J Allergy Clin Immunol 2018; 141(1): 94-103.e15.
[http://dx.doi.org/10.1016/j.jaci.2017.03.044] [PMID: 28479329]

[55]   Krysko O, Teufelberger A, Van Nevel S, Krysko DV, Bachert C. Protease/antiprotease network in allergy: The role of *Staphylococcus aureus* protease-like proteins. Allergy 2019; 74(11): 2077-86.
[http://dx.doi.org/10.1111/all.13783] [PMID: 30888697]

[56]   Stentzel S, Teufelberger A, Nordengrün M, *et al.* Staphylococcal serine protease–like proteins are pacemakers of allergic airway reactions to Staphylococcus aureus. J Allergy Clin Immunol 2017; 139(2): 492-500.e8.

[http://dx.doi.org/10.1016/j.jaci.2016.03.045] [PMID: 27315768]

[57]   Abdel-Aziz MI, Brinkman P, Vijverberg SJH, *et al.* Sputum microbiome profiles identify severe asthma phenotypes of relative stability at 12 to 18 months. J Allergy Clin Immunol 2021; 147(1): 123-34.
[http://dx.doi.org/10.1016/j.jaci.2020.04.018] [PMID: 32353491]

[58]   Huang YJ, Nariya S, Harris JM, *et al.* The airway microbiome in patients with severe asthma: Associations with disease features and severity. J Allergy Clin Immunol 2015; 136(4): 874-84.
[http://dx.doi.org/10.1016/j.jaci.2015.05.044] [PMID: 26220531]

[59]   Sokolowska M, Frei R, Lunjani N, Akdis CA, O'Mahony L. Microbiome and asthma. Asthma Res Pract 2018; 4(1): 1.
[http://dx.doi.org/10.1186/s40733-017-0037-y] [PMID: 29318023]

[60]   Min Z, Zhou J, Mao R, Cui B, Cheng Y, Chen Z. Pyrroloquinoline quinone administration alleviates allergic airway inflammation in mice by regulating the JAK-STAT signaling pathway. Mediators Inflamm 2022; 2022: 1-18.
[http://dx.doi.org/10.1155/2022/1267841] [PMID: 36345503]

[61]   Zhou Y, Hu L, Zhang H, *et al.* Guominkang formula alleviate inflammation in eosinophilic asthma by regulating immune balance of Th1/2 and Treg/Th17 cells. Front Pharmacol 2022; 13: 978421.
[http://dx.doi.org/10.3389/fphar.2022.978421] [PMID: 36330091]

[62]   Charrad R, Berraïes A, Hamdi B, Ammar J, Hamzaoui K, Hamzaoui A. Anti-inflammatory activity of IL-37 in asthmatic children: Correlation with inflammatory cytokines TNF-α, IL-β, IL-6 and IL-17A. Immunobiology 2016; 221(2): 182-7.
[http://dx.doi.org/10.1016/j.imbio.2015.09.009] [PMID: 26454413]

[63]   Seif F, Khoshmirsafa M, Aazami H, Mohsenzadegan M, Sedighi G, Bahar M. The role of JAK-STAT signaling pathway and its regulators in the fate of T helper cells. Cell Commun Signal 2017; 15(1): 23.
[http://dx.doi.org/10.1186/s12964-017-0177-y] [PMID: 28637459]

[64]   Seif F, Aazami H, Khoshmirsafa M, *et al.* JAK Inhibition as a New Treatment Strategy for Patients with COVID-19. Int Arch Allergy Immunol 2020; 181(6): 467-75.
[http://dx.doi.org/10.1159/000508247] [PMID: 32392562]

[65]   Xu L, Kitani A, Stuelten C, McGrady G, Fuss I, Strober W. Positive and negative transcriptional regulation of the Foxp3 gene is mediated by access and binding of the Smad3 protein to enhancer I. Immunity 2010; 33(3): 313-25.
[http://dx.doi.org/10.1016/j.immuni.2010.09.001] [PMID: 20870174]

[66]   Wuest TY, Willette-Brown J, Durum SK, Hurwitz AA. The influence of IL-2 family cytokines on activation and function of naturally occurring regulatory T cells. J Leukoc Biol 2008; 84(4): 973-80.
[http://dx.doi.org/10.1189/jlb.1107778] [PMID: 18653463]

[67]   Collison LW, Workman CJ, Kuo TT, *et al.* The inhibitory cytokine IL-35 contributes to regulatory T-cell function. Nature 2007; 450(7169): 566-9.
[http://dx.doi.org/10.1038/nature06306] [PMID: 18033300]

[68]   Amado T, Schmolka N, Metwally H, Silva-Santos B, Gomes AQ. Cross-regulation between cytokine and microRNA pathways in T cells. Eur J Immunol 2015; 45(6): 1584-95.
[http://dx.doi.org/10.1002/eji.201545487] [PMID: 25865116]

[69]   Chu M, Chu I, Yung E, *et al.* Aberrant expression of novel cytokine IL-38 and regulatory T lymphocytes in childhood asthma. Molecules 2016; 21(7): 933.
[http://dx.doi.org/10.3390/molecules21070933] [PMID: 27438823]

[70]   Hirota JA, Hirota SA, Warner SM, *et al.* The airway epithelium nucleotide-binding domain and leucine-rich repeat protein 3 inflammasome is activated by urban particulate matter. J Allergy Clin Immunol 2012; 129(4): 1116-1125.e6.
[http://dx.doi.org/10.1016/j.jaci.2011.11.033] [PMID: 22227418]

[71] Chen L, Hou W, Liu F, *et al.* Blockade of NLRP3/Caspase-1/IL-1β Regulated Th17/Treg immune imbalance and attenuated the neutrophilic airway inflammation in an ovalbumin-induced murine model of asthma. J Immunol Res 2022; 2022: 1-11.
[http://dx.doi.org/10.1155/2022/9444227] [PMID: 35664352]

[72] de Graaf DM, Teufel LU, Joosten LAB, Dinarello CA. Interleukin-38 in health and disease. Cytokine 2022; 152: 155824.
[http://dx.doi.org/10.1016/j.cyto.2022.155824] [PMID: 35220115]

[73] Tillie-Leblond I, Pugin J, Marquette CH, *et al.* Balance between proinflammatory cytokines and their inhibitors in bronchial lavage from patients with status asthmaticus. Am J Respir Crit Care Med 1999; 159(2): 487-94.
[http://dx.doi.org/10.1164/ajrccm.159.2.9805115] [PMID: 9927362]

[74] Hastie AT, Moore WC, Meyers DA, *et al.* Analyses of asthma severity phenotypes and inflammatory proteins in subjects stratified by sputum granulocytes. J Allergy Clin Immunol 2010; 125(5): 1028-1036.e13.
[http://dx.doi.org/10.1016/j.jaci.2010.02.008] [PMID: 20398920]

[75] Yang Y, Huang G, Xu Q, *et al.* miR-146a-5p attenuates allergic airway inflammation by inhibiting the NLRP3 inflammasome activation in macrophages. Int Arch Allergy Immunol 2022; 183(9): 919-30.
[http://dx.doi.org/10.1159/000524718] [PMID: 35660690]

[76] Mankan AK, Dau T, Jenne D, Hornung V. The NLRP3/ASC/Caspase-1 axis regulates IL-1β processing in neutrophils. Eur J Immunol 2012; 42(3): 710-5.
[http://dx.doi.org/10.1002/eji.201141921] [PMID: 22213227]

[77] Blomgran R, Patcha Brodin V, Verma D, *et al.* Common genetic variations in the NALP3 inflammasome are associated with delayed apoptosis of human neutrophils. PLoS One 2012; 7(3): e31326.
[http://dx.doi.org/10.1371/journal.pone.0031326] [PMID: 22403613]

[78] Shavandi M, Yazdani Y, Asar S, Mohammadi A, Mohammadi-Noori E, Kiani A. The Effect of Oral Administration of Silymarin on Serum Levels of Tumor Necrosis Factor-α and Interleukin-1ß in Patients with Rheumatoid Arthritis. Iran J Immunol 2022; 19(4): 427-35.
[PMID: 36585884]

[79] Xue B, Zhao Q, Chen D, *et al.* Network Pharmacology Combined with Molecular Docking and Experimental Verification Reveals the Bioactive Components and Potential Targets of Danlong Dingchuan Decoction against Asthma. Evid Based Complement Alternat Med 2022; 2022: 1-15.
[http://dx.doi.org/10.1155/2022/7895271] [PMID: 35186104]

[80] Stackowicz J, Gaudenzio N, Serhan N, *et al.* NeutrophiL-specific gain-of-function mutations in *Nlrp3* promote development of cryopyrin-associated periodic syndrome. J Exp Med 2021; 218(10): e20201466.
[http://dx.doi.org/10.1084/jem.20201466] [PMID: 34477811]

[81] Liu W, Xin M, Li Q, Sun L, Han X, Wang J. IL-17A promotes the migration, invasion and the emt process of lung cancer accompanied by NLRP3 activation. BioMed Res Int 2022; 2022: 1-14.
[http://dx.doi.org/10.1155/2022/7841279] [PMID: 36349316]

CHAPTER 9

Inflammasomes, Inflammation and Neuropathic Pain

Lokesh Sharan[1], Anubrato Pal[1], Priya Saha[2] and Ashutosh Kumar[2,*]

[1] *Department of Pharmacology and Toxicology, National Institute of Pharmaceutical Education and Research (NIPER), Kolkata 700054, West Bengal, India*

[2] *Department of Pharmacology and Toxicology, National Institute of Pharmaceutical Education and Research (NIPER)-SAS Nagar, Mohali, Punjab, 160062, India*

Abstract: Inflammasomes such as NOD-like receptor protein 1 (NLRP1), NLRP3, NLR family CARD domain-containing protein 4 (NLRC4) and absent in melanoma 2 (AIM2) are the primary mediators of inflammation and its associated neuropathic pain. These inflammasomes are activated leading to various autoimmune & metabolic disorders, cancer, and other inflammatory diseases. The activation of inflammasomes occurs due to molecular alterations like mitochondrial dysfunction, neuroinflammation, lysosomal damage, oxidative stress, sensitization, and disinhibition, which lead to proinflammatory pathways causing inflammasome-related neuropathic pain. Among these inflammasomes, NLRP3 has been widely studied and proven to be the key player in the development of neuropathy. In this chapter, we have summarized the role of inflammasome and how NLRP3 is involved in neuropathic pain. Therefore, based on the facts available, it has been suggested that focusing on inflammasome activity may be a cutting-edge and successful treatment approach for neuropathic pain.

Keywords: Inflammasomes, Inflammation, Neuropathy, Neuropathic Pain models, NLRP3.

INTRODUCTION

Inflammation is a pivotal physiological reaction/immune response to harmful substances. Inflammation can occur locally or systemically by activating the innate immune system to provide a protective response in the presence of disease-causing pathogens and sterile intrusions, such as trauma, cancer, ischemia and metabolic perturbations. Pathogen-associated molecular patterns (PAMPs), the infectious pathogens, and damage-associated molecular patterns (DAMPs), the

* **Corresponding author Ashutosh Kumar:** Department of Pharmacology and Toxicology, National Institute of Pharmaceutical Education and Research (NIPER)-SAS Nagar, Mohali, Punjab, 160062, India; E-mails: drashutoshniper@gmail.com, ashutosh@niper.ac.in

Puneetpal Singh (Ed.)
All rights reserved-© 2024 Bentham Science Publishers

indicators of host cellular distress, are two different categories of innate inflammatory response. An increasing number of highly conserved sensors, called pattern recognition receptors (PRRs), detect PAMPs and DAMPs to eradicate disease-causing or harmful substances [1].

Inflammasomes are the cytosolic multiprotein complex of basic processing units for sensing PAMPs and DAMPs and actively integrating their downstream signalling. Inflammasomes are basically composed of a sensor molecule called the pattern recognition receptor, an adaptor protein and an effector known as inflammatory caspases. A few sensor molecules recognized that take part in the assembly are nucleotide-binding oligomerization domain (NOD), leucine-rich repeat (LLR), NOD-like receptors (NLRs) family, absent in melanoma 2-(AIM2-) like receptors (ALRs) family, interferon-inducible protein 16 (IFI-16), and retinoic acid-inducible gene I (RIG-I). The inflammatory signal is attained by the assembly of hetero-oligomeric complex. After the activation of the sensor molecule, they promote the involvement of apoptosis-associated spec like protein containing caspase activation and recruitment domain (CARD). They trigger the proteolytic activity of proinflammatory caspases, which leads to the activation of proinflammatory mediators that stimulate systemic immunological responses and inflammation [2, 3].

The most important function of the inflammasome is the detection of stimuli and to respond against those stimuli to induce cellular responses and host defense. This control system for the inflammatory processes is inherent to effectively regulating inflammasomes. Inflammatory caspase activation is the principal mechanism of inflammasome signalling. This activity requires the formation of hetero-oligomeric complexes, such as the AIM2 protein and the NOD-like receptor-pyrin-containing proteins (NLRP). The activation of caspases due to inflammasomes causes the activation of interleukin-1β (IL-1β) and interleukin-18 (IL-18) proteolytically, causing an inflammatory response. In particular, IL-1β is a guardian for cytokine that plays a crucial role in several processes that activate and control inflammation [4, 5].

Currently, there are six inflammasomes that have been identified which include NLR protein family and AIM2. NLR (Leucine-rich repeat and pyrin domain-containing protein) protein family includes NLRP1, NLRP3, NLRP6, NLRP12 and NLRC4/IPAF inflammasome (NLR family CARD domain-containing protein). These NLR inflammasomes have a C-terminus LRR for ligand recognition and a Nucleotide-Binding Domain (NBD) for self-oligomerization. NLR family, being a crucial component of the innate immune system, is able to sense a variety of bacterial and viral stimuli. Among all the NLR inflammasomes, NLRP3 inflammasomes are widely present in the immune cells, such as macrophages, neutrophils and to some lesser extent in dendritic cells, microglial cells and dorsal root ganglia. Thus, the activation of NLRP3 leads to the release of proinflammatory mediators and contributes to the pathogenesis of several painful inflammatory conditions. Recently, AIM2 has also shown a significant connection to inflammation and pain-related pathways [6, 7] (Fig. **1**).

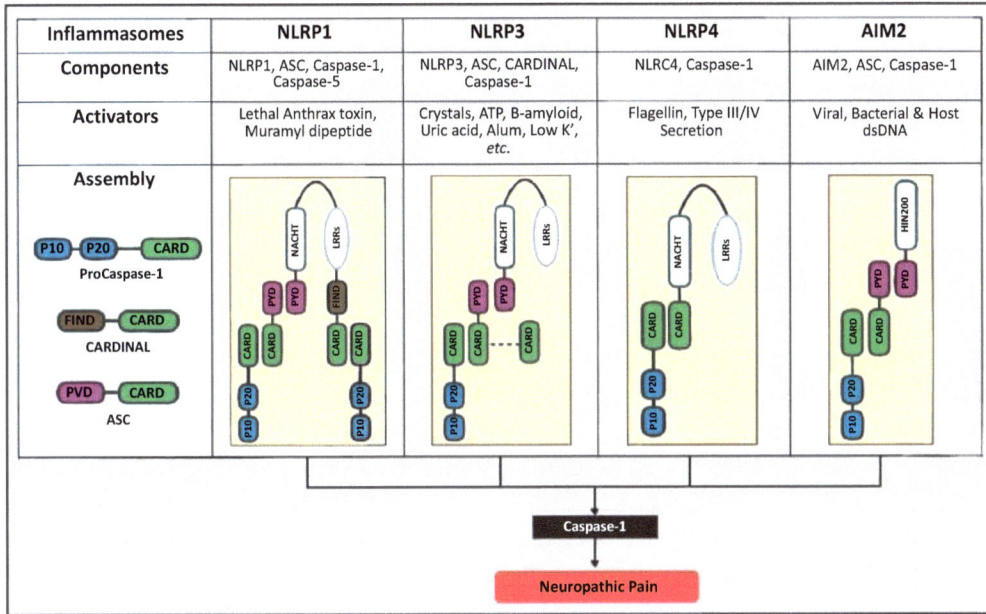

Fig. (1). NLRP1, leucine-rich repeat (LRR) and pyrin domain (PYD) containing protein 1; NLRP3, leucine-rich repeat (LRR) and pyrin domain (PYD) containing protein 3; NLRC4, NLR family CARD domain-containing protein 4; AIM2, absent in melanoma 2. All these Inflammasomes lead to the formation of caspase-1, followed by neuropathic Pain.

NLRP1 Inflammasomes

NLRP1 is the first cytosolic sensor discovered to construct a caspase-1-activated inflammasome response for the toxins produced by *Bacillus anthracis* [2]. NLRP1 connects to ASC *via* the PYD domain and caspase-1 *via* the CARD domain. Microbial ligands/bacterial toxins activate NLRP1, and these toxins, after entering the cytosol, play a pivotal role in the induction, assembly and activation of NLRP1 inflammasome [3, 4]. Numerous illnesses, including Vitiligo, Inflammatory Bowel Disease (IBD), Systemic Lupus Erythematosus (SLE), Human Mendelian Monogenic Disease, and Celiac disease are connected to NLRP1 inflammasomes [5, 6]. Recent studies have identified that the anti-apoptotic proteins Bcl-2 and Bcl-xL bind to NLRP1 and inhibit the activation. Apart from that, inhibiting the binding of ATP to NLRP1 has also been demonstrated to reduce NLRP1 oligomerization. As a result, it prevents caspase-1 from activating on its own and digesting proinflammatory cytokines. K^+ efflux also appears crucial for NLRP1 activation in addition to the possible NLRP1 activity regulators. Studies have indicated that rats with chronic constriction injury (CCI)-induced neuropathic pain had highly activated NLRP1 inflammasome in the hippocampus. In addition to reducing depressive-like behaviours, inhibiting the NLRP1 inflammasome product also reduced the amount of IL-1β produced in the hippocampus of CCI rats [7].

NLRC4 Inflammasomes

NLRC4 inflammasome is crucial in identifying and managing intracellular bacterial infections [8]. It is the only member of the NLRC family, and it has C-terminal LRRs, a central NBD domain, and an amino-terminal CARD. Without the assistance of an adaptor protein, NLRC4 interacts with procaspase-1 *via* its CARD domain. However, IL-1β secretion needs interaction with ASC. The Neural Apoptosis Inhibitor Proteins (NAIPs), a member of the non-NLR family, must bind to NLRC4 to activate, which makes it distinct from other inflammasomes. NAIPs serve as PAMP sensors, and upon direct ligand binding, they join forces with NLRC4 to create the NAIP/NLRC4 inflammasome. Caspase-1 is then drawn in and activated, which leads to the release of mature IL-1β and IL-18. NLRC4 activation also requires a conformational shift after being phosphorylated by protein kinase Cδ [9]. Intracellular bacterial flagellin or elements of the pathogen-produced type-3 secretion system are examples of ligands for NLRC4 inflammasome activation [10]. Evidence supports the protective effect of NLRC4 against respiratory melioidosis and Salmonella typhimurium infection *in vivo* [11 - 13].

NLRP3 Inflammasomes

The most extensively researched inflammasome is the NLRP3 inflammasome. NLRP3 inflammasomes include NLRP3, ASC, the CARD-containing Protein-CARDINAL, and caspase-1 [14]. NEK7, a serine/threonine kinase essential for advancing the mitotic cell cycle, is required to form the NLRP3 inflammasome. Direct binding between NEK7 and the LRR domain of NLRP3 during cell interphase promotes inflammasome assembly [15, 16]. Several molecular alterations like increased levels of glucose, cholesterol, low intracellular potassium, increased intracellular calcium, depletion of ATP, Cathepsin B released from damaged lysosomes, production of mitochondrial ROS, release of mitochondrial DNA or cardiolipin activate the NLRP3 inflammasome [17].

The activation of NLRP3 inflammasome is also helpful in developing innate and adaptive immunological responses and antimicrobial host defence against various pathogens [18, 19]. However, overexpression of the NLRP3 inflammasome under pathological circumstances causes various diseases, including autoimmune disorders, neurodegenerative, metabolic, neuroinflammatory, and neuropathic conditions [20 - 22]. Therefore, more research is necessary to fully comprehend the complex processes of NLRP3 activation, which will help to create therapeutics for disorders linked to the NLRP3 inflammasome.

AIM2 Inflammasome

AIM2 is the most recent and well-known non-NLR capable of generating an inflammasome [23] and is primarily present in the cytosol of neural and skin tissues. In contrast to NLRs, which connect indirectly to their ligands, AIM2 directly binds to double-stranded DNA (dsDNA). AIM2 can also interact with ASC through their PYD to create a caspase-1 stimulating inflammasome, which results in the release of IL-1β [24, 25]. Infections caused by intracellular bacterial and viral DNA activate the AIM2 inflammasome, which then coordinates the host response [26, 27]. AIM2 inflammasome detects self-DNA molecules and leads to activation. Activated AIM2 inflammasome causes disorders, such as carcinogenesis, psoriasis, and systemic lupus erythematosus [28, 29]. In type 2 diabetic patients, circulating mitochondrial DNA activates the AIM2 inflammasome, which indicates that AIM2 plays a significant role in the development of chronic inflammation in type 2 diabetes [30]. Understanding the controls over AIM2 inflammasome activation may help us prevent several human disorders.

Neuropathic Pain

According to the International Association for the Study of Pain (IASP), neuropathic pain is defined as "pain initiated or caused by the lesion or disease of the somatosensory nervous system" [31]. It has been estimated that approx 7–10% of the population experience persistent neuropathic pain. Neuropathic pain is characterized by paresthesia, dysesthesia, hyperalgesia, allodynia, tingling and burning sensations. Neuropathic pain occurs due to lesions or disorders of the somatosensory system, including central neurons, peripheral fibres (Aβ, Aδ, C fibres) and the spinal or supraspinal nervous system. Various disorders are linked to neuropathic pain, such as diabetic neuropathy, trigeminal neuralgia, radiculo-pathy, H.I.V. infection, stroke, post-herpetic neuropathy and amputation [32].

The progression of neuropathic pain involves alterations in the expression and function of voltage-gated sodium, potassium, and calcium channels, transient receptor potential channel (TRP) and in the activity of nociceptive neurons and inhibitory interneurons. Apart from these alterations, other inflammatory responses also present diverse cellular pathways in the setting of pathological circumstances for chronic neuropathic pain [33]. As a result of these alterations, the sensory pathways become hyperexcited, causing the brain to acquire altered sensory signals. This hyperexcitability may eventually lead to a neuropathic pain condition. Since neuropathic pain frequently coexists with other issues, including depression, anxiety, sleep disturbances, and heavy prescription medication usage, it can significantly lower quality of life. Patients with neuropathic pain report a much lower quality of life in terms of physical and emotional health than the general population.

Numerous pharmacological classes, including opioids, calcium channel blockers, antidepressants, and topical lidocaine, have been shown to exhibit consistent effectiveness in randomized controlled clinical studies [34]. Among available medications compared to monoamine reuptake inhibitors, tricyclic antidepressants show promising results in limiting the spread of pain. Tricyclic antidepressants can regulate the emotional elements of pain and their analgesic effects because depression is a common comorbidity with chronic neuropathy [35]. The opioid receptors on presynaptic and postsynaptic neurons are agonists in opioid analgesics. The use of opioids is limited due to concerns about long-term adverse effects, including immunological alterations, physical dependence, abuse, or violence [36]. Pregabalin and gabapentin bind to the calcium channel of afferent nociceptors and reduce neurotransmitter release. However, these drugs provide only short-term systematic relief due to the extensive range of adverse effects. Thus, their usage is closely monitored in patients with neuropathic pain [37]. Lidocaine blocks non-specific sodium channels without causing numbness on the injured skin, relieving strain on the peripheral afferent fibres. Topical therapy provides frequent relief of temporary pain by inhibiting pain signals from a particular body part when insufficient systemic absorption occurs. However, they also have local side effects, such as erythema or dermatitis [38]. Recently, some invasive therapies such as spinal cord stimulation, intrathecal pump implantation, and transcranial magnetic stimulation have been used in patients resistant to drug treatment [32]. These therapies are only limited to patients who are unresponsive to pharmacological interventions. Despite the wide range of available medications, treatment is ineffective due to various side effects and other factors [39]. Neuropathic pain is still a critical medical need that has gone unmet, and there are many great options, but their practicality and acceptability are less than ideal.

Pathophysiology of Neuropathic Pain

The pathophysiology of neuropathic pain is multifactorial, involving structural, physiological and functional changes along the neuroaxis. Neuropathic pain may be disease-induced, physical nerve injury during surgery or trauma and also drug-induced Table **1**. The main mechanisms underlying neuropathic pain include significant stimulation or alteration in the dorsal horn of the spinal cord, NMDA (N-methyl-D-aspartate) receptor activation, alteration in the expression and function of voltage-sensitive ion channels, stimulation of transcriptional factor - nuclear factor-kappa B (NF-κB), and generation of inflammatory cytokines *via* activation of inflammasomes like NLRP3, AIM2 *etc.*, which contribute to the neuropathic pain [101].

Table 1. Neuropathic Pain Models

S. No.	Model	Mode of Induction	Species	Advantage	Disadvantage	Refs.
A. Nerve Injury Models:						
1.	Axotomy	Complete transection of the sciatic nerve by removing a portion of the sciatic nerve.	Rats	Create pain from phantom limbs.	Absence of local inflammatory elements.	[40, 41]
2.	Brachial plexus avulsion	Brachial plexus dissection.	Rats	There is no autotomy. Neuropathy can be recognized at places other than the site of damage (in both hind paws).	Thermal Hyperalgesia is not observed.	[42, 43]
3.	Chronic constriction injury	Around the sciatic nerve, four loose ligatures spaced 1 mm apart.	Rats, Mice	Pain is created steadily. Easy procedure and within 24 hours following the operation, a reproducible response was noticed.	Variations in the reaction are associated with variations in the ligature and suture material's tightness.	[44, 45]
4.	Partial sciatic nerve ligation (Seltzer Model)	Tight ligation of the sciatic nerve, between one-third or one-half.	Rats, Mice	There is no autotomy. Simple surgical technique.	It is impossible to ligate the same number of axons at the same place of the nerve.	[46, 47]
5.	Spared nerve injury	Tibial and common peroneal nerve axotomy.	Rats, Mice	Strong response and reproducible.	Sural nerve injury can result in paralysis.	[48, 49]
6.	Spinal nerve ligation	A tight ligation of the spinal neurons at L5 and L6 segments.	Rats	Lower variation and higher repeatability.	Muscle injury due to intense operative procedure.	[50 - 52]

S. No.	Model	Mode of Induction	Species	Advantage	Disadvantage	Refs.
7.	Tibial and sural nerve transection	Tibial and sural nerve axotomy.	Rats	Used to investigate sympathetically independent pain.	Pain produced is only dependent on the sympathetic nervous system.	[53, 54]
8.	Ligation of common peroneal nerve	Suturing of the common peroneal nerve.	Mice	Long-lasting thermal hyperalgesia and allodynia.	Cannot be used to study motor function.	[55]
9.	Caudal trunk resection	Resection of the inferior caudal trunk between the S3 and S4 spinal nerves.	Rats, Mice	Allodynia and hyperalgesia produced last for weeks.	Surgical procedure is time consuming and post-operative care is required.	[56, 57]
10.	Sciatic cryoneurolysis	Sciatic Nerve freezing.	Rats	Distinct peripheral analgesic in that it does not cause sensory, motor, or proprioceptive impairments.	Employs extreme cold to reversibly ablate a peripheral nerve, resulting in acute analgesia.	[58]
11.	Photochemical model of spinal cord injury	Thrombosis of small arteries connecting the sciatic nerve using a photosensitizing dye and a laser.	Rats, Mice	Low mortality and little invasiveness.	Irregular infracts can arise as a result of poor illumination.	[59, 60]
12.	Sciatic inflammatory neuritis	Zymosan, HMG, and TNF-alpha injections around the sciatic nerve.	Rats, Mice	Mechanical allodynia develops within 3 hours of injection.	No Thermal Hyperalgesia.	[61, 62]
13.	Cuffing-induced sciatic nerve injury	Polyethylene cuff implantation around the sciatic nerve.	Rats, Mice	Variability is low, and genetically engineered organisms can be employed.	Infections might occur if the polyethylene cuff is of poor quality.	[63, 64]
14.	Trigeminal Neuralgia	Chronic compression of trigeminal ganglion or chronic constriction of infra-orbital nerve.	Rats	Due to various etiologies, disease-related pain may be classified as central as well as peripheral.	Hyperalgesia is mostly not observed.	[65, 66]

(Table 1) cont.....

S. No.	Model	Mode of Induction	Species	Advantage	Disadvantage	Refs.
15.	Weight drop or contusive spinal cord injury (Allen's Model)	Dropping heavy weight over exposed sciatic nerve.	Rats, Mice	Easy to perform. CNS-related pain is studied.	Chance of reproducibility is very low.	[67, 68]
16.	Excitotoxic spinal cord injury	Injections of excitatory amino acids into the spinal cord.	Rats, Mice	Helpful in researching the CNS-related pain.	Chemical interactions are one of the major concerns.	[69, 70]
17.	Spinal hemisection	Laminectomy is performed at T11–T12 segments.	Rats	By separating the damaged area from the intact side. CNS-related pain is studied.	Complicated surgical procedure.	[71, 72]
B. Disease-Induced Neuropathic Pain Models:						
1.	Diabetes-induced neuropathy	Streptozotocin injections result in prolonged hyperglycemia, which causes neuropathy in genetic models.	Rats, Mice	Clinical condition is mimicked.	It takes a long time to induce and it is challenging to measure spontaneous pain.	[73 - 78]
2.	Cancer pain model	By injecting cancer cells	Rats, Mice	Correlate discomfort from nerve compression in cancer patients.	Different cancer cell invasion results in variable effects.	[79 - 83]
3.	HIV-induced Neuropathy	Wrapping cellulose with HIV-1 envelope protein gp120 on the sciatic nerve.	Rats	Paraesthesis with symmetrical pain.	Workers may be unintentionally exposed to the HIV-1 envelope protein gp120.	[84, 85]
4.	Post-herpetic neuralgia (Varicella Zoster virus, Herpes simplex virus, Non-viral model)	Injection of virally-infected cells into the footpad, Depletion of capsaicin-sensitive afferents contaminated with resiniferotoxin.	Rats, Mice	All virus models are unique in that they have different advantages for disease conditions.	High facility is required to induce virus, and human safety should be taken care of.	[86 - 88]

(Table 1) cont.....

S. No.	Model	Mode of Induction	Species	Advantage	Disadvantage	Refs.
C. Drug-Induced Neuropathic Pain Models:						
1.	Anticancer Drug-Induced Neuropathic Pain	Drugs that cause direct damage to the nerves of the peripheral nervous system by injecting drugs like vincristine, cisplatin, oxaliplatin, and paclitaxel.	Rats, Mice, Guinea pigs	Similar to clinical symptoms and an excellent model for long-term research.	Autonomic and neurophysiological problems arise with increasing dosage.	[89 - 93]
2.	Anti-retroviral drugs induced neuropathic pain	By injecting antiviral drugs, such as didanosine, stavudine, and zalcitabine.	Rats, Rabbits	Useful in examining the function of aberrant mitochondrial and caspase-1 signalling in neuropathic pain behaviour.	Neuropathic pain behaviour is transient.	[94 - 96]
D. Miscellaneous Models:						
1.	Alcoholic neuropathy	Ethanol administration for an extended period of ~ 70 days.	Rats	Causes a painful, small-fiber neuropathy known as "dying back neuropathy" that is marked by distal axonal degeneration.	When alcohol was first consumed, some analgesia effects were observed.	[97, 98]
2.	Pyridoxine-induced neuropathy	Long-term administration of a high dosage of pyridoxine.	Rats, Dogs	A reversible sensory nerve axonopathy develops at low and intermediate dosages, while an irreversible sensory ganglion neuropathy develops at high doses.	Different doses produce different effects, so determination of dose is essential.	[99, 100]

Synaptic transmission plays a significant role in chronic pain conditions, which is usually facilitated by interacting non-nociceptive myelinated Aβ, Aδ fibers and nociceptive C-fibers with microglia. At the same time, GABAergic interneurons often have an inhibitory impact on the neuron. Peripheral sensitization of primary neurons, caused by nerve injury or partial nerve ligation, occurs when some axons degenerate and become damaged. In contrast, others are still functional and attached to the peripheral organs.

However, during injury, the activation of sodium channels is enhanced in injured neurons. In the area of spared fibers, a nerve growth factor linked to Wallerian degeneration is produced, which can increase the expression of channels and receptors on unharmed fibres, such as adrenoreceptors, sodium channels, and Transient receptor potential V1 (TRPV1) receptors. Mechanoreceptor of A-fiber input is translated into pain by hyperexcitation at the spinal cord, triggering the immediate activation at C-fibers [102]. Central sensitization involves both presynaptic and postsynaptic ligands, such as calcium channels, opioid receptors, GABA, glutamate, sodium/5HT, and AMPA/kainate receptors. Central sensitizations are increased after nerve injury because of decreased activity of inhibitory interneurons and descending pain modulatory systems. Chemokines are released from microglia in response to nerve damage and activate spinal cord glial cells, which in turn leads to the production of inflammasomes, interleukins, cytokines, and growth factors as well as rising glutamate concentrations [103]. Apart from these, oxidative stress, neuroinflammation, mitochondrial dysfunction, and lysosomal damage also contribute to the development and progression of neuropathic pain.

Neuroinflammation

Neuroinflammation plays an important role in the development of neuropathic pain *via* the interaction of the immune system with the sensory nervous system. It is characterized by increased vascular permeability, glial cell activation, immune cell infiltration, and increased synthesis of inflammasomes [104]. As a result of nerve damage, resident immune cells such as mast cells and macrophages react with Schwann cells to damage the axons. Then, these damaged axons activate the extracellular signal-related (ERK) mitogen-activated protein kinase (MAPK), which leads to the release of inflammatory mediators like cytokines, prostaglandins, chemokines, and reactive oxygen species (ROS) [105, 106], recruiting the immune cells at the site of injury. The blood-brain barrier (BBB) and the blood-spinal cord barrier become permeable due to peripheral nerve damage, which might promote the storming of peripheral immune cells into the central nervous system (CNS) [107]. Activated peripheral glia, such as Schwann cells in the nerve and satellite cells in the trigeminal and dorsal root ganglia, are involved in the progression of pain. The primary line of defence in the CNS is microglia, which actively scan their surroundings for possible disruptions while also helping to re-establish equilibrium. The released glial activators may cause several alterations in molecular mechanisms and gene expression in glial cells that result in nerve injury (Fig. **2**).

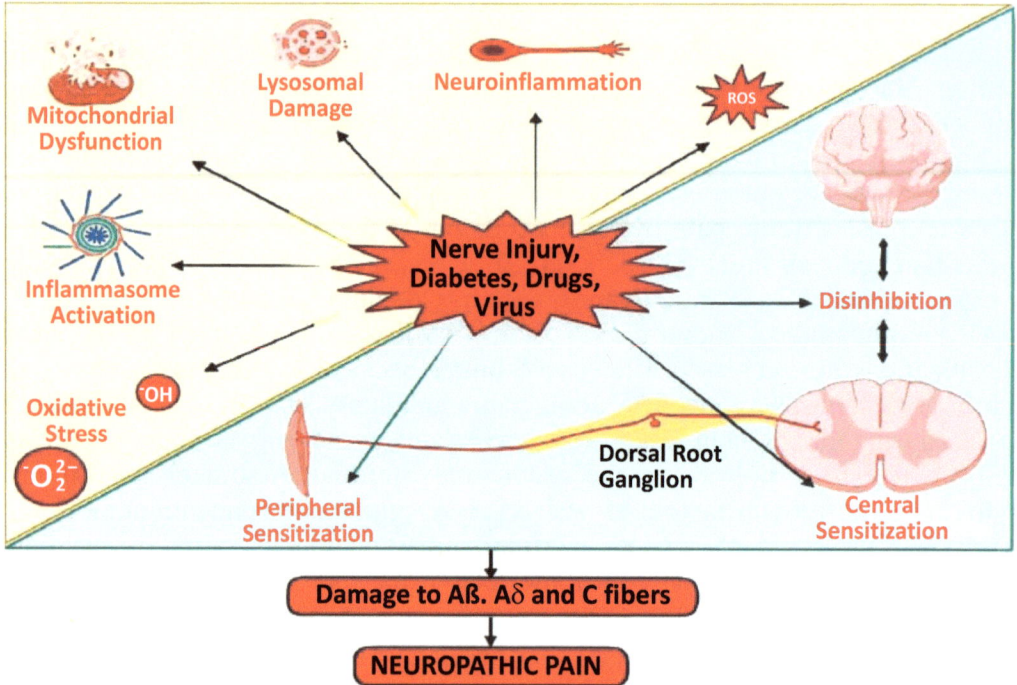

Fig. (2). Due to various factors such as enrve injury, diabetes, drugs, viruses, *etc.*, there is an alteration in the metabolic process, such as oxidative stress, mitochondrial dysfunction, lysosomal damage, neuroinflammation, ROS generation, disinhibition, and peripheral and central sensitization. These modifications damage the nerve fibres ending up in neuropathic conditions.

Furthermore, active microglia have been shown to activate astrocytes. In contrast, astrocyte stimulation produces signalling molecules that affect activated microglia—an essential aspect of the involvement of astrocytes-microglia in the pathophysiology of neuropathic pain [108 - 110]. Additionally, the activation of proinflammatory cytokines, inflammasomes, ROS, and growth factors can alter excitatory and inhibitory synaptic transmission and intensify pain through central and peripheral sensitization. In particular, the significance of proinflammatory cytokines in pain induction, including tumour necrosis factor (TNF), IL-1β, IL-18, and IL-6, has long been acknowledged. Various animal experiments have demonstrated that it causes neuropathy-like behaviour, therefore, inhibiting them in the CNS and PNS reduces neuropathic pain [111].

Sensitization and Disinhibition Mechanisms

According to the IASP, central sensitization is defined as "an increase in the responsiveness of nociceptive neurons in the central nervous system to normal or subthreshold afferent input" [112]. Central sensitization is distinguished from peripheral sensitization by tactile allodynia and hyperalgesia without harmful stimulations. Synaptic transfer in central sensitization has two activities, *i.e.*, short and long-lasting activities. Short-lasting activity occurs due to heterosynaptic potential, whereas long-lasting activity is due to alterations in astrocytes, microglia, excitation of membrane and gene transcription [104].

Peripheral sensitization is defined as a decrease in threshold followed by a sudden increased activity of the nociceptor's peripheral ends [113]. Once tissue damage occurs, there is an increase in the translocation of inflammasomes to the injury site. Following are the major processes involved in peripheral sensitization: (i) Posttranslational modification, such as phosphorylation, acetylation, ribosylates, nitrosylation, and ubiquitination [114] and (ii) Alterations in gene expression, such as chemical alterations to the DNA or DNA-associated proteins, production of noncoding RNAs, or chemical alterations to the RNA [115].

Afferent terminal sprouting, disinhibition, and central sensitization enhance Aβ fibre-mediated pain. During pain transmission, presynaptic modulation occurs at the synapses between the terminals of primary sensory neurons and inhibitory dorsal horn interneurons [116]. Additionally, spinal interneurons- GABAergic and glycinergic inhibition control the activity of postsynaptic transmission [117]. Symptoms such as tactile allodynia are caused by inhibiting GABAergic or glycinergic receptors, followed by increased synaptic currents to nociceptive lamina I neurons from Aβ fibres. The amygdala, anterior cingulate gyrus, and hypothalamus are the origins of several downstream pathways involved in modifying the spinal transmission of nociceptive information [118]. Additionally, the brain stem nuclei in the rostroventral medulla and periaqueductal grey convey the original descending routes to the spinal cord. These downstream pathways involve many inhibitory transmitters, including 5-hydroxytryptamine, norepinephrine, and endogenous opioids [119]. The tonic noradrenergic inhibition that affects α2-adrenoceptors appears to be halted after nerve damage, and the overall impact of descending serotoninergic input switches from inhibition to facilitation. These alterations cause this complex system of inhibitory regulation to change. Due to the decrease in the expression level of opioid μ receptors in primary afferent neurons brought on by nerve damage, dorsal horn neurons are found to be less sensitive to the inhibitory effects of opioid μ agonists [120]. Additionally, many processes are at play, including the loss of presynaptic and postsynaptic GABAergic inhibition in the spinal cord. However, in nociceptive lamina I neurons, increased transmembrane gradient for chloride ions leads to a reduction in GABA-A receptor activation-driven hyperpolarization.

As a result, this mechanism activates depolarization, resulting in paradoxical excitation and activation. This perplexing excitation is exacerbated further by the brain-derived neurotrophic factor (BDNF) production by active microglia, which causes potassium cotransporter isoform 2 to be downregulated [121]. In contrast, the loss of GABAergic interneurons (IPSCs) independently impairs the inhibition in the dorsal horn of the spinal cord, which results in a reduction in the activation of GABAergic inhibitory postsynaptic currents (IPSCs) induced by afferent stimulation. By stopping the apoptotic cell and restoring GABAergic IPSCs, mechanical allodynia, hyperalgesia, and cold allodynia caused by post-nerve damage can be reduced [122]. Loss of spinal inhibitory interneurons is cited as the leading cause of post-nerve injury and chronic pain. A potential technique for treating neuropathic pain is to modulate the GABA receptor [123].

Oxidative Stress

In response to environmental stress, most living organisms initiate sequences of molecular processes that include complicated alterations in cellular macromolecules, including proteins, lipids, and nucleic acids [124]. Such alterations result in DNA damage, followed by cellular apoptosis and necrosis [125].

The redox reactions control a wide range of neurological functions, including neurotransmission and degeneration, and help in maintaining the homeostasis of the nervous system [126]. The equilibrium is regularly maintained by removing substances like reactive oxygen species (ROS) and reactive nitrogen species (RNS). In neutralizing ROS/RNS, several endogenous antioxidants, including glutathione, superoxide dismutase (SOD), and catalase, play a crucial role [127]. Additionally, the transcription factor nuclear factor erythroid 2-related factor 2(Nrf2) is a crucial modulator of redox homeostasis that protects against damage by enhancing the formation of several antioxidants and detoxifying enzymes. Excessive ROS/RNS generation and impaired degradation can upset redox equilibrium, causing a buildup of nitroxidative species that harm the cellular environment. Reactive oxygen species majorly include superoxide ($O_2 \bullet$), hydroxyl radical ($HO \bullet$), and hydrogen peroxide (H_2O_2). Electron Transport Chain (*ETC*) and NOX enzymes are the primary endogenous producers of ROS. However, other enzymes can also produce ROS, including xanthine oxidase, cyclooxygenases, lipoxygenases, cytochrome P450 monooxygenases, and nitric oxide synthases (NOS). However, the only specific and controlled producers of ROS are NOXs. Nitric oxide ($NO \bullet$) and peroxynitrite ($ONOO-$) are two examples of reactive nitrogen species (RNS), which are engaged in redox signalling [128] and have the NOS as their primary sources. NO synthases convert L-arginine into nitric oxide (NO•), which then combines with oxygen to make peroxynitrite (ONOO–). Both H_2O_2 and NO• are crucial for physiological function. However, the disruption of redox balance can set off the pathophysiological processes linked to several illnesses, including neuropathy. The equilibrium between pro- and antioxidant processes is modulated by many drugs, such as opioids, NSAIDs and antidepressants, in a way that is important to both their clinical effectiveness and side effects. The CNS and PNS are particularly susceptible to nitroxidative species because of their high lipid content and weak antioxidant defence [129, 130]. Synaptic strength in the excitatory state is elevated and reduced inhibitory state at the spinal cord synapses in neuropathic conditions. The excitability of the strength of nociceptive neuronsand the plasticity of their synapses can be regulated by ROS, either actively or passively [131]. Oxidative stress results in mitochondrial dysfunction, which appears as cellular metabolic and functional deficiencies and may eventually induce the degeneration of primary afferents. Higher levels of radical leakage from dysfunctional mitochondria lead to a buildup of ROS and a mechanism of nitroxidative damage [132].

Additionally, nitroxidative species can alter the structure of the mitochondria and promote the production of pro-apoptotic factors [133]. Due to the suppression of MAPK phosphatases and oxidative alterations of MAPK signalling proteins, oxidative stress is also a significant contributor to neuroinflammation *via* modifying neuroinflammatory signalling, such as transcription factors like NF-κB and MAPK pathways [134]. Through TLRs, nitroxidative species and signals produced by damaged mitochondria also cause proinflammatory reactions. In several neuropathic pain models, ROS has been demonstrated to control cytokine production. Increased ROS levels are linked to proinflammatory cytokine upregulation [135], and concurrent anti-inflammatory cytokines are downregulated in the nervous system. Additionally, ROS reduce BBB permeability by activating NOX in a cytokine-dependent manner [136]. NLRP3 inflammasomes can also be triggered by oxidative stress. ROS may influence the priming of the NLRP3 inflammasome rather than its activation and help in the development of neuropathic pain [137].

Mitochondrial Dysfunction

Mitochondrial dysfunction is a common pathogenic mechanism linked to the development of many disorders defined by neurodegeneration and altered metabolic markers [138]. Maintaining a crucial pool of intact mitochondria may help in providing important ATP supply, appropriate metabolic control, and apoptosis prevention for neurons in metabolic imbalance and neurodegeneration.

This can be accomplished by modulating two mechanisms-mitochondrial dynamics and mitophagy pathways [139]. As a result, interventions focused on modulating these pathways are significantly studied , particularly for issues related to bioenergetic deficiency and mitochondrial dysfunction.

Mitophagy is critical for maintaining mitochondrial integrity and homeostasis. Several distinct effectors are known to engage in the mitophagy process. Among these effectors are PINK1/Parkin and several mitophagy receptors, including NIP3-like protein X (NIX; also known as BNIP3L), BNIP3, FK506 Binding Protein 8 (FKBP8), Syntaxin 17 (STX17), and FUN14 domain containing 1 (FUNDC1). A balance between mitophagy and inflammasome activities is necessary to prevent harmful inflammatory reactions against microbial or other dangerous signals and maintain a protective defence mechanism and overall health. Any imbalance between mitophagy and inflammasome induces mitochondrial stress, leading to pyroptosis, pathological inflammation and neuropathic pain [140].

Mitochondrial dynamics are essential in inflammasome activation, linked to persistent inflammation and discomfort in diabetic conditions. Furthermore, Drp1 inhibition and production of fusion proteins reduce inflammatory responses due to inflammasomes, indicating that elements in mitochondrial dynamics control inflammasome activation. However, during RNA virus infection, MFN2 interacts with NLRP3 and activates the inflammasome [141, 142].

Excess ROS production caused by Drp1-mediated mitochondrial fission is connected to the pathophysiology of neuropathic pain. Therefore, mitophagy, Drp1, and mtROS homeostasis disruption in the mitochondria play crucial roles in neuropathic pain [143].

Lysosomal Damage

Particles activate the NLRP3 inflammasome in macrophages, including silica, asbestos, amyloid-β, cholesterol crystals, and uric acids [144 - 146]. After phagocytosis, foreign debris damages lysosomes, which causes lysosomal contents to spill into the cytoplasm. Uncertainty persists regarding the exact mechanism that connects lysosomal damage to the activation of the NLRP3 inflammasome. Additionally, LPS and nicotine increase endothelial cell lysosomal membrane permeability and cause the release of cathepsin B and K^+ efflux from lysosomes, which increases NLRP3 inflammasome activation [147, 148].

Through the combined effects of lysosomal disruption, membrane permeabilization, and enhanced K^+ efflux, the soluble lysosomotropic drug leu-

leu-O-methyl ester (LLME) causes NLRP3 inflammasome activation [149]. The release of cathepsin B from lysosomes causes the NLRP3 inflammasome activation when treated with CA-074-Me (an inhibitor for cathepsin B), which shows a protective effect against cathepsin B [150].

Studies have shown that cathepsin B release is necessary for IL-1β and IL-18 release, suggesting that cathepsin B is involved in activating the NLRP3 inflammasome [151]. Cathepsin B also activates pro-caspase-1, which triggers the maturation and release of IL-1β and IL-18 by spinal microglia and is essential for producing chronic inflammatory pain. Cathepsin B inhibitors may be a valuable new target for treating pain caused by inflammation [152].

NLRP3 Activation and Diabetic Neuropathic Pain

Neuropathic pain caused by nerve injuries can produce a variety of DAMPs/PAMPs, which in turn trigger the activation of the NLRP3 inflammasome [153,-155]. During neuropathic pain, the NLRP3 inflammasome is expressed and activated in the sensory nervous system and its surrounding environment, including the spinal cord dorsal horn such as neurons, microglia, and astrocytes [156, 157]; peripheral inflamed cells such as mast cells, macrophages, and neutrophils [158, 159]; and peripheral nerves and DRG [160, 161]. Therefore, understanding the molecular mechanisms of NLRP3 implicated in neuropathic pain conditions is vital in the treatment and research aspect. According to widespread consensus, the activation of the NLRP3 inflammasome occurs *via* the Toll-like receptor (TLR) 4, IL-1 receptor (R), and TNF-R, and it is a two-step process that involves priming and secondary signal (assembly) [162, 163].

Innate immune cells must produce pro-IL-1, pro-IL-18, and NLRP3 as the initial signal for priming of inflammasomes. In reality, a variety of variables at the transcriptional level strictly control the inflammasome activity [164]. Interferon regulatory factor 1(IRF1), AP-1, and other transcriptional factors regulate the assembly of NLRP3 inflammasomes and NF-κB activation [165, 166]. For further activation of inflammasome complex formation, these priming signals also cause phosphorylation of ASC, deubiquitination and ubiquitination of NLRP3, among other post-translational changes of various inflammasome components [167]. The second signals are necessary for the NLRP3 inflammasome assembly, even though the inflammasome assembly is still not completely understood. Pro-caspase-1 is recruited and activated due to the binding between NLRP3 and ASC during the development of NLRP3 inflammasome complexes [168]. The second signal consists of bacterial pore-forming toxins, potassium efflux through ATP-dependent P2X7 receptor activation, mtROS production, and cathepsin B release from lysosomal damage [169]. An essential catalyst for ATP release during apoptosis is pannexin-1, a channel-forming glycoprotein. It is also involved in canonical or non-canonical NLRP3 inflammasome activation during apoptosis [170, 171]. Significantly, impaired mitophagy, increased mitochondrial fission protein Drp1 and increased mitochondrial ROS act as the second signal to activate NLRP3 and are vitally engaged in mitochondrial disturbance and dysfunction. The NLRP3 inflammasome is activated due to increased mitochondrial ROS production caused by mitochondrial Ca^{2+} excess and other mitochondrial alterations [172 - 174]. In this situation, the cytosolic translocation of mitochondrial DNA serves as a platform for inflammasome formation and the mitochondria-associated membrane functions as a signal for NLRP3 inflammasome activation [175]. Uncertainty exists about the molecular processes behind the upstream signals that activate NLRP3. Through interactions with NLPR3, mitochondrial outer membrane proteins such as mitochondrial antiviral signalling protein (MAVS) contribute to the activation of the NLRP3 inflammasome [176, 177]. Furthermore, the serine-threonine kinase NIMA-related kinase 7 (NEK7) activates the NLRP3 inflammasome *via* interactions with NLRP3 oligomerization [15, 178].

Pyroptosis is characterized by the production of proinflammatory cytokines (IL-1β and IL-18), an inflammatory form of programmed cell death. There are two recognized pyroptotic pathways: the canonical (mediated by caspase-1) and non-canonical (mediated by caspase-4/5/11) inflammasome pathways [179]. Gasdermin D (GSDMD) is a crucial precursor of inflammatory caspases (caspase-1/4/5/11) during pyroptosis. Notably, LPS from gram-negative bacteria may activate a non-canonical inflammasome to cause pyroptosis and release IL-1β and IL-18 through direct interaction with the mouse caspase-11 and human caspase-4 [180]. The development of cytotoxic pores on the cell membrane is an inherent property of the GSDMD N-terminal domain that allows it to induce pyroptosis [181, 182]. All the molecular mechanisms eventually disrupt the nervous system, leading to neuropathic conditions.

Studies have shown that symptoms in people with cryopyrin-associated periodic syndromes (CAPS), chemotherapy-induced peripheral neuropathy (CIPN), chronic constructive injury (CCI), and diabetic neuropathy are molecularly based on the elevated activity of the NLRP3 inflammasome. These works established that mutations or increased activation of NLRP3 result in caspase-1 activation and increased IL-1β and IL-18 production, leading to disease conditions [183 - 186] (Fig. **3**).

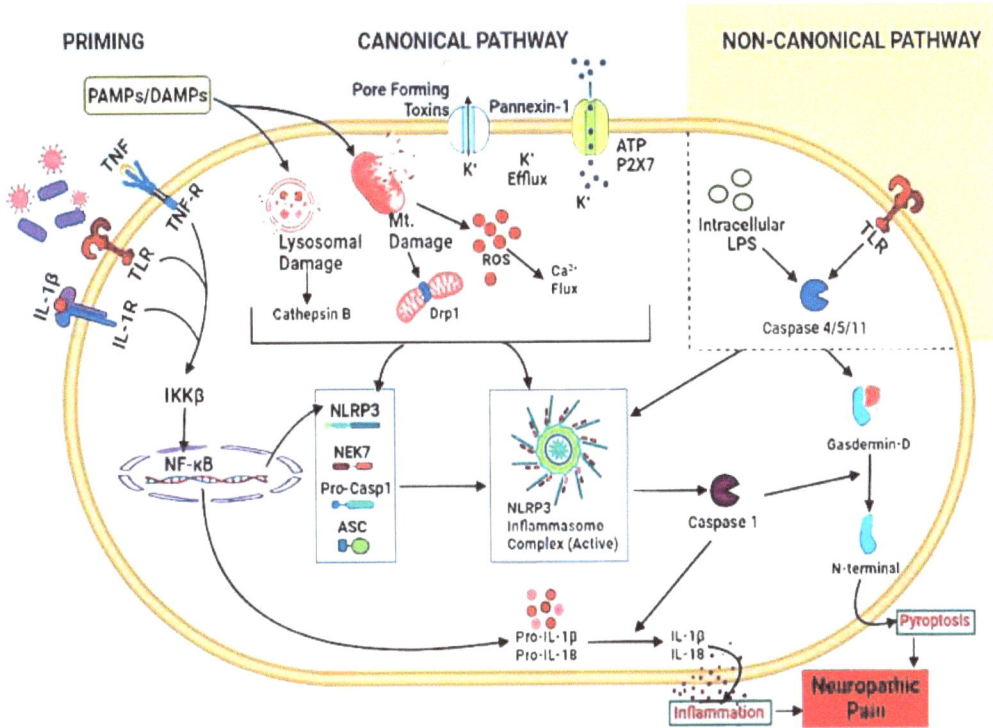

Fig. (3). NLRP3 inflammasome activation requires two stages. Priming, activated by PAMPs/DAMPs, is necessary to increase the production of pro-IL-1β, pro-IL-18, and NLRP3 *via* the nuclear factor-B (NF-κB). The second step is to activate the NLRP3 inflammasome, which comprises both canonical and noncanonical activation pathways. The canonical activation pathway involves activation signals such as ion fluxes by P2X7 receptors, lysosome damage, mitochondrial dysfunction, metabolic stress, and pore-forming toxins - all of which promote NLRP3 inflammasome assembly and activation, which cause caspase-1 activation, leading to the maturation and release of IL-1β/IL-18 and pyroptosis. The noncanonical activation pathway is mediated by caspase-4/5/11, which indirectly promotes the synthesis of interleukins and gasdermin D. All the inflammasome activations result in pyroptosis *via* gasdermin D, which serves as a significant substrate for inflammatory caspases.

Current research is focusing on a number of pharmacological inhibitors that inhibit the NLRP3 inflammasome to reduce neuropathic pain. These modulators work through a number of mechanisms, such as NLRP3-induced caspase 1 activation, inhibition of NLRP3-ASC binding, and alkalylation of NLRP3-ATPase domain cysteine residues. Table **2** provides a detailed description of these modulators.

Table 2. Pharmacological inhibitors of NLRP3.

S. No.	Drug	Target	Mechanism	Refs.
1.	MCC950	NLRP3 NACHT domain	By directly attaching to the Walker B motif of the NLRP3 NACHT domain, MCC950 inhibits ATP hydrolysis, NLRP3 activation, and inflammasome development.	[187, 188]
2.	MNS	NLRP3 LRR and NACHT domains	MNS interferes with ATPase action by targeting the cysteine residue on NLRP3.	[189]
3.	CY-09	NLRP3 NACHT domain	Inhibits ASC, Caspase-1, NLRP3 ATPase activity and blocks NLRP3 inflammasome activation.	[190]
4.	OLT1177 (Dapansutrile)	NLRP3 NACHT domain (ATPase region)	NLRP3-ASC contact is blocked by an ATPase inhibitor.	[191]
5.	Tranilast	NLRP3 NACHT domain	Blocks by binding to the NLRP3 NACHT domain.	[192]
6.	Oridonin	NLRP3 NACHT domain (cysteine 279)	Suppresses NLRP3 inflammasome activation by interacting with cysteine 279 of NLRP3 to eliminate NLRP3-NEK7 interaction.	[193]
7.	Bay 11–7082	NLRP3 NACHT domain (ATPase region), IKK, E2/3 enzymes, PTPs	Suppresses NLRP3 ATPase function by alkylating the cysteines in the ATPase domain.	[194 - 196]
8.	INF39	NLRP3 domain	Irreversibly inhibits the NLRP3 inflammasome.	[197, 198]
9.	β-carotene	NLRP3 PYD domain	Directly binds to NLRP3 and blocks.	[199, 200]
10.	Parthenolide	NLRP3 NACHT domain (cysteine modifcation), NLRP1, Caspase-1, NF-κB, IKKβ kinase activity	Caspase-1 and the NLRP3 ATPase domain cysteine residues are alkylated, which reduces the function of the NLRP3 ATPase.	[201 - 203]

CONCLUSION

The innate immune system generates inflammation locally or systemically to protect the biological system from harmful substances and to maintain homeostasis. The initial inflammatory response induces various cellular and molecular pathways to reduce the impact of pathological circumstances. The main participants in the inflammatory reactions are the complex molecular structures known as inflammasomes. After discovering inflammasomes, a new line of research on the molecular processes underlying the activation of the innate immune system in metabolic, infectious, autoinflammatory, and neurodegenerative illnesses has been opened. These diseases or metabolic alterations lead to chronic neuropathic pain characterized by paraesthesia, hyperalgesia, allodynia, tingling, and burning sensations. IL-1β and IL-18 operate as intermediate inflammatory mediators, directly or indirectly upregulating cytokines and activating nociceptive neurons. Although four inflammasome subtypes (NLRP1, NLRP3, NLRC4, and AIM2) have been found to contribute to pain, targeting specific inflammasomes might be beneficial in treating inflammasome-activating neuropathic pain. Existing medications for neuropathy need to be improved; therefore, they require even more precise and advanced approaches to solve issues like extensive side effects and ineffective mechanisms. There are many opinions on improving neuropathy medication, but its practicality and acceptance are still under discussion.

REFERENCES

[1]   Zindel J, Kubes P. DAMPs, PAMPs, and LAMPs in immunity and sterile inflammation. Annu Rev Pathol 2020; 15(1): 493-518.
[http://dx.doi.org/10.1146/annurev-pathmechdis-012419-032847] [PMID: 31675482]

[2]   Levinsohn JL, Newman ZL, Hellmich KA, *et al.* Anthrax lethal factor cleavage of Nlrp1 is required for activation of the inflammasome. PLoS Pathog 2012; 8(3): e1002638.
[http://dx.doi.org/10.1371/journal.ppat.1002638] [PMID: 22479187]

[3]   Franchi L, Eigenbrod T, Muñoz-Planillo R, Nuñez G. The inflammasome: A caspase-1-activation platform that regulates immune responses and disease pathogenesis. Nat Immunol 2009; 10(3): 241-7.
[http://dx.doi.org/10.1038/ni.1703] [PMID: 19221555]

[4]   Faustin B, Lartigue L, Bruey JM, *et al.* Reconstituted NALP1 inflammasome reveals two-step mechanism of caspase-1 activation. Mol Cell 2007; 25(5): 713-24.
[http://dx.doi.org/10.1016/j.molcel.2007.01.032] [PMID: 17349957]

[5]   Grandemange S, Sanchez E, Louis-Plence P, *et al.* A new autoinflammatory and autoimmune syndrome associated with NLRP1 mutations: NAIAD (*NLRP1-* associated autoinflammation with arthritis and dyskeratosis). Ann Rheum Dis 2017; 76(7): 1191-8.
[http://dx.doi.org/10.1136/annrheumdis-2016-210021] [PMID: 27965258]

[6]   Zhong FL, Mamaï O, Sborgi L, *et al.* Germline NLRP1 mutations cause skin inflammatory and cancer susceptibility syndromes *via* inflammasome activation. Cell 2016; 167(1): 187-202.e17.
[http://dx.doi.org/10.1016/j.cell.2016.09.001] [PMID: 27662089]

[7]   Li Q, Liu S, Zhu X, *et al.* Hippocampal PKR/NLRP1 inflammasome pathway is required for the depression-like behaviors in rats with neuropathic pain. Neuroscience 2019; 412: 16-28.
[http://dx.doi.org/10.1016/j.neuroscience.2019.05.025] [PMID: 31125603]

[8]   Andrade WA, Zamboni DS. NLRC4 biology in immunity and inflammation. J Leukoc Biol 2020; 108(4): 1117-27.
[http://dx.doi.org/10.1002/JLB.3MR0420-573R] [PMID: 32531834]

[9]   Qu Y, Misaghi S, Izrael-Tomasevic A, *et al.* Phosphorylation of NLRC4 is critical for inflammasome activation. Nature 2012; 490(7421): 539-42.
[http://dx.doi.org/10.1038/nature11429] [PMID: 22885697]

[10]   Bauer R, Rauch I. The NAIP/NLRC4 inflammasome in infection and pathology. Mol Aspects Med 2020; 76: 100863.
[http://dx.doi.org/10.1016/j.mam.2020.100863] [PMID: 32499055]

[11]   West TE, Myers ND, Chantratita N, *et al.* NLRC4 and TLR5 each contribute to host defense in respiratory melioidosis. PLoS Negl Trop Dis 2014; 8(9): e3178.
[http://dx.doi.org/10.1371/journal.pntd.0003178] [PMID: 25232720]

[12]   Hausmann A, Böck D, Geiser P, *et al.* Intestinal epithelial NAIP/NLRC4 restricts systemic dissemination of the adapted pathogen Salmonella Typhimurium due to site-specific bacterial PAMP expression. Mucosal Immunol 2020; 13(3): 530-44.
[http://dx.doi.org/10.1038/s41385-019-0247-0] [PMID: 31953493]

[13]   Tenthorey JL, Chavez RA, Thompson TW, Deets KA, Vance RE, Rauch I. NLRC4 inflammasome activation is NLRP3- and phosphorylation-independent during infection and does not protect from melanoma. J Exp Med 2020; 217(7): e20191736.
[http://dx.doi.org/10.1084/jem.20191736] [PMID: 32342103]

[14]   Martinon F, Tschopp J. NLRs join TLRs as innate sensors of pathogens. Trends Immunol 2005; 26(8): 447-54.
[http://dx.doi.org/10.1016/j.it.2005.06.004] [PMID: 15967716]

[15]   He Y, Zeng MY, Yang D, Motro B, Núñez G. NEK7 is an essential mediator of NLRP3 activation downstream of potassium efflux. Nature 2016; 530(7590): 354-7.
[http://dx.doi.org/10.1038/nature16959] [PMID: 26814970]

[16]   Schmid-Burgk JL, Chauhan D, Schmidt T, *et al.* A genome-wide CRISPR (clustered regularly interspaced short palindromic repeats) screen identifies NEK7 as an essential component of NLRP3 inflammasome activation. J Biol Chem 2016; 291(1): 103-9.
[http://dx.doi.org/10.1074/jbc.C115.700492] [PMID: 26553871]

[17]   Zhu S, Ding S, Wang P, *et al.* Nlrp9b inflammasome restricts rotavirus infection in intestinal epithelial cells. Nature 2017; 546(7660): 667-70.
[http://dx.doi.org/10.1038/nature22967] [PMID: 28636595]

[18]   Kuriakose T, Kanneganti TD. Regulation and functions of NLRP3 inflammasome during influenza virus infection. Mol Immunol 2017; 86: 56-64.
[http://dx.doi.org/10.1016/j.molimm.2017.01.023] [PMID: 28169000]

[19]   Kim JJ, Jo EK. NLRP3 inflammasome and host protection against bacterial infection. J Korean Med Sci 2013; 28(10): 1415-23.
[http://dx.doi.org/10.3346/jkms.2013.28.10.1415] [PMID: 24133343]

[20]   Christgen S, Kanneganti TD. Inflammasomes and the fine line between defense and disease. Curr Opin Immunol 2020; 62: 39-44.
[http://dx.doi.org/10.1016/j.coi.2019.11.007] [PMID: 31837596]

[21]   Awad F, Assrawi E, Louvrier C, *et al.* Inflammasome biology, molecular pathology and therapeutic implications. Pharmacol Ther 2018; 187: 133-49.
[http://dx.doi.org/10.1016/j.pharmthera.2018.02.011] [PMID: 29466702]

[22]   Kesavardhana S, Kanneganti TD. Mechanisms governing inflammasome activation, assembly and pyroptosis induction. Int Immunol 2017; 29(5): 201-10.
[http://dx.doi.org/10.1093/intimm/dxx018] [PMID: 28531279]

[23]   Wang B, Bhattacharya M, Roy S, Tian Y, Yin Q. Immunobiology and structural biology of AIM2 inflammasome. Mol Aspects Med 2020; 76: 100869.
[http://dx.doi.org/10.1016/j.mam.2020.100869] [PMID: 32660715]

[24]   Wang B, Yin Q. AIM2 inflammasome activation and regulation: A structural perspective. J Struct Biol 2017; 200(3): 279-82.
[http://dx.doi.org/10.1016/j.jsb.2017.08.001] [PMID: 28813641]

[25]   Sharma BR, Karki R, Kanneganti TD. Role of AIM2 inflammasome in inflammatory diseases, cancer and infection. Eur J Immunol 2019; 49(11): 1998-2011.
[http://dx.doi.org/10.1002/eji.201848070] [PMID: 31372985]

[26] Marim FM, Franco MM, Gomes MT, Miraglia MC, Giambartolomei GH, Oliveira SC. The role of NLRP3 and AIM2 in inflammasome activation during Brucella abortus infection. InSeminars in immunopathology 2017; 39: 215-23.
[http://dx.doi.org/10.1007/s00281-016-0581-1]

[27] Rathinam VAK, Jiang Z, Waggoner SN, *et al.* The AIM2 inflammasome is essential for host defense against cytosolic bacteria and DNA viruses. Nat Immunol 2010; 11(5): 395-402.
[http://dx.doi.org/10.1038/ni.1864] [PMID: 20351692]

[28] Man SM, Zhu Q, Zhu L, *et al.* Critical role for the DNA sensor AIM2 in stem cell proliferation and cancer. Cell 2015; 162(1): 45-58.
[http://dx.doi.org/10.1016/j.cell.2015.06.001] [PMID: 26095253]

[29] Dombrowski Y, Peric M, Koglin S, *et al.* Cytosolic DNA triggers inflammasome activation in keratinocytes in psoriatic lesions. Sci Transl Med 2011; 3(82): 82ra38.
[http://dx.doi.org/10.1126/scitranslmed.3002001] [PMID: 21562230]

[30] Bae JH, Jo SII, Kim SJ, *et al.* Circulating cell-free mtDNA contributes to AIM2 inflammasome-mediated chronic inflammation in patients with type 2 diabetes. Cells 2019; 8(4): 328.
[http://dx.doi.org/10.3390/cells8040328] [PMID: 30965677]

[31] Alles SRA, Smith PA. Etiology and pharmacology of neuropathic pain. Pharmacol Rev 2018; 70(2): 315-47.
[http://dx.doi.org/10.1124/pr.117.014399] [PMID: 29500312]

[32] Colloca L, Ludman T, Bouhassira D, *et al.* Neuropathic pain. Nat Rev Dis Primers 2017; 3(1): 17002.
[http://dx.doi.org/10.1038/nrdp.2017.2] [PMID: 28205574]

[33] Naranjo C, Ortega-Jiménez P, del Reguero L, Moratalla G, Failde I. Relationship between diabetic neuropathic pain and comorbidity. Their impact on pain intensity, diabetes complications and quality of life in patients with type-2 diabetes mellitus. Diabetes Res Clin Pract 2020; 165: 108236.
[http://dx.doi.org/10.1016/j.diabres.2020.108236] [PMID: 32470476]

[34] Alles SRA, Cain SM, Snutch TP. Pregabalin as a pain therapeutic: Beyond calcium channels. Front Cell Neurosci 2020; 14: 83.
[http://dx.doi.org/10.3389/fncel.2020.00083] [PMID: 32351366]

[35] Peretti S, Judge R, Hindmarch I. Safety and tolerability considerations: tricyclic antidepressants vs. selective serotonin reuptake inhibitors. Acta Psychiatr Scand 2000; 101(S403): 17-25.
[http://dx.doi.org/10.1111/j.1600-0447.2000.tb10944.x] [PMID: 11019931]

[36] McNicol ED, Midbari A, Eisenberg E. Opioids for neuropathic pain. Cochrane Database of Systematic Reviews 2013; 8.
[http://dx.doi.org/10.1002/14651858.CD006146.pub2]

[37] Muthuraman A, Singh N, Jaggi AS, Ramesh M. Drug therapy of neuropathic pain: Current developments and future perspectives. Curr Drug Targets 2014; 15(2): 210-53.
[PMID: 24093749]

[38] Meier T, Wasner G, Faust M, *et al.* Efficacy of lidocaine patch 5% in the treatment of focal peripheral neuropathic pain syndromes: A randomized, double-blind, placebo-controlled study. Pain 2003; 106(1): 151-8.
[http://dx.doi.org/10.1016/S0304-3959(03)00317-8] [PMID: 14581122]

[39] Woolf CJ, Mannion RJ. Neuropathic pain: Aetiology, symptoms, mechanisms, and management. Lancet 1999; 353(9168): 1959-64.
[http://dx.doi.org/10.1016/S0140-6736(99)01307-0] [PMID: 10371588]

[40] Wall PD, Devor M, Inbal R, *et al.* Autotomy following peripheral nerve lesions: Experimental anesthesia dolorosa. Pain 1979; 7(2): 103-13.
[http://dx.doi.org/10.1016/0304-3959(79)90002-2] [PMID: 574931]

[41]   Zeltser R, Beilin BZ, Zaslansky R, Seltzer Z. Comparison of autotomy behavior induced in rats by various clinically-used neurectomy methods. Pain 2000; 89(1): 19-24.
[http://dx.doi.org/10.1016/S0304-3959(00)00342-0] [PMID: 11113289]

[42]   Anand P, Birch R. Restoration of sensory function and lack of long-term chronic pain syndromes after brachial plexus injury in human neonates. Brain 2002; 125(1): 113-22.
[http://dx.doi.org/10.1093/brain/awf017] [PMID: 11834597]

[43]   Rodrigues-Filho R, Santos ARS, Bertelli JA, Calixto JB. Avulsion injury of the rat brachial plexus triggers hyperalgesia and allodynia in the hindpaws: a new model for the study of neuropathic pain. Brain Res 2003; 982(2): 186-94.
[http://dx.doi.org/10.1016/S0006-8993(03)03007-5] [PMID: 12915254]

[44]   Bennett GJ, Xie YK. A peripheral mononeuropathy in rat that produces disorders of pain sensation like those seen in man. Pain 1988; 33(1): 87-107.
[http://dx.doi.org/10.1016/0304-3959(88)90209-6] [PMID: 2837713]

[45]   Martucci C, Trovato AE, Costa B, *et al.* The purinergic antagonist PPADS reduces pain related behaviours and interleukin-1β, interleukin-6, iNOS and nNOS overproduction in central and peripheral nervous system after peripheral neuropathy in mice. Pain 2008; 137(1): 81-95.
[http://dx.doi.org/10.1016/j.pain.2007.08.017] [PMID: 17900807]

[46]   Seltzer Z, Dubner R, Shir Y. A novel behavioral model of neuropathic pain disorders produced in rats by partial sciatic nerve injury. Pain 1990; 43(2): 205-18.
[http://dx.doi.org/10.1016/0304-3959(90)91074-S] [PMID: 1982347]

[47]   Malmberg AB, Basbaum AI. Partial sciatic nerve injury in the mouse as a model of neuropathic pain: Behavioral and neuroanatomical correlates. Pain 1998; 76(1): 215-22.
[http://dx.doi.org/10.1016/S0304-3959(98)00045-1] [PMID: 9696476]

[48]   Decosterd I, Woolf CJ. Spared nerve injury: An animal model of persistent peripheral neuropathic pain. Pain 2000; 87(2): 149-58.
[http://dx.doi.org/10.1016/S0304-3959(00)00276-1] [PMID: 10924808]

[49]   Shields SD, Eckert WA III, Basbaum AI. Spared nerve injury model of neuropathic pain in the mouse: A behavioral and anatomic analysis. J Pain 2003; 4(8): 465-70.
[http://dx.doi.org/10.1067/S1526-5900(03)00781-8] [PMID: 14622667]

[50]   Ho Kim S, Mo Chung J. An experimental model for peripheral neuropathy produced by segmental spinal nerve ligation in the rat. Pain 1992; 50(3): 355-63.
[http://dx.doi.org/10.1016/0304-3959(92)90041-9] [PMID: 1333581]

[51]   Carlton SM, Lekan HA, Kim SH, Chung JM. Behavioral manifestations of an experimental model for peripheral neuropathy produced by spinal nerve ligation in the primate. Pain 1994; 56(2): 155-66.
[http://dx.doi.org/10.1016/0304-3959(94)90090-6] [PMID: 8008406]

[52]   Komori N, Takemori N, Kim HK, *et al.* Proteomics study of neuropathic and nonneuropathic dorsal root ganglia: altered protein regulation following segmental spinal nerve ligation injury. Physiol Genomics 2007; 29(2): 215-30.
[http://dx.doi.org/10.1152/physiolgenomics.00255.2006] [PMID: 17213366]

[53]   Lee BH, Won R, Baik EJ, Lee SH, Moon CH. An animal model of neuropathic pain employing injury to the sciatic nerve branches. Neuroreport 2000; 11(4): 657-61.
[http://dx.doi.org/10.1097/00001756-200003200-00002] [PMID: 10757496]

[54]   Jain V, Jaggi AS, Singh N. Ameliorative potential of rosiglitazone in tibial and sural nerve transection-induced painful neuropathy in rats. Pharmacol Res 2009; 59(6): 385-92.
[http://dx.doi.org/10.1016/j.phrs.2009.02.001] [PMID: 19429470]

[55]   Vadakkan KI, Jia YH, Zhuo M. A behavioral model of neuropathic pain induced by ligation of the common peroneal nerve in mice. J Pain 2005; 6(11): 747-56.
[http://dx.doi.org/10.1016/j.jpain.2005.07.005] [PMID: 16275599]

[56]   Na HS, Han JS, Ko KH, Hong SK. A behavioral model for peripheral neuropathy produced in rat's tail by inferior caudal trunk injury. Neurosci Lett 1994; 177(1-2): 50-2.
[http://dx.doi.org/10.1016/0304-3940(94)90042-6] [PMID: 7824181]

[57]   Sung B, Sik Na H, In Kim Y, *et al.* Supraspinal involvement in the production of mechanical allodynia by spinal nerve injury in rats. Neurosci Lett 1998; 246(2): 117-9.
[http://dx.doi.org/10.1016/S0304-3940(98)00235-3] [PMID: 9627194]

[58]   DeLeo JA, Coombs DW, Willenbring S, *et al.* Characterization of a neuropathic pain model: sciatic cryoneurolysis in the rat. Pain 1994; 56(1): 9-16.
[http://dx.doi.org/10.1016/0304-3959(94)90145-7] [PMID: 8159445]

[59]   Gazelius B, Cui JG, Svensson M, Meyerson B, Linderoth B. Photochemically induced ischaemic lesion of the rat sciatic nerve. A novel method providing high incidence of mononeuropathy. Neuroreport 1996; 7(15): 2619-24.
[http://dx.doi.org/10.1097/00001756-199611040-00042] [PMID: 8981434]

[60]   Hao JX, Blakeman KH, Yu W, Hultenby K, Xu XJ, Wiesenfeld-Hallin Z. Development of a mouse model of neuropathic pain following photochemically induced ischemia in the sciatic nerve. Exp Neurol 2000; 163(1): 231-8.
[http://dx.doi.org/10.1006/exnr.2000.7373] [PMID: 10785462]

[61]   Chacur M, Milligan ED, Gazda LS, *et al.* A new model of sciatic inflammatory neuritis (SIN): induction of unilateral and bilateral mechanical allodynia following acute unilateral peri-sciatic immune activation in rats. Pain 2001; 94(3): 231-44.
[http://dx.doi.org/10.1016/S0304-3959(01)00354-2] [PMID: 11731060]

[62]   Gazda LS, Milligan ED, Hansen MK, *et al.* Sciatic inflammatory neuritis (SIN): Behavioral allodynia is paralleled by peri-sciatic proinflammatory cytokine and superoxide production. J Peripher Nerv Syst 2001; 6(3): 111-29.
[http://dx.doi.org/10.1046/j.1529-8027.2001.006001111.x] [PMID: 11817330]

[63]   Mosconi T, Kruger L. Fixed-diameter polyethylene cuffs applied to the rat sciatic nerve induce a painful neuropathy: Ultrastructural morphometric analysis of axonal alterations. Pain 1996; 64(1): 37-57.
[http://dx.doi.org/10.1016/0304-3959(95)00077-1] [PMID: 8867246]

[64]   Benbouzid M, Pallage V, Rajalu M, *et al.* Sciatic nerve cuffing in mice: A model of sustained neuropathic pain. Eur J Pain 2008; 12(5): 591-9.
[http://dx.doi.org/10.1016/j.ejpain.2007.10.002] [PMID: 18006342]

[65]   Ahn DK, Lim EJ, Kim BC, *et al.* Compression of the trigeminal ganglion produces prolonged nociceptive behavior in rats. Eur J Pain 2009; 13(6): 568-75.
[http://dx.doi.org/10.1016/j.ejpain.2008.07.008] [PMID: 18774318]

[66]   Imamura Y, Kawamoto H, Nakanishi O. Characterization of heat-hyperalgesia in an experimental trigeminal neuropathy in rats. Exp Brain Res 1997; 116(1): 97-103.
[http://dx.doi.org/10.1007/PL00005748] [PMID: 9305818]

[67]   Siddall P, Xu CL, Cousins M. Allodynia following traumatic spinal cord injury in the rat. Neuroreport 1995; 6(9): 1241-4.
[http://dx.doi.org/10.1097/00001756-199506090-00003] [PMID: 7669978]

[68]   Drew GM, Siddall PJ, Duggan AW. Responses of spinal neurones to cutaneous and dorsal root stimuli in rats with mechanical allodynia after contusive spinal cord injury. Brain Res 2001; 893(1-2): 59-69.
[http://dx.doi.org/10.1016/S0006-8993(00)03288-1] [PMID: 11222993]

[69]   Yezierski RP, Park SH. The mechanosensitivity of spinal sensory neurons following intraspinal injections of quisqualic acid in the rat. Neurosci Lett 1993; 157(1): 115-9.
[http://dx.doi.org/10.1016/0304-3940(93)90656-6] [PMID: 8233021]

[70]   Aanonsen LM, Wilcox GL. Muscimol, gamma-aminobutyric acidA receptors and excitatory amino

acids in the mouse spinal cord. J Pharmacol Exp Ther 1989; 248(3): 1034-8.
[PMID: 2467978]

[71]   Christensen MD, Everhart AW, Pickelman JT, Hulsebosch CE. Mechanical and thermal allodynia in chronic central pain following spinal cord injury. Pain 1996; 68(1): 97-107.
[http://dx.doi.org/10.1016/S0304-3959(96)03224-1] [PMID: 9252004]

[72]   Kim J, Yoon YW, Hong SK, Na HS. Cold and mechanical allodynia in both hindpaws and tail following thoracic spinal cord hemisection in rats: Time courses and their correlates. Neurosci Lett 2003; 343(3): 200-4.
[http://dx.doi.org/10.1016/S0304-3940(03)00377-X] [PMID: 12770696]

[73]   Courteix C, Eschalier A, Lavarenne J. Streptozocin-induced diabetic rats: Behavioural evidence for a model of chronic pain. Pain 1993; 53(1): 81-8.
[http://dx.doi.org/10.1016/0304-3959(93)90059-X] [PMID: 8316394]

[74]   Grover VS, Sharma A, Singh M. Role of nitric oxide in diabetes-induced attenuation of antinociceptive effect of morphine in mice. Eur J Pharmacol 2000; 399(2-3): 161-4.
[http://dx.doi.org/10.1016/S0014-2999(00)00343-5] [PMID: 10884515]

[75]   Khan N, Bakshi KS, Jaggi AS, Singh N. Ameliorative potential of spironolactone in diabetes induced hyperalgesia in mice. Yakugaku Zasshi 2009; 129(5): 593-9.
[http://dx.doi.org/10.1248/yakushi.129.593] [PMID: 19420890]

[76]   Oltman CL, Coppey LJ, Gellett JS, Davidson EP, Lund DD, Yorek MA. Progression of vascular and neural dysfunction in sciatic nerves of Zucker diabetic fatty and Zucker rats. Am J Physiol Endocrinol Metab 2005; 289(1): E113-22.
[http://dx.doi.org/10.1152/ajpendo.00594.2004] [PMID: 15727946]

[77]   Drel VR, Mashtalir N, Ilnytska O, *et al.* Leptin-deficient (ob/ob) mouse-a new animal model of peripheral neuropathy of Type 2 diabetes and obesity.

[78]   Kumar A, Negi G, Sharma SS. Suppression of NF-κB and NF-κB regulated oxidative stress and neuroinflammation by BAY 11-7082 (IκB phosphorylation inhibitor) in experimental diabetic neuropathy. Biochimie 2012; 94(5): 1158-65.
[http://dx.doi.org/10.1016/j.biochi.2012.01.023] [PMID: 22342224]

[79]   Schwei MJ, Honore P, Rogers SD, *et al.* Neurochemical and cellular reorganization of the spinal cord in a murine model of bone cancer pain. J Neurosci 1999; 19(24): 10886-97.
[http://dx.doi.org/10.1523/JNEUROSCI.19-24-10886.1999] [PMID: 10594070]

[80]   Walker K, Medhurst SJ, Kidd BL, *et al.* Disease modifying and anti-nociceptive effects of the bisphosphonate, zoledronic acid in a model of bone cancer pain. Pain 2002; 100(3): 219-29.
[http://dx.doi.org/10.1016/S0304-3959(02)00040-4] [PMID: 12467993]

[81]   Shimoyama M, Tanaka K, Hasue F, Shimoyama N. A mouse model of neuropathic cancer pain. Pain 2002; 99(1): 167-74.
[http://dx.doi.org/10.1016/S0304-3959(02)00073-8] [PMID: 12237194]

[82]   Hald A, Nedergaard S, Hansen RR, Ding M, Heegaard AM. Differential activation of spinal cord glial cells in murine models of neuropathic and cancer pain. Eur J Pain 2009; 13(2): 138-45.
[http://dx.doi.org/10.1016/j.ejpain.2008.03.014] [PMID: 18499488]

[83]   Andoh T, Sugiyama K, Fujita M, *et al.* Pharmacological evaluation of morphine and non-opioid analgesic adjuvants in a mouse model of skin cancer pain. Biol Pharm Bull 2008; 31(3): 520-2.
[http://dx.doi.org/10.1248/bpb.31.520] [PMID: 18310922]

[84]   Herzberg U, Sagen J. Peripheral nerve exposure to HIV viral envelope protein gp120 induces neuropathic pain and spinal gliosis. J Neuroimmunol 2001; 116(1): 29-39.
[http://dx.doi.org/10.1016/S0165-5728(01)00288-0] [PMID: 11311327]

[85]   Wallace VCJ, Blackbeard J, Pheby T, *et al.* Pharmacological, behavioural and mechanistic analysis of HIV-1 gp120 induced painful neuropathy. Pain 2007; 133(1): 47-63.

[http://dx.doi.org/10.1016/j.pain.2007.02.015] [PMID: 17433546]

[86]   Fleetwood-Walker SM, Quinn JP, Wallace C, *et al.* Behavioural changes in the rat following infection with varicella-zoster virus. J Gen Virol 1999; 80(9): 2433-6.
[http://dx.doi.org/10.1099/0022-1317-80-9-2433] [PMID: 10501498]

[87]   Takasaki I, Andoh T, Shiraki K, Kuraishi Y. Allodynia and hyperalgesia induced by herpes simplex virus type-1 infection in mice. Pain 2000; 86(1): 95-101.
[http://dx.doi.org/10.1016/S0304-3959(00)00240-2] [PMID: 10779666]

[88]   Pan HL, Khan GM, Alloway KD, Chen SR. Resiniferatoxin induces paradoxical changes in thermal and mechanical sensitivities in rats: mechanism of action. J Neurosci 2003; 23(7): 2911-9.
[http://dx.doi.org/10.1523/JNEUROSCI.23-07-02911.2003] [PMID: 12684478]

[89]   Siau C, Bennett GJ. Dysregulation of cellular calcium homeostasis in chemotherapy-evoked painful peripheral neuropathy. Anesth Analg 2006; 102(5): 1485-90.
[http://dx.doi.org/10.1213/01.ane.0000204318.35194.ed] [PMID: 16632831]

[90]   Contreras PC, Vaught JL, Gruner JA, *et al.* Insulin-like growth factor-I prevents development of a vincristine neuropathy in mice. Brain Res 1997; 774(1-2): 20-6.
[http://dx.doi.org/10.1016/S0006-8993(97)81682-4] [PMID: 9452187]

[91]   Szilvássy J, Sziklai I, Racz T, Horvath P, Rabloczky G, Szilvassy Z. Impaired bronchomotor responses to field stimulation in guinea-pigs with cisplatin-induced neuropathy. Eur J Pharmacol 2000; 403(3): 259-65.
[http://dx.doi.org/10.1016/S0014-2999(00)00488-X] [PMID: 10973628]

[92]   Cavaletti G, Tredici G, Petruccioli MG, *et al.* Effects of different schedules of oxaliplatin treatment on the peripheral nervous system of the rat. Eur J Cancer 2001; 37(18): 2457-63.
[http://dx.doi.org/10.1016/S0959-8049(01)00300-8] [PMID: 11720843]

[93]   Flatters SJL, Bennett GJ. Studies of peripheral sensory nerves in paclitaxel-induced painful peripheral neuropathy: Evidence for mitochondrial dysfunction. Pain 2006; 122(3): 245-57.
[http://dx.doi.org/10.1016/j.pain.2006.01.037] [PMID: 16530964]

[94]   Anderson TD, Davidovich A, Arceo R, Brosnan C, Arezzo J, Schaumburg H. Peripheral neuropathy induced by 2′,3′-dideoxycytidine. A rabbit model of 2′,3′-dideoxycytidine neurotoxicity. Lab Invest 1992; 66(1): 63-74.
[PMID: 1309930]

[95]   Schmued LC, Albertson CM, Andrews A, Sandberg JA, Nickols J, Slikker W Jr. Evaluation of brain and nerve pathology in rats chronically dosed with ddI or isoniazid. Neurotoxicol Teratol 1996; 18(5): 555-63.
[http://dx.doi.org/10.1016/0892-0362(96)00088-8] [PMID: 8888020]

[96]   Joseph EK, Chen X, Khasar SG, Levine JD. Novel mechanism of enhanced nociception in a model of AIDS therapy-induced painful peripheral neuropathy in the rat. Pain 2004; 107(1): 147-58.
[http://dx.doi.org/10.1016/j.pain.2003.10.010] [PMID: 14715401]

[97]   Dina OA, Barletta J, Chen X, *et al.* Key role for the epsilon isoform of protein kinase C in painful alcoholic neuropathy in the rat. J Neurosci 2000; 20(22): 8614-9.
[http://dx.doi.org/10.1523/JNEUROSCI.20-22-08614.2000] [PMID: 11069970]

[98]   Dina OA, Messing RO, Levine JD. Ethanol withdrawal induces hyperalgesia mediated by PKCε. Eur J Neurosci 2006; 24(1): 197-204.
[http://dx.doi.org/10.1111/j.1460-9568.2006.04886.x] [PMID: 16800864]

[99]   Chung JY, Choi JH, Hwang CY, Youn HY. Pyridoxine induced neuropathy by subcutaneous administration in dogs. J Vet Sci 2008; 9(2): 127-31.
[http://dx.doi.org/10.4142/jvs.2008.9.2.127] [PMID: 18487933]

[100]   Perry TA, Weerasuriya A, Mouton PR, Holloway HW, Greig NH. Pyridoxine-induced toxicity in rats: A stereological quantification of the sensory neuropathy. Exp Neurol 2004; 190(1): 133-44.

[http://dx.doi.org/10.1016/j.expneurol.2004.07.013] [PMID: 15473987]

[101] Wu LJ, Zhuo M. Targeting the NMDA receptor subunit NR2B for the treatment of neuropathic pain. Neurotherapeutics 2009; 6(4): 693-702.
[http://dx.doi.org/10.1016/j.nurt.2009.07.008] [PMID: 19789073]

[102] Kiguchi N, Kobayashi Y, Kishioka S. Chemokines and cytokines in neuroinflammation leading to neuropathic pain. Curr Opin Pharmacol 2012; 12(1): 55-61.
[http://dx.doi.org/10.1016/j.coph.2011.10.007] [PMID: 22019566]

[103] Hoffmann S, Beyer C. A fatal alliance between microglia, inflammasomes, and central pain. Int J Mol Sci 2020; 21(11): 3764.
[http://dx.doi.org/10.3390/ijms21113764] [PMID: 32466593]

[104] Ji RR, Nackley A, Huh Y, Terrando N, Maixner W. Neuroinflammation and central sensitization in chronic and widespread pain. Anesthesiology 2018; 129(2): 343-66.
[http://dx.doi.org/10.1097/ALN.0000000000002130] [PMID: 29462012]

[105] Ji RR, Chamessian A, Zhang YQ. Pain regulation by non-neuronal cells and inflammation. Science 2016; 354(6312): 572-7.
[http://dx.doi.org/10.1126/science.aaf8924] [PMID: 27811267]

[106] Echeverry S, Shi XQ, Rivest S, Zhang J. Peripheral nerve injury alters blood-spinal cord barrier functional and molecular integrity through a selective inflammatory pathway. J Neurosci 2011; 31(30): 10819-28.
[http://dx.doi.org/10.1523/JNEUROSCI.1642-11.2011] [PMID: 21795534]

[107] Ji RR, Xu ZZ, Gao YJ. Emerging targets in neuroinflammation-driven chronic pain. Nat Rev Drug Discov 2014; 13(7): 533-48.
[http://dx.doi.org/10.1038/nrd4334] [PMID: 24948120]

[108] Ji RR, Donnelly CR, Nedergaard M. Astrocytes in chronic pain and itch. Nat Rev Neurosci 2019; 20(11): 667-85.
[http://dx.doi.org/10.1038/s41583-019-0218-1] [PMID: 31537912]

[109] Li T, Chen X, Zhang C, Zhang Y, Yao W. An update on reactive astrocytes in chronic pain. J Neuroinflammation 2019; 16(1): 140.
[http://dx.doi.org/10.1186/s12974-019-1524-2] [PMID: 31288837]

[110] Jha MK, Jo M, Kim JH, Suk K. Microglia-astrocyte crosstalk: An intimate molecular conversation. Neuroscientist 2019; 25(3): 227-40.
[http://dx.doi.org/10.1177/1073858418783959] [PMID: 29931997]

[111] Hung AL, Lim M, Doshi TL. Targeting cytokines for treatment of neuropathic pain. Scand J Pain 2017; 17(1): 287-93.
[http://dx.doi.org/10.1016/j.sjpain.2017.08.002] [PMID: 29229214]

[112] Nijs J, Leysen L, Vanlauwe J, *et al.* Treatment of central sensitization in patients with chronic pain: Time for change? Expert Opin Pharmacother 2019; 20(16): 1961-70.
[http://dx.doi.org/10.1080/14656566.2019.1647166] [PMID: 31355689]

[113] Song H, Zhu Z, Zhou Y, *et al.* MIF/CD74 axis participates in inflammatory activation of Schwann cells following sciatic nerve injury. J Mol Histol 2019; 50(4): 355-67.
[http://dx.doi.org/10.1007/s10735-019-09832-0] [PMID: 31197516]

[114] Chen G-L, Chen Q, Lin L-J, *et al.* Protein post-translational modifications after spinal cord injury. Neural Regen Res 2021; 16(10): 1935-43.
[http://dx.doi.org/10.4103/1673-5374.308068] [PMID: 33642363]

[115] Luo D, Li X, Tang S, *et al.* Epigenetic modifications in neuropathic pain. Mol Pain 2021; 17.
[http://dx.doi.org/10.1177/17448069211056767] [PMID: 34823400]

[116] Lee KY, Ratté S, Prescott SA. Excitatory neurons are more disinhibited than inhibitory neurons by

chloride dysregulation in the spinal dorsal horn. eLife 2019; 8: e49753.
[http://dx.doi.org/10.7554/eLife.49753] [PMID: 31742556]

[117]   Yin Y, Yi MH, Kim DW. Impaired autophagy of GABAergic interneurons in neuropathic pain. Pain Research and Management 2018.
[http://dx.doi.org/10.1155/2018/9185368]

[118]   White K, Targett M, Harris J. Gainfully employing descending controls in acute and chronic pain management. Vet J 2018; 237: 16-25.
[http://dx.doi.org/10.1016/j.tvjl.2018.05.005] [PMID: 30089540]

[119]   Lv Q, Wu F, Gan X, *et al.* The involvement of descending pain inhibitory system in electroacupuncture-induced analgesia. Front Integr Nuerosci 2019; 13: 38.
[http://dx.doi.org/10.3389/fnint.2019.00038] [PMID: 31496944]

[120]   Martínez-Navarro M, Maldonado R, Baños JE. Why mu-opioid agonists have less analgesic efficacy in neuropathic pain? Eur J Pain 2019; 23(3): 435-54.
[http://dx.doi.org/10.1002/ejp.1328] [PMID: 30318675]

[121]   Akhter ET, Griffith RW, English AW, Alvarez FJ. Removal of the potassium chloride co-transporter from the somatodendritic membrane of axotomized motoneurons is independent of BDNF/TrkB signaling but is controlled by neuromuscular innervation. Eneuro 2019; 6: 5.

[122]   Alsaqati M, Heine VM, Harwood AJ. Pharmacological intervention to restore connectivity deficits of neuronal networks derived from ASD patient iPSC with a TSC2 mutation. Mol Autism 2020; 11(1): 80.
[http://dx.doi.org/10.1186/s13229-020-00391-w] [PMID: 33076974]

[123]   Lorenzo LE, Godin AG, Ferrini F, *et al.* Enhancing neuronal chloride extrusion rescues α2/α3 GABA$_A$-mediated analgesia in neuropathic pain. Nat Commun 2020; 11(1): 869.
[http://dx.doi.org/10.1038/s41467-019-14154-6] [PMID: 32054836]

[124]   Jacobs AT, Marnett LJ. Systems analysis of protein modification and cellular responses induced by electrophile stress. Acc Chem Res 2010; 43(5): 673-83.
[http://dx.doi.org/10.1021/ar900286y] [PMID: 20218676]

[125]   Chen R, Hou R, Hong X, Yan S, Zha J. Organophosphate flame retardants (OPFRs) induce genotoxicity *in vivo*: A survey on apoptosis, DNA methylation, DNA oxidative damage, liver metabolites, and transcriptomics. Environ Int 2019; 130: 104914.
[http://dx.doi.org/10.1016/j.envint.2019.104914] [PMID: 31226563]

[126]   Franco R, Vargas MR. Redox biology in neurological function, dysfunction, and aging. Antioxid Redox Signal 2018; 28(18): 1583-6.
[http://dx.doi.org/10.1089/ars.2018.7509] [PMID: 29634346]

[127]   Ighodaro OM, Akinloye OA. First line defence antioxidants-superoxide dismutase (SOD), catalase (CAT) and glutathione peroxidase (GPX): Their fundamental role in the entire antioxidant defence grid. Alex J Med 2018; 54(4): 287-93.
[http://dx.doi.org/10.1016/j.ajme.2017.09.001]

[128]   Sies H, Berndt C, Jones DP. Oxidative stress. Annu Rev Biochem 2017; 86(1): 715-48.
[http://dx.doi.org/10.1146/annurev-biochem-061516-045037] [PMID: 28441057]

[129]   Areti A, Yerra VG, Naidu VGM, Kumar A. Oxidative stress and nerve damage: Role in chemotherapy induced peripheral neuropathy. Redox Biol 2014; 2: 289-95.
[http://dx.doi.org/10.1016/j.redox.2014.01.006] [PMID: 24494204]

[130]   Cobley JN, Fiorello ML, Bailey DM. 13 reasons why the brain is susceptible to oxidative stress. Redox Biol 2018; 15: 490-503.
[http://dx.doi.org/10.1016/j.redox.2018.01.008] [PMID: 29413961]

[131]   Bittar A, Jun J, La JH, Wang J, Leem JW, Chung JM. Reactive oxygen species affect spinal cell type-specific synaptic plasticity in a model of neuropathic pain. Pain 2017; 158(11): 2137-46.

[http://dx.doi.org/10.1097/j.pain.0000000000001014] [PMID: 28708760]

[132] Lim TKY, Rone MB, Lee S, Antel JP, Zhang J. Mitochondrial and bioenergetic dysfunction in trauma-induced painful peripheral neuropathy. Mol Pain 2015; 11: s12990-015-0057.
[http://dx.doi.org/10.1186/s12990-015-0057-7] [PMID: 26376783]

[133] Chen XJ, Wang L, Song XY. Mitoquinone alleviates vincristine-induced neuropathic pain through inhibiting oxidative stress and apoptosis *via* the improvement of mitochondrial dysfunction. Biomed Pharmacother 2020; 125: 110003.
[http://dx.doi.org/10.1016/j.biopha.2020.110003] [PMID: 32187955]

[134] Son Y, Cheong YK, Kim NH, Chung HT, Kang DG, Pae HO. Mitogen-activated protein kinases and reactive oxygen species: How can ROS activate MAPK pathways. J Signal Transduct 2011; 2011.

[135] Miao H, Xu J, Xu D, Ma X, Zhao X, Liu L. Nociceptive behavior induced by chemotherapeutic paclitaxel and beneficial role of antioxidative pathways. Physiol Res 2019; 68(3): 491-500.
[http://dx.doi.org/10.33549/physiolres.933939] [PMID: 30433798]

[136] Rochfort KD, Collins LE, Murphy RP, Cummins PM. Downregulation of blood-brain barrier phenotype by proinflammatory cytokines involves NADPH oxidase-dependent ROS generation: consequences for interendothelial adherens and tight junctions. PLoS One 2014; 9(7): e101815.
[http://dx.doi.org/10.1371/journal.pone.0101815] [PMID: 24992685]

[137] Arruri VK, Gundu C, Kalvala AK, Sherkhane B, Khatri DK, Singh SB. Carvacrol abates NLRP3 inflammasome activation by augmenting Keap1/Nrf-2/p62 directed autophagy and mitochondrial quality control in neuropathic pain. Nutr Neurosci 2022; 25(8): 1731-46.
[http://dx.doi.org/10.1080/1028415X.2021.1892985] [PMID: 33641628]

[138] Islam MT. Oxidative stress and mitochondrial dysfunction-linked neurodegenerative disorders. Neurol Res 2017; 39(1): 73-82.
[http://dx.doi.org/10.1080/01616412.2016.1251711] [PMID: 27809706]

[139] Ni HM, Williams JA, Ding WX. Mitochondrial dynamics and mitochondrial quality control. Redox Biol 2015; 4: 6-13.
[http://dx.doi.org/10.1016/j.redox.2014.11.006] [PMID: 25479550]

[140] Yuk JM, Silwal P, Jo EK. Inflammasome and mitophagy connection in health and disease. Int J Mol Sci 2020; 21(13): 4714.
[http://dx.doi.org/10.3390/ijms21134714] [PMID: 32630319]

[141] Chang YH, Lin HY, Shen FC, *et al.* The causal role of mitochondrial dynamics in regulating innate immunity in diabetes. Front Endocrinol 2020; 11: 445.
[http://dx.doi.org/10.3389/fendo.2020.00445] [PMID: 32849261]

[142] Ichinohe T, Yamazaki T, Koshiba T, Yanagi Y. Mitochondrial protein mitofusin 2 is required for NLRP3 inflammasome activation after RNA virus infection. Proc Natl Acad Sci 2013; 110(44): 17963-8.
[http://dx.doi.org/10.1073/pnas.1312571110] [PMID: 24127597]

[143] Dai CQ, Guo Y, Chu XY. Neuropathic pain: The dysfunction of Drp1, mitochondria, and ROS homeostasis. Neurotox Res 2020; 38(3): 553-63.
[http://dx.doi.org/10.1007/s12640-020-00257-2] [PMID: 32696439]

[144] Kool M, Pétrilli V, De Smedt T, *et al.* Cutting edge: Alum adjuvant stimulates inflammatory dendritic cells through activation of the NALP3 inflammasome. J Immunol 2008; 181(6): 3755-9.
[http://dx.doi.org/10.4049/jimmunol.181.6.3755] [PMID: 18768827]

[145] Martinon F, Pétrilli V, Mayor A, Tardivel A, Tschopp J. Gout-associated uric acid crystals activate the NALP3 inflammasome. Nature 2006; 440(7081): 237-41.
[http://dx.doi.org/10.1038/nature04516] [PMID: 16407889]

[146] Dostert C, Pétrilli V, Van Bruggen R, Steele C, Mossman BT, Tschopp J. Innate immune activation through Nalp3 inflammasome sensing of asbestos and silica. Science 2008; 320(5876): 674-7.

[http://dx.doi.org/10.1126/science.1156995] [PMID: 18403674]

[147]   Zhang Y, Chen Y, Zhang Y, Li PL, Li X. Contribution of cathepsin B-dependent Nlrp3 inflammasome activation to nicotine-induced endothelial barrier dysfunction. Eur J Pharmacol 2019; 865: 172795.
[http://dx.doi.org/10.1016/j.ejphar.2019.172795] [PMID: 31733211]

[148]   Corrêa R, Silva LFF, Ribeiro DJS, *et al.* Lysophosphatidylcholine induces NLRP3 inflammasome-mediated foam cell formation and pyroptosis in human monocytes and endothelial cells. Front Immunol 2020; 10: 2927.
[http://dx.doi.org/10.3389/fimmu.2019.02927] [PMID: 31998284]

[149]   Katsnelson MA, Lozada-Soto KM, Russo HM, Miller BA, Dubyak GR. NLRP3 inflammasome signaling is activated by low-level lysosome disruption but inhibited by extensive lysosome disruption: Roles for K$^+$ efflux and Ca^{2+} influx. Am J Physiol Cell Physiol 2016; 311(1): C83-C100.
[http://dx.doi.org/10.1152/ajpcell.00298.2015] [PMID: 27170638]

[150]   Barry R, John SW, Liccardi G, *et al.* SUMO-mediated regulation of NLRP3 modulates inflammasome activity. Nat Commun 2018; 9(1): 3001.
[http://dx.doi.org/10.1038/s41467-018-05321-2] [PMID: 30069026]

[151]   Weber K, Schilling JD. Lysosomes integrate metabolic-inflammatory cross-talk in primary macrophage inflammasome activation. J Biol Chem 2014; 289(13): 9158-71.
[http://dx.doi.org/10.1074/jbc.M113.531202] [PMID: 24532802]

[152]   Sun L, Wu Z, Hayashi Y, *et al.* Microglial cathepsin B contributes to the initiation of peripheral inflammation-induced chronic pain. J Neurosci 2012; 32(33): 11330-42.
[http://dx.doi.org/10.1523/JNEUROSCI.0677-12.2012] [PMID: 22895716]

[153]   Widerström-Noga E. Neuropathic pain and spinal cord injury: Phenotypes and pharmacological management. Drugs 2017; 77(9): 967-84.
[http://dx.doi.org/10.1007/s40265-017-0747-8] [PMID: 28451808]

[154]   Donnelly CR, Chen O, Ji RR. How do sensory neurons sense danger signals? Trends Neurosci 2020; 43(10): 822-38.
[http://dx.doi.org/10.1016/j.tins.2020.07.008] [PMID: 32839001]

[155]   Liu S, Mi WL, Li Q, *et al.* Spinal IL-33/ST2 signaling contributes to neuropathic pain *via* neuronal CaMKII–CREB and astroglial JAK2–STAT3 cascades in mice. Anesthesiology 2015; 123(5): 1154-69.
[http://dx.doi.org/10.1097/ALN.0000000000000850] [PMID: 26352378]

[156]   Chen SP, Zhou YQ, Wang XM, *et al.* Pharmacological inhibition of the NLRP3 inflammasome as a potential target for cancer-induced bone pain. Pharmacol Res 2019; 147: 104339.
[http://dx.doi.org/10.1016/j.phrs.2019.104339] [PMID: 31276771]

[157]   Grace PM, Strand KA, Galer EL, *et al.* Morphine paradoxically prolongs neuropathic pain in rats by amplifying spinal NLRP3 inflammasome activation. Proc Natl Acad Sci 2016; 113(24): E3441-50.
[http://dx.doi.org/10.1073/pnas.1602070113] [PMID: 27247388]

[158]   Goldberg EL, Asher JL, Molony RD, *et al.* β-Hydroxybutyrate deactivates neutrophil NLRP3 inflammasome to relieve gout flares. Cell Rep 2017; 18(9): 2077-87.
[http://dx.doi.org/10.1016/j.celrep.2017.02.004] [PMID: 28249154]

[159]   Reber LL, Marichal T, Sokolove J, *et al.* Contribution of mast cell-derived interleukin-1β to uric acid crystal-induced acute arthritis in mice. Arthritis Rheumatol 2014; 66(10): 2881-91.
[http://dx.doi.org/10.1002/art.38747] [PMID: 24943488]

[160]   Jia M, Wu C, Gao F, *et al.* Activation of NLRP3 inflammasome in peripheral nerve contributes to paclitaxel-induced neuropathic pain. Mol Pain 2017; 13.
[http://dx.doi.org/10.1177/1744806917719804] [PMID: 28714351]

[161]   Liu CC, Huang ZX, Li X, *et al.* Upregulation of NLRP3 *via* STAT3-dependent histone acetylation contributes to painful neuropathy induced by bortezomib. Exp Neurol 2018; 302: 104-11.

[http://dx.doi.org/10.1016/j.expneurol.2018.01.011] [PMID: 29339053]

[162] Howrylak JA, Nakahira K. Inflammasomes: Key mediators of lung immunity. Annu Rev Physiol 2017; 79(1): 471-94.
[http://dx.doi.org/10.1146/annurev-physiol-021115-105229] [PMID: 28192059]

[163] Lee S, Suh GY, Ryter SW, Choi AMK. Regulation and function of the nucleotide binding domain leucine-rich repeat-containing receptor, pyrin domain-containing-3 inflammasome in lung disease. Am J Respir Cell Mol Biol 2016; 54(2): 151-60.
[http://dx.doi.org/10.1165/rcmb.2015-0231TR] [PMID: 26418144]

[164] Christgen S, Place DE, Kanneganti TD. Toward targeting inflammasomes: Insights into their regulation and activation. Cell Res 2020; 30(4): 315-27.
[http://dx.doi.org/10.1038/s41422-020-0295-8] [PMID: 32152420]

[165] Yen WC, Wu YH, Wu CC, *et al.* Impaired inflammasome activation and bacterial clearance in G6PD deficiency due to defective NOX/p38 MAPK/AP-1 redox signaling. Redox Biol 2020; 28: 101363.
[http://dx.doi.org/10.1016/j.redox.2019.101363] [PMID: 31707353]

[166] Chen H, Jiang Z. The essential adaptors of innate immune signaling. Protein Cell 2013; 4(1): 27-39.
[http://dx.doi.org/10.1007/s13238-012-2063-0] [PMID: 22996173]

[167] Elliott EI, Sutterwala FS. Initiation and perpetuation of NLRP 3 inflammasome activation and assembly. Immunol Rev 2015; 265(1): 35-52.
[http://dx.doi.org/10.1111/imr.12286] [PMID: 25879282]

[168] Broz P, Dixit VM. Inflammasomes: Mechanism of assembly, regulation and signalling. Nat Rev Immunol 2016; 16(7): 407-20.
[http://dx.doi.org/10.1038/nri.2016.58] [PMID: 27291964]

[169] Yang Y, Wang H, Kouadir M, Song H, Shi F. Recent advances in the mechanisms of NLRP3 inflammasome activation and its inhibitors. Cell Death Dis 2019; 10(2): 128.
[http://dx.doi.org/10.1038/s41419-019-1413-8] [PMID: 30755589]

[170] Chen KW, Demarco B, Broz P. Pannexin-1 promotes NLRP3 activation during apoptosis but is dispensable for canonical or noncanonical inflammasome activation. Eur J Immunol 2020; 50(2): 170-7.
[http://dx.doi.org/10.1002/eji.201948254] [PMID: 31411729]

[171] Chen KW, Demarco B, Heilig R, *et al.* Extrinsic and intrinsic apoptosis activate pannexin-1 to drive NLRP 3 inflammasome assembly. EMBO J 2019; 38(10): e101638.
[http://dx.doi.org/10.15252/embj.2019101638] [PMID: 30902848]

[172] Yu JW, Lee MS. Mitochondria and the NLRP3 inflammasome: Physiological and pathological relevance. Arch Pharm Res 2016; 39(11): 1503-18.
[http://dx.doi.org/10.1007/s12272-016-0827-4] [PMID: 27600432]

[173] Tschopp J. Mitochondria: Sovereign of inflammation? Eur J Immunol 2011; 41(5): 1196-202.
[http://dx.doi.org/10.1002/eji.201141436] [PMID: 21469137]

[174] Liu R, Wang SC, Li M, *et al.* An inhibitor of DRP1 (Mdivi-1) alleviates LPS-induced septic AKI by inhibiting NLRP3 inflammasome activation. BioMed Res Int 2020; 2020.

[175] Liu Q, Zhang D, Hu D, Zhou X, Zhou Y. The role of mitochondria in NLRP3 inflammasome activation. Mol Immunol 2018; 103: 115-24.
[http://dx.doi.org/10.1016/j.molimm.2018.09.010] [PMID: 30248487]

[176] Mohanty A, Tiwari-Pandey R, Pandey NR. Mitochondria: The indispensable players in innate immunity and guardians of the inflammatory response. J Cell Commun Signal 2019; 13(3): 303-18.
[http://dx.doi.org/10.1007/s12079-019-00507-9] [PMID: 30719617]

[177] Subramanian N, Natarajan K, Clatworthy MR, Wang Z, Germain RN. The adaptor MAVS promotes NLRP3 mitochondrial localization and inflammasome activation. Cell 2013; 153(2): 348-61.

[http://dx.doi.org/10.1016/j.cell.2013.02.054] [PMID: 23582325]

[178] Shi H, Wang Y, Li X, *et al.* NLRP3 activation and mitosis are mutually exclusive events coordinated by NEK7, a new inflammasome component. Nat Immunol 2016; 17(3): 250-8.
[http://dx.doi.org/10.1038/ni.3333] [PMID: 26642356]

[179] Lu F, Lan Z, Xin Z, *et al.* Emerging insights into molecular mechanisms underlying pyroptosis and functions of inflammasomes in diseases. J Cell Physiol 2020; 235(4): 3207-21.
[http://dx.doi.org/10.1002/jcp.29268] [PMID: 31621910]

[180] Yi YS. Caspase-11 non-canonical inflammasome: A critical sensor of intracellular lipopolysaccharide in macrophage-mediated inflammatory responses. Immunology 2017; 152(2): 207-17.
[http://dx.doi.org/10.1111/imm.12787] [PMID: 28695629]

[181] He W, Wan H, Hu L, *et al.* Gasdermin D is an executor of pyroptosis and required for interleukin-1β secretion. Cell Res 2015; 25(12): 1285-98.
[http://dx.doi.org/10.1038/cr.2015.139] [PMID: 26611636]

[182] Shi J, Zhao Y, Wang K, *et al.* Cleavage of GSDMD by inflammatory caspases determines pyroptotic cell death. Nature 2015; 526(7575): 660-5.
[http://dx.doi.org/10.1038/nature15514] [PMID: 26375003]

[183] Mortimer L, Moreau F, MacDonald JA, Chadee K. NLRP3 inflammasome inhibition is disrupted in a group of auto-inflammatory disease CAPS mutations. Nat Immunol 2016; 17(10): 1176-86.
[http://dx.doi.org/10.1038/ni.3538] [PMID: 27548431]

[184] Fumagalli G, Monza L, Cavaletti G, Rigolio R, Meregalli C. Neuroinflammatory process involved in different preclinical models of chemotherapy-induced peripheral neuropathy. Front Immunol 2021; 11: 626687.
[http://dx.doi.org/10.3389/fimmu.2020.626687] [PMID: 33613570]

[185] Derangula K, Javalgekar M, kumar Arruri V, Gundu C, kumar Kalvala A, kumar A. Probucol attenuates NF-κB/NLRP3 signalling and augments Nrf-2 mediated antioxidant defence in nerve injury induced neuropathic pain. Int Immunopharmacol 2022; 102: 108397.
[http://dx.doi.org/10.1016/j.intimp.2021.108397] [PMID: 34891000]

[186] Zheng T, Wang Q, Bian F, *et al.* Salidroside alleviates diabetic neuropathic pain through regulation of the AMPK-NLRP3 inflammasome axis. Toxicol Appl Pharmacol 2021; 416: 115468.
[http://dx.doi.org/10.1016/j.taap.2021.115468] [PMID: 33639149]

[187] Coll RC, Hill JR, Day CJ, *et al.* MCC950 directly targets the NLRP3 ATP-hydrolysis motif for inflammasome inhibition. Nat Chem Biol 2019; 15(6): 556-9.
[http://dx.doi.org/10.1038/s41589-019-0277-7] [PMID: 31086327]

[188] Tapia-Abellán A, Angosto-Bazarra D, Martínez-Banaclocha H, *et al.* MCC950 closes the active conformation of NLRP3 to an inactive state. Nat Chem Biol 2019; 15(6): 560-4.
[http://dx.doi.org/10.1038/s41589-019-0278-6] [PMID: 31086329]

[189] He Y, Varadarajan S, Muñoz-Planillo R, Burberry A, Nakamura Y, Núñez G. 3,4-methylenedioxy-β-nitrostyrene inhibits NLRP3 inflammasome activation by blocking assembly of the inflammasome. J Biol Chem 2014; 289(2): 1142-50.
[http://dx.doi.org/10.1074/jbc.M113.515080] [PMID: 24265316]

[190] Jiang H, He H, Chen Y, *et al.* Identification of a selective and direct NLRP3 inhibitor to treat inflammatory disorders. J Exp Med 2017; 214(11): 3219-38.
[http://dx.doi.org/10.1084/jem.20171419] [PMID: 29021150]

[191] Marchetti C, Swartzwelter B, Gamboni F, *et al.* OLT1177, a β-sulfonyl nitrile compound, safe in humans, inhibits the NLRP3 inflammasome and reverses the metabolic cost of inflammation. Proc Natl Acad Sci USA 2018; 115(7): E1530-9.
[http://dx.doi.org/10.1073/pnas.1716095115] [PMID: 29378952]

[192] Huang Y, Jiang H, Chen Y, *et al.* Tranilast directly targets NLRP 3 to treat inflammasome-driven

diseases. EMBO Mol Med 2018; 10(4): e8689.
[http://dx.doi.org/10.15252/emmm.201708689] [PMID: 29531021]

[193]   He H, Jiang H, Chen Y, *et al.* Oridonin is a covalent NLRP3 inhibitor with strong anti-inflammasome activity. Nat Commun 2018; 9(1): 2550.
[http://dx.doi.org/10.1038/s41467-018-04947-6] [PMID: 29959312]

[194]   Strickson S, Campbell DG, Emmerich CH, *et al.* The anti-inflammatory drug BAY 11-7082 suppresses the MyD88-dependent signalling network by targeting the ubiquitin system. Biochem J 2013; 451(3): 427-37.
[http://dx.doi.org/10.1042/BJ20121651] [PMID: 23441730]

[195]   Meng X, Martinez MA, Raymond-Stintz MA, Winter SS, Wilson BS. IKK inhibitor bay 11-7082 induces necroptotic cell death in precursor-B acute lymphoblastic leukaemic blasts. Br J Haematol 2010; 148(3): 487-90.
[http://dx.doi.org/10.1111/j.1365-2141.2009.07988.x] [PMID: 19958360]

[196]   Krishnan N, Bencze G, Cohen P, Tonks NK. The anti-inflammatory compound BAY -11-7082 is a potent inhibitor of protein tyrosine phosphatases. FEBS J 2013; 280(12): 2830-41.
[http://dx.doi.org/10.1111/febs.12283] [PMID: 23578302]

[197]   Cocco M, Pellegrini C, Martínez-Banaclocha H, *et al.* Development of an acrylate derivative targeting the NLRP3 inflammasome for the treatment of inflammatory bowel disease. J Med Chem 2017; 60(9): 3656-71.
[http://dx.doi.org/10.1021/acs.jmedchem.6b01624] [PMID: 28410442]

[198]   Shi Y, Lv Q, Zheng M, Sun H, Shi F. NLRP3 inflammasome inhibitor INF39 attenuated NLRP3 assembly in macrophages. Int Immunopharmacol 2021; 92: 107358.
[http://dx.doi.org/10.1016/j.intimp.2020.107358] [PMID: 33508701]

[199]   Yang G, Lee HE, Moon SJ, *et al.* Direct binding to NLRP3 pyrin domain as a novel strategy to prevent NLRP3-driven inflammation and Gouty Arthritis. Arthritis Rheumatol 2020; 72(7): 1192-202.
[http://dx.doi.org/10.1002/art.41245] [PMID: 32134203]

[200]   Clarke J. β-carotene blocks the inflammasome. Nat Rev Rheumatol 2020; 16(5): 248-8.
[http://dx.doi.org/10.1038/s41584-020-0415-3] [PMID: 32231303]

[201]   D'anneo A, Carlisi D, Lauricella M, *et al.* Parthenolide generates reactive oxygen species and autophagy in MDA-MB231 cells. A soluble parthenolide analogue inhibits tumour growth and metastasis in a xenograft model of breast cancer. Cell death & disease 2013; 4(10): 891.

[202]   Chinta PK, Tambe S, Umrani D, Pal AK, Nandave M. Effect of parthenolide, an NLRP3 inflammasome inhibitor, on insulin resistance in high-fat diet-obese mice. Can J Physiol Pharmacol 2022; 100(3): 272-81.
[http://dx.doi.org/10.1139/cjpp-2021-0116] [PMID: 35119950]

[203]   Ou Y, Sun P, Wu N, *et al.* Synthesis and biological evaluation of parthenolide derivatives with reduced toxicity as potential inhibitors of the NLRP3 inflammasome. Bioorg Med Chem Lett 2020; 30(17): 127399.
[http://dx.doi.org/10.1016/j.bmcl.2020.127399] [PMID: 32738997]

SUBJECT INDEX

Puneetpal Singh (Ed.)
All rights reserved-© 2024 Bentham Science Publishers

www.ingramcontent.com/pod-product-compliance
Lightning Source LLC
Chambersburg PA
CBHW050832220326
41598CB00006B/361

* 9 7 8 9 8 1 5 2 2 3 9 6 5 *